RETHINKING OBESITY

Theoretically informed and empirically grounded, *Rethinking Obesity* invites readers to reconsider the medical and public health framing of population weight (gain) as a massive global problem, epidemic or crisis. Attentive to social values, scientific uncertainty and possible harms, the book furthers critique of the weight-centred health paradigm and world war on obesity. Building upon existing international literature from critical weight studies, fat studies and critical obesity research, the book advances scholarship with reference to body politics and health policy, epidemiology and obesity science, media reporting and weight-related stigma.

The authors resist the common moralised narrative that 'the overweight majority' are lazy, gluttonous, and personally responsible for their actual or potential ills and the solution ultimately necessitates individual lifestyle change. Critique is also extended to seemingly compassionate public health interventions that putatively avoid victim-blaming through an appeal to 'the obesogenic environment', a consequence of modern living. Empirical case studies are grounded in women's repeated and often frustrating experiences of dieting and schoolgirls' encounters with fat pedagogy, which challenges dominant obesity discourse. Recognising that declared public health crises may become layered and cascade through society, this book also includes timely research on the COVID-19 pandemic response amidst concerns about lockdown weight-gain, heightened risk of infection and death among people deemed overweight and obese.

Rethinking Obesity interrogates how social injustice is reproduced not only through cruelty but also through seemingly benevolent representations, pedagogies and policies. Alternative approaches and action, ranging from weight-inclusive health paradigms to broader social change, are also considered when seeking to foster collective hope in crisis times. This is valuable reading for students and researchers in medical sociology, social and population health sciences, physical education, critical weight and fat studies, and the social dimensions of the body.

Lee F. Monaghan is Associate Professor of Sociology, University of Limerick, Ireland. His research and teaching largely fall within the areas of medical sociology and sociological theory. Besides advancing critical weight studies, Lee has published qualitative research on drug use among bodybuilders, physical violence in the night-time leisure economy, chronic illness among children and the embodiment of masculinities and heterosexualities.

Emma Rich is Professor of Physical Activity and Health Pedagogy, University of Bath, UK. Her research examines sport, physical activity and physical/health education from critical/socio-cultural perspectives. Working across sociology and education, her work around critical pedagogies of health and physical education has informed research projects addressing obesity policy, health education in schools, eating disorders and digital health technologies.

Andrea E. Bombak is currently Assistant Professor, University of New Brunswick, Canada. She is a social and population health scientist who leads provincially and federally funded studies on intersectional health inequities, weight stigmatisation and post-secondary food pedagogies.

Critical Approaches to Health

The Routledge *Critical Approaches to Health* series aims to present critical, inter-disciplinary books around psychological, social and cultural issues related to health. Each volume in the series provides a critical approach to a particular issue or important topic, and is of interest and relevance to students and practitioners across the social sciences. The series is produced in association with the International Society of Critical Health Psychology (ISCHP).

Series Editors: Kerry Chamberlain & Antonia Lyons

Titles in the series:

Disability and Sexual Health
A Critical Exploration of Key Issues
Poul Rohleder, Stine Hellum Braathen, and Mark T. Carew

Postfeminism and Health
Critical Psychology and Media Perspectives
Sarah Riley, Adrienne Evans, and Martine Robson

Health at Work
Critical Perspectives
Leah Tomkins and Katrina Pritchard

Complementary and Alternative Medicine
Containing and Expanding Therapeutic Possibilities
Kevin Dew

Selling Immunity
Self, Culture and Economy in Healthcare and Medicine
Mark Davis

Embodied Trauma and Healing
Critical Conversations on the Concept of Health
Anna Westin

For more information about this series, please visit: https://www.routledge.com/ Critical-Approaches-to-Health/book-series/CRITHEA

RETHINKING OBESITY

Critical Perspectives in Crisis Times

*Lee F. Monaghan, Emma Rich and
Andrea E. Bombak*

Routledge
Taylor & Francis Group

LONDON AND NEW YORK

Cover image: © Getty Images

First published 2022
by Routledge
4 Park Square, Milton Park, Abingdon, Oxon OX14 4RN

and by Routledge
605 Third Avenue, New York, NY 10158

Routledge is an imprint of the Taylor & Francis Group, an informa business

British Library Cataloguing-in-Publication Data
A catalogue record for this book is available from the British Library

Library of Congress Cataloging-in-Publication Data
Names: Monaghan, Lee F., 1972- author. | Rich, Emma, 1977- author. |
Bombak, Andrea E., 1986- author.
Title: Rethinking obesity : critical perspectives in crisis times / Lee F.
Monaghan, Emma Rich, Andrea E. Bombak.
Description: Milton Park, Abingdon, Oxon ; New York, NY : Routledge, 2022.
| Series: Critical approaches to heath | Includes bibliographical
references and index.
Identifiers: LCCN 2021050021 (print) | LCCN 2021050022 (ebook) | ISBN
9781138999718 (hardback) | ISBN 9781138999749 (paperback) | ISBN
9781315658087 (ebook)
Subjects: LCSH: Obesity. | Obesity--Social aspects.
Classification: LCC RC628 .M597 2022 (print) | LCC RC628 (ebook) | DDC
362.1963/98--dc23/eng/20211015
LC record available at https://lccn.loc.gov/2021050021
LC ebook record available at https://lccn.loc.gov/2021050022

ISBN: 978-1-138-99971-8 (hbk)
ISBN: 978-1-138-99974-9 (pbk)
ISBN: 978-1-315-65808-7 (ebk)

DOI: 10.4324/9781315658087

Typeset in Bembo
by SPi Technologies India Pvt Ltd (Straive)

CONTENTS

TABLES

ABBREVIATIONS

ASDAH	Association for Size Diversity and Health
BMI	Body Mass Index
CDC	Centers for Disease Control and Prevention
CCF	Center for Consumer Freedom
DHHS	Department of Health and Human Services
DHSC	Department of Health and Social Care
DOH	Department of Health
DPP	Diabetes Prevention Program
HAES	Health At Every Size
NAAFA	National Association to Advance Fat Acceptance
NHS	National Health Service
OECD	Organization for Economic Co-operation and Development
ORF	Official Recontextualising Field
PE	Physical Education
PHE	Public Health England
PHSA	Provisional Health Service Authority
PM	Prime Minister
PRF	Pedagogic Recontextualising Field
PSHE	Personal, Social and Health Education
TARA	There Are Reasonable Alternatives
TINA	There Is No Alternative
US DHHS	United States Department of Health and Human Services
WCHP	Weight-Centred Health Paradigm
WHO	World Health Organization
WOF	World Obesity Federation

SERIES EDITORS' PREFACE

Health is a major issue for people all around the world, and is fundamental to individual well-being, personal achievements and satisfaction, as well as to families, communities and societies. It is also embedded in social notions of participation and citizenship. Much has been written about health, from a variety of perspectives and disciplines, but a lot of this writing takes a biomedical and causally positivist approach to health matters, neglecting the historical, social and cultural contexts and environments within which health is experienced, understood and practiced. It is pertinent to present a series of books offering critical, social science perspectives on important health topics.

The *Critical Approaches to Health* series aims to provide new critical writing on health. The series advances critical, interdisciplinary and theoretical writing about broad aspects of health. The series seeks to include books that range across important health topics, including general health-related issues (such as gender and media), major social issues for health (such as medicalisation, obesity and palliative care), particular health concerns (such as pain, doctor–patient interaction, health services and health technologies) and health problems (such as diabetes, autoimmune disease and medically unexplained illness), or health for specific groups of people (such as migrants, the homeless and the aged), or combinations of these.

The series seeks, above all, to promote critical consideration of health topics. By critical, we mean going beyond the critique of the topic and work in the field, to more general considerations of power and benefit, and in particular, to addressing concerns about whose understandings and interests are upheld and whose are marginalised by the approaches, findings and practices in these various domains of health. Such critical agendas involve reflections on what constitutes knowledge, how it is created and how it is used. Accordingly, critical approaches consider epistemological and theoretical positioning, as well as issues of methodology and practice, and seek to examine how health is enmeshed within broader social relations and structures. Books within this series take up this challenge and seek to provide new insights and understandings by applying a critical agenda to their topics.

In this book, *Rethinking Obesity: Critical Perspectives in Crisis Times*, Lee Monaghan, Emma Rich and Andrea Bombak provide insightful, wide-ranging and original views that unsettle and challenge dominant understandings and conceptualisations of obesity and its precursor, overweight. The book is presented in three interrelated parts. In Part 1, the authors deliver a critical analysis of how weight or fatness is positioned and understood in different contexts, including in contemporary societies where the 'war on obesity' is waged, in epidemiological and social research, in mass media, in social marketing and the pedagogy of obesity knowledge, in policy initiatives and by neoliberalism. This part also discusses how 'excess' weight/fatness is positioned and shaped by discursive frames, and documents resistance and alternatives that are made available through competing frames, including those of the fat rights movement with those produced by the fashion and food industries, and through the contradictions of policy initiatives invoking healthy choices as solutions. Notably, the authors critically examine how obesity is stigmatised, considered a health threat and a 'crisis', legitimated as a major public health problem, and how these issues are enhanced by the COVID-19 pandemic. They highlight the contradictions and uncertainties involved and open considerations of how these issues might be responded to, anticipating the third part of their book.

Part 2 of the book offers three chapters, each focussed on a research project by the three authors. The first examines obesity in the context of bodily change and health identity, focussing on the 'body-as-project', dieting, the embodiment of identity and the trajectories of bodies across the lifecourse. This chapter argues that critical weight and fat studies scholarship would gain from more nuanced considerations of bodily transformation and embodied identity. The second chapter in this part takes up the concern with body pedagogies, and critically interrogates how school-based programmes to prevent body dissatisfaction and eating disorders are situated within neoliberalism and the war on obesity, and promoted with little attention to their evaluation. The third chapter in this part takes up the issue of weight stigma, which is examined though a case study of activities on a right-wing media platform, and addressed by applying recent scholarship on fatness and media to the weaponising of stigma, health fascism and political cruelty.

Part 3 offers a more optimistic perspective on obesity discourse, with a critical discussion of Health At Every Size® as the best-known weight-neutral intervention, and the premises and tensions underpinning this approach. The authors point towards more radical alternatives which address the politicisation of health, and reject stigmatisation of fatness, personal responsibilisation and weight as a proxy for societal ills. They then turn to a consideration of obesity in pandemic times, arguing for ways to advance knowledge and counter pandemic psychology with its accounts of fear and moralising, the divide between obesity scholarship and policymaking, and the reproduction of inequalities via a 'dual crisis' frame pertaining to obesity and COVID-19. This part concludes with an Epilogue, which picks up and extends the major themes of previous chapters. Here, the authors argue for alternatives to weight-centred health paradigms that reflect the need to rethink not only obesity but also health and society. In closing, they promote the need to foster collective hope and collaborative action to ensure the achievement of a fairer society.

Monaghan, Rich and Bombak offer a wide-ranging and critical coverage of research, theory and societal perspectives on what biomedicine terms 'obesity', fully delivering on the promise of the book's title, *Rethinking Obesity*. Their presentation takes a sociological focus but offers broad-ranging arguments that establish a convincing case for why and how we need to rethink this issue and respond to contemporary dominant understandings of weight and fatness, as well as rethink the implications of these, both for health practice and policy and for society at large. This book is far-reaching in its coverage of obesity issues and thought-provoking in its approach, especially given the current crises faced by society. As such, it provides a timely and highly significant contribution to the *Critical Approaches to Health* series.

Kerry Chamberlain & Antonia Lyons
September 2021

ACKNOWLEDGEMENTS

This book took longer than expected to complete, under challenging circumstances. We are grateful to Kerry Chamberlain and Antonia Lyons, editors of Routledge's *Critical Approaches to Health* series, for their understanding and patience. Lee's scholarship on weight-related issues has received funding from the Economic and Social Research Council (grant numbers: RES-000-22-0784, RES-451-26-0768-A). He would also like to thank Brendan Halpin, former Head of Sociology, University of Limerick, for facilitating a sabbatical and Darcy Thoune, who made the research reported in Chapter 6 possible. He dedicates this book to Millie and Ewa, in the hope of a better world. Emma would like to dedicate this book to her dear mum, Sylvia Rich, who sadly lost her protracted battle with cancer in 2020; her love, guidance and support have and always will have a profound influence. Emma also wishes to acknowledge the school and students who kindly participated in the research reported in Chapter 5 and the Public Engagement Unit at the University of Bath for funding. She is grateful to friends and colleagues around the world with whom she has worked and who have also provided inspiration and support, in particular lifelong friend and mentor, John Evans. Andrea thanks her research assistants and colleagues at the University of New Brunswick and Central Michigan University, those who participated in and oversaw the research reported in Chapter 4, and her collaborator, Natalie Riediger. Some of the chapters in this book draw from, or are revised versions of, previously published articles; namely:

Bombak, A.E. and Monaghan, L.F. (2017) Obesity, bodily change and health identities: a qualitative study of Canadian women, *Sociology of Health & Illness*, 39(6): 923–940.

Bombak, A.E., Monaghan, L.F. and Rich, E. (2019) Dietary approaches to weight-loss, Health At Every Size® and beyond: rethinking the war on obesity, *Social Theory & Health*, 17(1): 89–108.

Monaghan, L.F. (2021) Degrading bodies in pandemic times: politicizing cruelty during the COVID-19 and obesity crises, *Journal of Communication Inquiry*. Advance online publication: https://doi.org/10.1177/01968599211043403.

Monaghan, L.F., Rich, E. and Bombak, A.E. (2019) Media, 'fat panic' and public pedagogy: mapping contested terrain, *Sociology Compass*, 13(1): e12651.

Rich, E., Monaghan, L.F. and Bombak, A.E. (2020) A discourse analysis of schoolgirls engagement with fat pedagogy and critical health education: rethinking the childhood 'obesity scandal', *Sport, Education and Society*, 25(2): 127–142.

INTRODUCTION

These are troubling times. Whether the crises confronting today's world are real, manufactured or exaggerated, they are consequential. Disorientation and shock seem endemic as people struggle to interpret and respond to disturbing and rapidly shifting events. Publics are continually 'informed' by governments and other authorities of their vulnerability to multiple dangers and the need for responsible risk avoidance and management. As we were close to finishing this book in early 2020 the SARS-CoV-2 coronavirus (COVID-19) pandemic 'shook the world' (Žižek, 2020), incorporating waves of fear, panic, moralising action and other corrosive responses (Dingwall, 2022; Monaghan, 2020). However, the world was already in crisis mode. Whilst there are grounds for tracing the gyrations of the world-system to an ongoing structural crisis of capitalism (Wallerstein, 2011), relatively recent events heightened a general sense of dis-ease. Besides the aftershocks of the 2008 Great Financial Crisis, which paved the way for austerity and related political economic problems (Dinerstein et al., 2014), many other threats were generating concern. When we initiated this book in 2015, an Ebola outbreak and its potential spread outside of Africa were causing alarm in the Global North. Other threats to hit the headlines included terrorism, notably the November Paris terror attacks that left over 100 people dead and many others seriously injured. Shortly thereafter Northwest Europe was hit by a devastating storm, causing widespread flooding and costly damage. The storm coincided with the United Nations Climate Change Conference in Paris as world leaders sought to agree a plan to fight rising global temperatures and predictions of a dire future.

Seizing upon such events and associated fears, England's Chief Medical Officer, Professor Dame Sally Davies, expressed alarm about obesity among women when launching her annual health report. A popular British news source, the *MailOnline*, recounted the views of the 'health chief' under the headline 'Obesity in women "as dangerous as terror threat"', followed by statements such as 'Davies wants the

DOI: 10.4324/9781315658087-1

obesity crisis in women to be classed alongside flooding and major outbreaks of disease – as well as the threat from violent extremism' (Borland, 2015). According to this 'extraordinary' narrative, obesity in women 'may lead to them being teased as teenagers' whilst also increasing health risks during their reproductive years (especially when pregnant) and thereafter in the form of post-menopausal cancer and heart disease. Hence, Davies is reported calling upon the UK Government to add obesity 'to its National Register of Civil Emergencies. This is an official list of major possible threats to public health which includes terrorism, war, flooding and disease pandemics'. Fuelling what has been termed 'fat panic' (LeBesco, 2010), the article adds that the government will publish 'a new obesity strategy amid accusations they have failed to tackle the crisis' (Borland, 2015).

Although rhetoric about 'the global obesity epidemic' (World Health Organization [WHO], 1998) is now more than 20 years old, concerns persist. Indeed, they have been advanced with an amalgam of declared crises and efforts to find solutions. For *The Lancet* Commission on Obesity, the world is in the grip of a 'syndemic' or 'synergy of pandemics' not only comprising 'excess' weight/fatness but also 'climate change' and 'undernutrition' (Swinburn et al., 2019). Influential US media seem to be on the same page. *The New York Times* warns: 'Climate change is not the only source of dire projections for the coming decade. Perhaps just as terrifying from both a health and an economic perspective is a predicted continued rise in obesity, including severe obesity, among American adults' (Brody, 2020). The so-called obesity crisis has also been discursively amplified via authoritative calls that conflate it with overweight, centre children (implying heightened vulnerability and future problems) and include the Global South (comprising nations typically deemed to be at greater risk from starvation). According to the WHO (2016), low- and middle-income countries now have more overweight and obese children than high-income countries, prompting melodramatic media reporting: 'childhood obesity "an exploding nightmare", says health expert' (Siddique, 2016).

Referring to media, governments and medical authorities, Gailey and Harjunen (2019: 377) state such actors 'frequently tout that "obesity" is quickly becoming the number one threat facing global citizens, and that the growing number of fat persons is a global crisis'. Of course, particular health issues peak and decline, notably in news media that require 'new' material or a novel angle (Lupton, 2018). Nonetheless, Gailey and Harjunen's (2019) statement cannot be dismissed amidst governments' fiscal concerns and rhetoric about 'sugar addiction' that have helped 'fan the flames of crisis surrounding the "obesity epidemic"' (Throsby, 2020: 11). Myriad actors continue to warn about and demand policy solutions to 'the obesity crisis'. The Organization for Economic Co-operation and Development (OECD), for instance, published an updated report proclaiming 'more than one in two adults and nearly one in six children are overweight or obese' in the region, an 'epidemic' best tackled by 'new policy strategies' or 'communication policies' that 'empower people to make healthier choices' (2017: 1).

Now add COVID-19 to this mix. Early in the pandemic mass media claimed: 'Obese and overweight coronavirus patients most in need of critical care' and 'Seven in 10 patients admitted to intensive care units in the UK with coronavirus were overweight or obese' (Donnelly and Newey, 2020). The World Obesity Federation (WOF) promptly added to these concerns. Their 'Obesity and COVID-19 policy statement' cited, inter alia, an international study suggesting '99% of deaths have been in patients with pre-existing conditions, including those which are commonly seen in people with obesity such as hypertension, cancer, diabetes and heart diseases' (WOF, 2020). Thereafter, in line with a 'paradigm of preparedness' (David and Le Dévédec, 2019) and concerns about further 'waves' of COVID-19, the UK Government launched an obesity strategy that sought to 'empower' citizens to live 'healthier lives' (Department of Health and Social Care [DHSC], 2020). Even in this changed world (Lupton, 2020), 'obesity discourse' prevails, defined as a:

> [F]ramework of thought, talk and action concerning the body in which 'weight' is privileged not only as a primary determinant but as a manifest index of well-being surpassing all antecedent and contingent dimensions of 'health'.
>
> *(Evans et al., 2008: 13)*

Obesity discourse, or what Kwan and Graves (2013) term the 'fat as fatal' frame, has shaped public health concerns and policy over several decades (Chapter 1). Although this is a globally circulating discourse, national anxieties also find expression amidst entangled concerns about multiple (costly) chronic health conditions typically associated with ageing populations and growing socio-economic inequalities. For example, before COVID-19, *The Telegraph*, following a report from Diabetes UK, proclaimed that the National Health Service (NHS) 'could collapse under the strain of Britain's weight problem' (Donnelly, 2019). The UK Government also warned that 'obesity-related conditions' not only burdened the NHS but also estimated that they cost society 'around £27 billion each year, with some estimates placing this figure much higher' (DHSC, 2019: 4). Such claims echo earlier medicalised and parliamentary concerns about a 'ticking time bomb' requiring 'a war on obesity' (Monaghan, 2008).

Although women and children are often targeted in this metaphorical 'war' (Herndon, 2014), weight-related concerns ricochet throughout society. Even high-profile privileged White men – those in a position to shape national policy, public discourse and pedagogy – report 'struggling' with their weight and have urged everybody to slim down. Conservative Prime Minister (PM) Boris Johnson is a case in point, not only after falling ill with COVID-19 and being admitted to Intensive Care (Maidment, 2020a) but also before his premiership amidst anxieties about Brexit and moral leadership (Knibbs, 2019). Entwined with clinical practices, economics and 'the imperative of health' (Lupton, 1995), men's weight has also been invoked when denying couples NHS fertility treatment (Pidd, 2018), followed by an announcement that NHS England would trial very low-calorie diets in order to 'tackle obesity' and 'related' diseases (Boseley, 2018). Citing a similar intervention, demonstrating *short-term* success, the article's headline declared general practitioners would prescribe diets 'in the hope of reversing diabetes'. The NHS would be 'ramping up practical action' to help people 'avoid obesity-induced heart attacks, strokes, cancers and type 2 diabetes'. For NHS England's Chief Executive, such action was vital '[b]ecause what is good for our waistlines is also good for our wallets, given the huge costs to all of us as taxpayers from these largely preventable illnesses' (cited by Boseley, 2018).

In short, concerns about 'excess' weight or fatness, defined on the cusp of the twenty-first century as a 'global epidemic' (WHO, 1998), persist and warrant interrogation as a public issue and potentially private trouble. Indeed, what Saguy (2013) calls a 'public health crisis frame' expands the issue beyond the Western cultural aesthetic, wherein fatness is deemed ugly and especially problematic for women and girls (Bordo, 2003; Kwan and Graves, 2013). We are all warned about our Body Mass Index (BMI), or waistlines, with 'everyone everywhere' (Gard and Wright, 2005: 19) urged to take responsibility in combatting this. O'Hara and Taylor (2018: 1) explain that this 'war on obesity' is premised on a weight-centred health paradigm (WCHP), comprising several (contentious) tenets (see Table 0.1).

One might equivocate on whether the term 'paradigm' or 'problematic' is more useful (Moore, 2013: 4), especially when seeking to build bridges in pedagogically significant fields. Whatever term is preferred, weight-related concerns demand critical investigation alongside *alternative approaches* to health in broader social context. This undertaking matters not least because authoritative anti-obesity messages, policies and interventions appear increasingly untenable, if not unethical (Evans et al., 2008; Lupton, 2018; Monaghan, 2014a; Pausé et al., 2021; Rich et al., 2011; Warin, 2020). For instance, O'Hara and Taylor (2018: 14), in a narrative review of critical literature, state the war on obesity contributes to 'an enhanced adipophobicogenic environment' characterised by 'fat phobia and oppression, including weight bias, prejudice, stigma, discrimination, bullying,

TABLE 0.1 Tenets of the Weight-Centred Health Paradigm (WCHP)

- Body weight is increasing rapidly around the world
- BMI and other measures of body weight or fatness are good indicators of current and future health status
- A BMI over 24.9 is a direct cause of disease and premature death
- Increases or decreases in body weight are caused by a simple imbalance between an individual's energy intake and energy expenditure
- Body weight is at least partly volitional and within the control of the individual
- Methods for successful and sustained weight-loss for individuals are well known to science
- Changes in the environment in the past few decades have created an 'obesogenic' environment
- Creating a less 'obesogenic' environment will reduce the prevalence of 'obesity'
- Focusing on body weight for all people, and losing weight for 'overweight' and 'obese' people, will result in achieving better health and reduce the personal, social and economic costs associated with higher than average body weight

Adapted from O'Hara and Taylor (2018: 4)

violence, and cultural imperialism'. They warn 'physical, mental, social and spiritual health and well-being' are potentially eroded by this environment, not only for people typified as fat but also for those who 'fear becoming fat' (p. 14).

An invitation to rethink obesity

This book invites readers to rethink what medicine terms obesity and its precursor, overweight. Such a task entails critically examining associated knowledge claims and, to use the language of pedagogy scholarship, their contexts of reproduction and recontextualisation (dislocation, relocation and refocusing) (Evans et al., 2008). *Rethinking Obesity* scrutinises received 'truths' about 'the obesity crisis' in a theoretically and empirically informed manner, evaluating the current state of knowledge and practices in contexts of power and inequality. In short, what medicine and public health policy define as the problem of overweight and obesity, or others term 'fatness' (see below), will be subject to careful deliberation. In so doing, we may also be in a better position to use this declared public health problem as a lens on other layered crises that include, but also go beyond, the COVID-19 pandemic (Pausé et al., 2021).

In this book we employ 'the sociological imagination' that locates possible personal private troubles within broader social structures (Mills, 1959), such as class, gender and ethnicity. At the same time, we invite transdisciplinary dialogue insofar as human embodiment is irreducible to any specific discourse or discipline (Yoshizawa, 2012). *Rethinking Obesity* proffers sociological insights whilst also going beyond disciplinary silos with reference to 'lived bodies' (Williams and Bendelow, 1998). This means that whilst we will scrutinise discourse, including the capacity of language to reflect and shape the world, we remain attuned to the reciprocal relationship between bodies and society (Williams and Monaghan, 2022). Accordingly, our effort to rethink obesity proceeds without writing out body materiality and structured social relations, emotions, organisation, culture, power and difference. Drawing from scholars such as Shilling (2008, 2012) and others (e.g. Scambler, 2018, 2020a; Williams, 2003), we accept that natural and social realities comprise interdependent and mind-independent processes. And, whilst these realities can only be known through socially constructed frameworks, pursuing such knowledge should not be at the expense of conflating ontology with epistemology (what exists with knowledge of what we think exists). As part of this critical or 'corporeal realist' (Shilling, 2012) approach, we will review and evaluate fact-based assertions. We remain attentive to but also question 'the evidence' and its uptake, reframing or silencing in a contentious arena.

As part of our invitation and efforts to develop ethically justifiable health-enhancing approaches, we will pose and seek to address, if not always fully answer, many questions. For instance, how is weight or fat 'framed', contested and experienced (Kwan and Graves, 2013)? Why does the war on obesity proceed with authority and certainty when the primary scientific field comprises many uncertainties (Bombak, 2014a)? Is widespread concern about obesity explicable in terms of a media-fuelled moral panic (Campos et al., 2006)? Are there better ways to understand this field without denigrating emotions as polluting, feminising and reactionary (Fraser et al., 2010)? What are the social structural mechanisms that recontextualise and pedagogise otherwise contested obesity knowledges, turning them into a potential 'symbolic ruler for consciousness' (Bernstein, 2000: 36)? What are the conditions under which weight-related stigma is 'weaponised' (Scambler, 2018)? What about the politics of health, life and cruelty as they intersect with obesity discourse and nationalist concerns, especially in the COVID-19 era? Why do ostensibly equity-centred public health policies lament the 'upstream' social determinants of health but drift 'downstream' towards lifestyles (Popay et al., 2010)? Why are calorie-restrictive diets repeatedly endorsed, despite over 60 years of damning evidence on their efficacy and safety (Rothblum, 2018)? When seeking to advance critical perspectives, how might we respond to those who castigate some of our work as an uninformed attempt to impugn the intentions of medics, obesity scientists and proponents of the new public health (Monaghan, 2013)?

There is plenty to digest and others to whom we will turn when contemplating these and other questions. For instance, Aphramor (2020a), a radical dietician who has spearheaded alternative thinking and action, urges critics to avoid 'glorifying Western science' not least because it 'normalizes Eurocentric values'. Their argument could be applied not only to the natural sciences but also to the social sciences; the global dynamics of such knowledge production have, after all, been entangled historically with violence and anxiety (Connell, 2007; Rebughini, 2021). Indebted to but also expanding upon the work of such critics, our position is more nuanced than simply being for or against science, medicine and public health. Rather, *Rethinking Obesity* aims to foster productive dialogue and reflexively develop better informed collaborative approaches to weight-related issues, health and society. In so doing, we eschew alarmist, individualising and depoliticising calls to 'fight the fat' whilst remaining attentive to lived bodies as multidimensional processes (affective, symbolic, biological and pragmatic) (Shilling, 2008; Watson, 2000), co-constituting a social world that is itself increasingly strained, if not 'fractured' (Scambler, 2018, 2020a). The putative obesity crisis is too big an issue to be left to the biomedical sciences independent of insights from the social sciences, critical weight and fat studies (see the next section).

Although we have extensively critiqued the anti-obesity offensive (e.g. Bombak, 2014a, 2014b, 2015; Bombak et al., 2016, 2020; Monaghan, 2005a, 2007a, 2007b, 2008, 2014a, 2014b, 2017; Monaghan et al., 2010, 2014, 2018, 2019; Rich, 2011, 2016; Rich and Evans, 2005; Rich et al., 2011, 2015), we eschew abstract criticism, or attempted destruction, of well-intended and informed health promotion. We are not 'against health', though, following Metzl and Kirkland (2010) and LeBesco (2010), we maintain that current conceptions of health (e.g. something that can be reduced to weight or the BMI) are problematic and warrant careful consideration of alternatives (e.g. Aphramor, 2016, 2019a; Bacon, 2010; Brady et al., 2013). Despite arguments from some detractors, we have never been anti-science nor against medicine and health workers (Monaghan, 2013; Chapter 2). Certainly, anti-fat bias, weight-related stigma and fatphobia are documented problems in the health professions, undermining the ethical delivery of effective care (Cooper Stoll, 2019; Lee and Pausé, 2016). Furthermore, scrutinising obesity orthodoxy can be challenging given various entrepreneurs' investments in defining weight/ fatness as a correctable or preventable public health problem (Monaghan et al., 2010). However, amidst such constraints and typically polarising positions, this problem field need not be construed as a case of angels versus devils, or friends versus enemies, as portrayed by some writing on the cultural politics of obesity scholarship (Gard, 2009a). Indeed, we have collaborated with health profession-als (Rich et al., 2011) and delivered health modules over three decades to student clinicians in our roles as educators working across university faculties, including nursing and medical schools. There is much scope to work *with* others, as also explained by Mykhalovskiy et al. (2019) in the context of critical public health scholarship.

Unfortunately, though, many obstacles hinder constructive critique, advancing alternatives to the WCHP and, more radically, challenging the conditions under which 'healthy lifestyle' prescriptions prevail. For instance, what Crawford (1980) terms 'healthism' elevates individual well-being to a 'super value' and it is reflec-tive of the globally circulating neoliberal ideology of personal responsibility (see also Overend et al., 2020). Whilst many individuals are understandably seduced by healthism, which would simply have us all choose health, health organisations and others exercising power over people's lives must also act ethically and on the basis of evidence. In contrast to the individualising and moralising features of healthism, 'The weight of scientific evidence supports a socioeconomic explana-tion of health inequalities' (DHSC, 1998: 8). The patterning of morbidity and mortality is irreducible to personal behaviours (Marmot, 2004a), or bodyweight as a crude proxy or imprecise marker for lifestyles. Rather, the socio-economic model demonstrates the massive influence of social structures; the 'fundamental causes' of health inequalities are societal (McCartney et al., 2021). For instance, Nazroo (2013: 13) explains that socio-economic inequalities or 'material fac-tors make the key contribution to differences in health between ethnic groups'. The causal efficacy of socio-economic factors, more so than lifestyles, for mor-bidity and mortality is recognised in earlier British state-funded health research and policy (e.g. DHSC, 1980, 1998), but this has since been eclipsed by obesity discourse (e.g. DOH, 2008; DHSC, 2020). To the extent that elements of the social structure do figure within hegemonic discourse, they are misrecognised as behavioural bodily matters among groups of individuals who have failed or risk failing as dutiful citizens. Whilst problematic, such reasoning resonates in neoliberal times when real crises (financial, economic, fiscal, political and demo-cratic) cascade through society but are often misrepresented in ways that protect powerful interests (Walby, 2015).

We would not be so naive as to appeal to a single element when proffering sociological explanations. However, under current material conditions of exis-tence a war on obesity (rather than, say, poverty) is politically expedient. By locating health problems and their promised solution in putatively deficient bodies that have failed to act appropriately, obesity discourse elides profound social transformations and market-oriented policies that favour financial capitalism and elites. Such groups include 'the governing oligarchy' or 'plutocracy' (Scambler, 2018: 75), comprising approximately 0.1 per cent of the population in neoliberal nations. Described by Scambler as 'surfers' of existing 'social structures and relations of class and command' (p. 100), these actors are dedicated to the capitalist project of ongoing accumulation (Wallerstein, 2011) and benefit most from what McGoey (2019) terms 'strategic ignorance', i.e. offensive and defensive actions tied to 'unknowing' and the perpetuation of injustice. Such processes, which have a history (e.g. in terms of garnering support for free-market ideologies over the past two centuries), have increased social inequalities and consequently health inequalities *independent* of common 'risk factors' for disease and early mortality (Scambler, 2013a, 2018). One might add to this reading Popay et al.'s (2010: 148) critique of 'lifestyle drift' in public health policy amidst a broad 'consumerist', 'personalization agenda'. There is also a multibillion-dollar weight-loss industry – part of what Clarke et al. (2010) term 'the Biomedical TechnoService Complex Inc.' – that persists despite failing in its promises to make and keep people slim (Bacon and Aphramor, 2014; Rothblum, 2018). The reproduction, amplification and legitimisation of obesity discourse (and associated privileges within a hierarchy of dis/credited bodies) do not require conspiracy (Evans et al., 2008; Monaghan, 2013; Monaghan et al., 2010). Rather, privilege tends to be reproduced in a habitus consisting of collective interests and 'tacit co-ordination' (Mills, 1959: 69; cited by Scambler, 2018: 71).

Yet, alternative approaches exist amidst mounting ethical, empirical and technical objections to the war on obesity (O'Hara and Taylor, 2018). Responding to unsuccessful, iatrogenic public health interventions – and the marginalisation or silencing of evidence from disciplines such as sociology and anthropology – Bombak (2014a: 1) asserts that 'a powerful role may exist for applied social scientists' in furthering research, policy and practice. She contends that only when more varied, inclusive and often complex forms of knowledge are credited will we be able to develop a 'nonstigmatizing, salutogenic approach to public health that accurately reflects the health priorities of all individuals'. *Rethinking Obesity* builds upon such arguments, in support of academic knowledge, health-related practices and ultimately a fairer society.

Such a project necessitates shared learning and democratic dialogue that is attentive to our vulnerabilities as thinking and feeling bodies. In so doing *Rethinking Obesity* gives due weight to the embodied effects and 'subtle but potentially more intrusive psychosocial *affects*' (Evans et al., 2013: 323, emphasis in original) of living in unequal societies wherein 'health concerns' provide a vehicle for myriad injustices and disadvantages (Fox and Powell, 2021). Also mindful of pedagogues' efforts to promote effective clinical practice and 'structural competency' (see Metzl and Hansen, 2014), our invitation foregrounds the need to explore the consequences of living in societies that are divided according to relatively enduring axes of power, such as: social class, gender, ethnicity and age. Such power relations infuse processes ranging from stigma and managing spoiled identity (Goffman, 1968 [1963]; Williams and Annandale, 2020) to social gradients in population health (Marmot et al., 2020a; Scambler, 2018). Hence, and in demonstrating the relevance and intersections of the social and health sciences, *Rethinking Obesity* grapples with the structural conditions under which weight-related issues are produced, interpreted or ignored, the pedagogical modalities of anti-obesity policies and their embodied yet frequently misrecognised effects and affects. On the latter point, note, for example, how contributors to a medical journal issued a call to the media to avoid weight stigma and discrimination (Flint et al., 2018). Yet, these authors ignored how high-profile physicians, including England's Chief Medical Officer, publicly enacted such stigma. Problems have persisted following the outbreak of COVID-19, ranging from the biomedical framing of viral infection as a 'lifestyle disease' to urging weight-loss as a protective measure (O'Connell et al., 2021; Pausé et al., 2021). Accordingly, in addition to underscoring the need for reflexivity, we contend that knowledge must be attentive to ethical, moral, political and experiential concerns. Going from measurements to meanings, 'well rounded' knowledge must incorporate not only biological but also social realities.

Rethinking Obesity offers readers a means of orienting to and evaluating conflicting arguments as formulated within and across disciplines, health professions, policy discourses and popular media (including social media). Theoretically informed and empirically grounded, it also *critically* reviews social scientific contributions to the obesity debate and weight-inclusive paradigms, notably Health At Every Size (HAES®), defined as an evidence-based social justice approach to health and well-being (Bacon, 2010; Bacon and Aphramor, 2011; Mensinger et al., 2016; O'Hara and Taylor, 2018; Tylka et al., 2014). Critically reviewing not only anti-obesity interventions but also alternatives is important amidst calls by social scientists to go beyond discursive realms and interrogate bodies, health issues/practices, social structures and their patterned effects in the material world (Warin, 2015; Williams, 2003).

The remainder of this introduction is structured as such. First, we clarify our use of terms (overweight, obese, weight, fatness) and our understanding of critical weight studies as a distinctive approach in this problem field. Second, we outline the chapter content.

Clarifying terms and delineating approaches

Attuned to the role of language and power in constructing social realities, social scientists writing on the putative obesity crisis usually offer some introductory remarks on their choice of words (e.g. Kwan and Graves, 2013; Lupton, 2018; Saguy, 2013). This is important because words matter, serving as tools whilst also embodying the emotional dimensions of group life (Crossley, 2001; cited by Monaghan, 2008: 22). Referring to somebody as 'fat' in everyday life, for instance, may cause offense and result in 'spoiled identity' (Goffman, 1968 [1963]), though responses can and do vary depending upon social context. Indeed, there are positive appropriations as seen among members of the size acceptance and admiration communities who urge 'fat people' to call themselves 'fatso' in order to 'turn fat hatred back on itself' (Wann, 1998: 28). The acceptability or otherwise of terms to describe body weight, size, shape and composition is a sociological matter. Much depends upon what 'frame' (Kwan and Graves, 2013; Saguy, 2013; see Chapter 1) is used by actors with diverse interests, such as asserting the beauty of fatness or medicalising it using, for example, the BMI that treats weight as a proxy for adiposity and disease (risk). In all of this, a crucial point is that even medical terms describing body mass and composition cannot simply be assumed to be technical and objective; rather, they carry a weight of meanings that are consequential in society (Murray, 2005a).

Similar to Monaghan (2008), Saguy (2013) offers a section early in her book defining and qualifying her use of terms such as 'overweight', 'obesity', 'fat' and 'fatness'. Drawing from dictionary definitions, authoritative health reports, fat activism and representations from popular culture, Saguy explains that there is no widely accepted term for levels of body mass that medicine deems 'excessive'. However, '[i]n the spirit of the budding fat studies subfield' she employs 'the terms *fat* and *fatness*' in contradistinction to medicalised categories (overweight, obesity) that 'explicitly affirm a specific interpretation of bigger bodies as *medical problems*' (2013: 7, emphasis in original). Kwan and Graves (2013) offer similar reasoning. They state, 'the term "fat" often signifies stigma and deviance (particularly when it is pitted against the term "normal"), but it is a term that fat acceptance activists readily accept', whilst the word 'obesity' 'indicates an extreme form of body deviance, both aesthetically and medically' (p. 18). These authors also prefer the term 'fat' in line with fat acceptance activists' efforts to 'reclaim' the word in response to 'a culture where fat bias, discrimination, and stigma are prevalent' (p. 18). Lupton (2018) is another scholar who acknowledges these concerns and defers to a politicised framing. This is amidst much prejudice which, as documented elsewhere, can even negatively impact academics who seek to advance critical perspectives on 'the obesity crisis' (Cameron, 2016; Cameron and Russell, 2016; Chapter 2).

We share the concerns of fat studies scholars, pedagogues and activists (Cooper, 2010; Rothblum and Solovay, 2009) who challenge the pathological connotations of what medicine terms overweight and obesity. Similar to Saguy (2013), Kwan and Graves (2013) and Lupton (2018), we nonetheless have to use biomedical words when, for example, engaging the work of obesity scientists, journalists and policymakers who are diagnosing, lamenting and seeking to remedy the putative crisis. Terms such as 'overweight' and 'obesity' should, however, be read throughout our book with an implicit 'so-called' preceding them and in scare quotes. For presentational purposes, we will not repeatedly insert scare quotes around these terms, but readers should note that we retain a critical distance from them. Our reasoning will likely resonate with others who exercise critical judgement, including at least some health professionals. Aphramor (2018), a dietician and poet with a knack for coining mordant neologisms, denounces the diagnosis of people as overweight or obese as 'obgobbing', defined as using language that 'thoughtlessly, inadvertently or intentionally' fosters 'oppression and/ or impede[s] justice'. Their ethical objections are grounded in the lifeworld. The word 'obesity' is often offensive to laity (Aphramor, 2009; Monaghan, 2008), which is unsurprising in societies wherein public health anti-obesity campaigns utilise 'the pedagogy of disgust' (Lupton, 2015).

When naming our approach, we prefer critical weight studies as a descriptor. Weight in this context is *not* treated as a euphemism for fatness, though weight can and often does include fatness in evaluations of human bodies. In anticipating possible objections from fat studies scholars, it should be clear from what we have already written that our use of the word 'weight' does not mean we are shunning 'fat' – an act that could 'validate and perpetuate the stigma' that we, along with other critics, want to challenge (Calogero et al., 2019: 23). Rather, in a rationalised or McDonaldized society, organised around the core principles of efficient calculability and technological control (Ritzer, 2010), *weight is a crucial definer and measure of 'the obesity epidemic' and the WCHP that we seek to critique*. Whilst supplementary measures (notably waist size) are sometimes used in public health (campaigns) (Dukelow, 2017; Lupton, 2014), the BMI is a calculation based on *weight* and height and it is favoured by those claiming there is an obesity crisis. Weight is often officially credited and preferred. At the population level, it is easily recorded, inexpensive and also deemed more accurate when monitoring larger bodies (i.e. those with a BMI ≥40 kg/m^2), recently defined as increasingly prevalent and 'a high demand epidemic' (K. Williamson et al., 2020b). Our view is that the ubiquitous use of weight – as a proxy for fat and health (risk) – warrants careful scrutiny because it spawns various irrationalities, including an emphasis upon big numbers (e.g. two-thirds of the population are too heavy and are burdening society) (Monaghan, 2007a).

We also prefer 'critical weight studies' because people medically categorised as overweight or obese might be subjects of social research in body-oriented cultures, but they are not necessarily seen as fat or identify as such in everyday life. Obvious examples include strength athletes, to echo Monaghan's (2007b) study of 'big fellas' who sought to slim down whilst justifying levels of body mass that medicine labels excessive. We also need to be mindful of other, potentially vulnerable, groups across the weight spectrum. These groups include schoolgirls who are subjected to obesity discourse via state-sponsored policies and pedagogies, which may fuel disordered eating (Evans et al., 2008). Self-identified 'weight stigma' researchers likely have such concerns in mind when they 'suggest that best practice in research, publishing, and healthcare would be to use neutral terms, with "weight" and "higher weight" likely to be suitable in the majority of situations' (Meadows and Daníelsdóttir, 2016: 3). Lee has previously written with others on such matters when advancing critical weight studies (Monaghan et al., 2010). As an aside, the following excerpt was written when critical obesity research and fat studies, cognate approaches in this nascent field, were also fledgling areas of scholarship. Hence, critical weight studies cannot be dismissed as, for example, the appropriation and whitewashing of fat studies (Cooper, 2016a); they are different, albeit overlapping, projects:

> Contributors come from a range of disciplines and have different ideas about what their work is doing and what it should be called. Although some term this literature 'critical obesity studies' (Gard, 2009a), others substitute 'weight' for 'obesity' since the latter term, like 'overweight', is a medicalised and pathologizing label that could be seen to jar with critical social science. Other scholars, such as Murray (2008) who critiques the 'moral panic' surrounding female fatness, term their work 'fat studies'. This emergent field has been described as 'an interdisciplinary, cross-disciplinary area of study that confronts and critiques cultural constraints against notions of "fatness" and "the fat body"' (Pop Culture Association, 2007). Academic fat activists, identifying as fat and proud, sometimes use the term 'fat studies' (Cooper, forthcoming).

> While endorsing the politicization of the body and fatness, and critiquing obesity epidemic thinking, we refer to our work and the area we seek to develop as 'critical weight studies' because: (a) the social construction of an obesity epidemic depends on the idea of weight (as a proxy for fatness); (b) while biomedical words, such as obesity, are a necessary part of our empirical research, we seek to distance our critical analytical approach from pathologizing labels that medicalize fatness; (c) like obesity, 'fat' is often offensive to people in everyday life (people who might be participants in our ethically informed studies); and (d) we are not simply concerned with 'the fat body' but rather heterogeneous bodies that do not necessarily fit or place themselves on a fat/thin dichotomy or continuum despite being medically categorized as overweight, obese or even morbidly obese.
>
> *(Monaghan et al., 2010: 39–40)*

Following the above and drawing from Cooper (2010), Bombak (2014b) also delineates these three approaches, noting points of overlap and possible connections. She explains that fat studies scholarship 'tends to focus on the embodiment and subjectivities of fat persons' (p. 509). Additionally, 'fat studies scholars are often aligned with critical obesity researchers' who are primarily focused on 'obesity epidemic discourse' (p. 509) including: the scientific arguments upon which the so-called epidemic is based, anti-obesity messaging and an ethically informed critique of the consequences of this discourse. Within critical obesity research the pathologisation and medicalisation of fatness tend to receive more attention than the embodied experiences of living in fatphobic culture. Bombak (2014b: 510) adds:

> A potential bridge for the fields of fat studies and critical obesity scholars may be Monaghan et al.' (2010) proposed discipline of critical weight studies, so termed to acknowledge the medicalization and stigmatization of

fatness implicit in the term 'obesity'. This may best suit researchers, like myself, who choose to interrogate the science of the 'obesity epidemic', while concurrently adopting a politicized view of the effects of such discourse on the embodied, lived experiences, and subjectivities of individuals. Situated as I am in a Faculty of Medicine, I follow Monaghan's (2013) focus on using critical weight studies to produce reflexive, politicized, ethical discussions of health concerns relevant to applied knowledge and practice.

Bombak's (2014b) use of the word 'bridge' is apposite and would likely resonate with others who use the same metaphor in the hope of making a difference in societies fractured by, inter alia, cultural disorientation and disconnected fatalism (Scambler, 2020a). In delineating our approach to health research, policy and practice, none of us would dismiss fat studies which, like fat activism, cannot be assumed to be 'about obesity and health' (Cooper, 2016a: 24). On the contrary, our work has benefitted from an explicit engagement with fat studies and activism (e.g. Monaghan et al., 2014; Rich et al., 2011), including participation in Fat Studies and HAES workshops funded by the UK's Economic and Social Research Council. Emma also recently co-edited a special issue of the *Fat Studies* journal (Rich and Mansfield, 2019). We similarly remain open to critical obesity research. Indeed, our book draws extensively from these approaches, in line with O'Hara and Taylor's (2018: 2) point that critical weight studies, critical obesity studies and fat studies 'share common ground in critiquing' dominant, pathologising claims. And, despite some inter-group contestation and meta-critique (Monaghan, 2013; Chapter 2), we are open to learning more from those publishing under the banner of critical obesity studies (e.g. Gard, 2016) and advancing their work (Fullagar et al., 2022).

On one level, and to draw from pedagogical scholarship on forms of knowledge and intellectual work (Bernstein, 2000), our priority is to systematically address a problematic more so than defend a specific approach (see Moore, 2013). Even so, we do not abandon critical weight studies as a referent and, following on from our previous contributions, there are several reasons why we prefer this descriptor over fat studies, etc. These reasons cannot be reduced to presumed 'professional power' that is allegedly tied to what fat activists might regard as our 'normative embodiment and sense of entitlement to define the terms of being fat' (Cooper, 2016a: 177). Nor are they a consequence of shying away from politicised concerns that include, but also go way beyond, fatness in neoliberal times (Monaghan and O'Flynn, 2017; Monaghan et al., 2018), or the abrasive meanings of the 'F-word'. On the latter point see, for example, Monaghan and Hardey (2011) on everyday responses to the term 'fat bastard'. Our reasoning is hopefully clear from what we have already written and in subsequent chapters where we explore ways of framing the discussion, including how politics, epistemology and ontology figure in this 'contested field' (Kwan and Graves, 2013: 1). However, rather than assume we have adequately cleared the decks, we will finish this section with some further reflections on what we see as the distinctiveness of critical weight studies vis-à-vis other cognate approaches.

Wann (2009: xv) proposes that 'fat studies is not concerned with a small sub-group of people'. Nonetheless, for many fat studies scholars and activists, 'fat people' are typically depicted as an oppressed minority who have a privileged take on 'fat culture' (Gingras and Cooper, 2013), comprising distinct embodied experiences and claims pertaining to social injustice and discrimination (Kwan and Graves, 2013; Saguy, 2013). Reference to fat people and fat culture likely has pragmatic and emotional value for fat activists who experience oppression and, understandably enraged by this (Mitchell, 2005), engage in identity politics and related practices in an attempt to make life more bearable. Nash and Warin (2017) provide a cogent account of why identity politics matter to fat activists, 'especially if the goal is gaining political and/or legal rights' (p. 72), and why any hint at ambiguity and contingency is anathema. Yet, and crucially, weight also serves as a proxy for fatness in dominant (bio)medicalised discourse *that defines the majority as overweight or obese* (ill, deficient, deviant, pathological, costly, etc.), regardless of whether most people identify as such or have actually become (significantly) fatter or heavier (Campos et al., 2006). Our concern, then, is with scrutinising a problematic as it pertains to widely circulating and officially legitimated *knowledges* that are irreducible to the specialised concerns, experiences and voices of 'fat people' qua 'situated' *knowers* – a distinction elaborated upon by Bernstein (2000) with reference to different knowledge structures and grammars in an attempt to avoid the reductive and exclusionary pitfalls associated with identity-based approaches (see also Moore, 2013).

The above 'problematisation of the normal' in obesity discourse is an expression of what Armstrong (1995) terms 'Surveillance Medicine' that 'attempts to bring *everyone* within its network of visibility' (p. 139, emphasis added). Other medical sociologists interrogate expansive medical power using the concept of 'biomedicalization', comprising processes ranging from 'risk and surveillance' to 'transformations of bodies and subjectivities' in a commodifying, technoscientific era (Clarke et al., 2010). Regardless of the specific concept, and in drawing inspiration from Goffman (1968 [1963]) on stigma, the above prompts us to view 'fat people' and 'normal people' (*sic*) as perspectives *not* distinct groups. We will therefore avoid reifying these categorisations or pitching them as rivals in the increasingly competitive neoliberal academy. Following Harvey (2005), we understand neoliberalism as part of a divisive class project that champions market logics and competitive individualism over social solidarity, interdependency and reciprocity. Neoliberalism is deservedly critiqued within fat activism (Cooper, 2016a) whilst, we would suggest, still exerting corrosive effects.

Our avoidance of a dichotomising approach to human bodies and reductive claims about who can legitimately contribute to these debates is also rooted in an appreciation of corporeal indeterminacy. To draw from symbolic interactionism (Waskul and Vannini, 2006), the body, as with any object in society, is not a self-existing entity with an intrinsic nature; rather, its nature is dependent upon the actions and orientations of people towards it (Monaghan, 2006). More specifically, the meanings and consequences of fatness depend upon contingent social judgements rather than unmediated biological reality, technoscientific 'truths' or a predefined political agenda. Yet, at least in Western culture, such judgements are embedded within a broader 'obesity assemblage' (Rich, 2010) that democratises 'excess' weight in accord with biomedical, public health, government and media endorsed regimes of surveillance, bodily measurement, control, discipline, healthism, profiteering, affect and public pedagogy that 'teaches' individuals to embody certain values (e.g. to be healthy, productive, competitive, self-reliant, responsible, efficient, entrepreneurial) (Evans et al., 2008; Guthman, 2009; Rich, 2011). Such considerations are pertinent when exploring issues such as gendered resistances to the BMI (Monaghan, 2007b) or scapegoating whole populations as costly deviants following the 2008 crisis (O'Flynn et al., 2014). To return to Nash and Warin (2017: 75), we would suggest such concerns are pertinent when seeking to offer 'a more nuanced reading of the complexities of power' and for 'shifts to occur in the cultural meanings attached to differing body sizes'.

In view of the above, the question 'who are these fat people' or 'obese people' (*sic*) in fat studies and critical obesity research respectively might be supplemented, if not replaced, by the question: 'when are people labelled overweight, obese or fat, or when do they identify as such and to what end?' In that regard, there are good reasons to 'expand the obesity debate' (Rich et al., 2011) through the lens of critical weight studies, which is irreducible to fat or obese individuals, in favour of *an emphasis upon society as a network of power relations that is potentially corrosive for all bodies across the weight spectrum*. Accordingly, our approach critically incorporates and synthesises diverse perspectives, understandings and theories without conflating ontology with epistemology, or being with knowing (Williams, 2003). Rethinking what biomedicine and public health term obesity is a much broader and inclusive endeavour than implied by the study of 'the fat' or 'obese' body if for no other reason than that all bodies contain various and varying proportions of adiposity, muscle, bone, tendons and other organic material that may or may not matter to people within their contexts of everyday life. Of course, 'fat people', similar to 'obese people', remain useful 'fabrications' (Evans et al., 2008) for different groups depending upon their values, interests, practices, politics and audiences. As with our reference to biomedical labels, we will also use these constructs where necessary albeit in a qualified, or ideal typical, sense.

Finally, we invite potential critics to rethink how they have imagined critical weight scholarship. For instance, our work is not naively premised on the goal of befriending 'obese people' (*sic*) in contrast to medical practitioners who might be hateful towards them (see also Monaghan, 2013). Rather, our fundamental goal as academic researchers and educators is to advance knowledge and critical pedagogy that could have applied value in the health field and, more ambitiously, support debate on macro-social change in crisis times.

Structure and content

Rethinking Obesity is divided into three parts: (1) The Politics of a 'Public Health Problem', (2) Researching Matters of Fat, and (3) Critically Exploring

Alternatives, Fostering Collective Hope. Part 2 reports and analyses data from three empirical studies that were undertaken independently by the authors. Part 3 is followed by an epilogue. We will outline the book's content below.

Part 1 contains three chapters. Chapter 1 situates critique in a broader context. After establishing that 'excess' weight/fatness continues to be authoritatively defined as a global problem, we outline the signature elements of various frames, ranging from health and aesthetic concerns to social justice. We also discuss the politics of health, embodied sociology and the influence of neoliberalism. Chapter 2 provides a map of critical perspectives on the obesity crisis. It includes a critique of obesity science and epidemiology; analyses of popular media (including digital media), 'fat panic' and body pedagogies; the stigmatising effects and affects of obesity discourse; and meta-critique. Chapter 3 explores anti-obesity policy as knowledges move from obesity science to the official recontextualising field of government and pedagogy, notably public health campaigns. We dissect the pedagogising of policy and stigmatising affects/effects, critiquing concepts such as 'lifestyle drift', 'nudging' and 'the obesogenic environment'.

Part 2 presents empirically grounded qualitative studies on 'matters of fat'. Chapter 4, researched by Andrea, draws from repeat interviews with Canadian women identifying as (formerly) obese. Core themes include participants' desire to embody a thin(ner) future and a better life, the harms of intentional weight-loss and resignation to living as a fat woman whilst nonetheless challenging stigma. Conceptually, the chapter contributes to studies of bodily change and the embodiment of health identities. Chapter 5, researched by Emma, uses a poststructuralist feminist perspective to analyse data generated during focus groups and classroom-based activities with girls in an English state secondary school. It explores how the girls conceptualised and represented health in postfeminist times but also their receptiveness to fat pedagogies that challenge obesity discourse. Barriers and constraints on the uptake of alternative pedagogies are also discussed, such as the contradictions between school-based interventions promoting self-acceptance versus those informed by obesity discourse. Chapter 6, researched by Lee, explores weight-related stigma during the initial COVID-19 lockdown. It draws from an online US right-wing news media platform, Campus Reform, and readers' comments denouncing fat studies professors. Such practices constituted an online status degradation ceremony that also targeted academic disciplines, expertise, universities and social justice agenda. The analysis is informed by ethnomethodology plus literature on media and bodyweight, weaponised stigma, health fascism and the politics of cruelty. A case is also made for vigilance at a time when 'big money' underpins ideologically motivated attacks on faculty.

Part 3, consisting of two chapters, builds on the promise of alternative approaches to health. Chapter 7 critically explores HAES, the most well-known weight-inclusive health paradigm. Reviewing scientific evidence, the chapter first questions the efficacy and safety of dieting before explicating HAES in social context. Discussion includes HAES principles plus tensions, resonance and controversies within the movement, including calls for a more radical approach towards the body politic and its impact upon health outcomes independent of people's weight and/or lifestyles. Chapter 8 seeks to pave the way for more 'rounded' knowledge and collective action in the (post) COVID society. Written at a time when responses to the COVID-19 pandemic had significantly disrupted everyday life, the chapter underscores the value of the social sciences and humanities before describing an ideal typical model on pandemic psychologies, the relationship between uncertain science and policymaking, and, finally, pandemic inequalities or how social divisions were being exacerbated. To the extent that COVID-19 and obesity were being framed as a dual crisis, Chapter 8 notes how we were perhaps entering a watershed moment for rethinking public health and society. Accordingly, Chapter 8 is followed by an epilogue that leaves space open for further dialogue and possible action. It offers a pithy way of distinguishing two distinct 'ideal typical' ways of orienting to obesity, health and society before making a case *with* others for critique, hope and change.

We will finish this introduction with a reflexive note on what is often termed 'thin privilege' within fat activism, fat pedagogy and HAES. Thin privilege refers to how people may undeservedly enjoy greater respect and opportunities because of their 'normative' physicality (Bacon et al., 2016; Kannen, 2016; Nash and Warin, 2017). The concept, intended to draw attention to weight stigma or fat oppression, is surrounded by ambivalence, but it also relates to the thorny issue of who has the right to discuss the sort of topics that we address in this book. We hinted at this above when delineating critical weight studies, which includes, but is not confined to, the study of fat people, fat culture and identity politics. As Nash and Warin (2017) explain with reference to reactions on Twitter to one of their presentations at a fat studies conference, a perceived 'failure' to acknowledge 'thin privilege' by scholars with bodies considered 'normative' may arouse much consternation. Rather than being drawn into these heated debates and associated 'confessionals' (e.g. whether we are entitled to rethink obesity based on our current physicality), we would state that our embodied biographies, identities and relations with food, fat and self-acceptance are diverse. Yet, all three of us understand and appreciate that lived bodies and subjectivities are constantly in flux or processual. Suffice to say, there have been times when our weight has or has not been especially important to us and/or other people, sometimes our body mass might fluctuate (e.g. during periods of intense study or through physical activity) and we see little point in reducing what follows to where we might have been, currently are or where we might end up on some arbitrary measure. In addition, just as it cannot be assumed that thinness is associated with privilege (e.g. especially in masculine cultures that expect robust physicality and promised action: see Monaghan, 2001, 2002), there may be other, more significant privileges at play. For example, our White ethnicity and status as university faculty within what Connell (2007) terms 'the global metropole' (Europe and North America) are likely to be more important than what our current BMI or body composition might be. Even so, we also seek to offer critical, reflexive commentary on how, inter alia, obesity discourse reproduces myriad social inequalities in 'fractured societies' (Scambler, 2018) such as the UK and kindred nations. We do not presume to speak for and on behalf of multiple oppressed groups (similarly, Kannen, 2016). However, that does not bar us from critically exploring different frames, evidence, politics, policies, pedagogies, media, dietary practices, health interventions and theoretical frameworks on weight-related issues.

PART 1

The politics of a 'public health problem'

1
THE GLOBAL OBESITY CRISIS

Situating critique in a broader context

The authoritative definition of obesity as a global public health crisis not only raises questions about what kind of problem weight/fat/obesity might be and where responsibility lies but also serves to mobilise actions and proposed interventions. Drawing on critical perspectives of health and other overlapping approaches outlined in our introduction (critical weight studies, fat studies and critical obesity research), this book furthers reflexive, ethically informed discussion on obesity discourse and the WCHP (O'Hara and Taylor, 2018). Building on earlier critical contributions (e.g. Bombak, 2014b; Evans et al., 2008; Gard and Wright, 2005; Kwan and Graves, 2013; Monaghan et al., 2014; Rich et al., 2011; Saguy, 2013), our challenge has been to rethink obesity and ask how this issue is or might be interpreted and approached within research, policy and practice. Ensuing chapters posit that amidst considerable uncertainty, complexity and contestation there remains a pressing need to scrutinise this problem field.

Before examining some of the theoretical traditions that shape the way obesity is constructed and critiqued in research, and how certain framings or narratives dominate the design of contemporary public health strategies and programmes (issues explored respectively in Chapters 2 and 3), this chapter situates our critique in a broader context. Discussion is divided into three main sections. First, we outline dominant representations of 'the global obesity crisis' in societies wherein an institutionalised war on fat or 'excess' weight tends to be strongest. As we will see, concerns about population weight (gain) have been recurrent in public health circles, government reports, mass media, academic journals and consumer culture. Second, we elaborate upon the 'signature elements' of the 'fat as fatal' frame (Kwan and Graves, 2013) or what Evans et al. (2008) term 'obesity discourse'. This section also opens up alternative spaces by outlining overlapping and competing frames or 'organizational premises' (Goffman, 1974: 247), including those produced by the fashion and food industries and fat rights movement. Third, we

DOI: 10.4324/9781315658087-3

position our critical scholarship within studies of body politics and embodied sociology, clarifying that we are not only interested in discourses and identity but also the materiality of flesh and blood bodies in contexts of power, inequality and pedagogy. This literature supports our goal to reconceptualise the putative obesity crisis and call for a broader rethink of health and society. Chapter 1 ends with a summary and preliminary reflections, including on the influence of neo-liberalism within politicised debates.

The ongoing world war on obesity

We began this book by referring to dire claims about obesity, expressed by England's Chief Medical Officer and other authoritative sources in a global context (e.g. WHO, 2016, 2018). According to these actors, obesity is in the same league as terrorism, climate change and pandemics of infectious disease (Borland, 2015; Brody, 2020; Swinburn et al., 2019). Defining obesity as a threat and calling for government action – bolstered in 'the COVID society' (Lupton, 2020) via a 'paradigm of preparedness' (David and Le Dévédec, 2019; see also Chapter 8) – are hardly original. Rather, these are recycled concerns that have been expressed by leading public health officials and their allies for decades. For example, US Surgeon General C. Everett Koop popularised the expression 'war on obesity' in 1997, citing an alleged annual death toll of 300,000 Americans (Mayer, 2004: 999). His call was preceded by a study in the *Journal of the American Medical Association*, reporting a large increase in the prevalence of overweight (Kuczmarski et al., 1994) alongside an editorial featuring the term 'epidemic' (Saguy, 2013: 107–8). As Saguy explains, the media then helped to 'spread' the idea that an 'obesity epidemic' was afoot. Whilst the 1990s could be viewed as the beginning of a distinct obesity 'epidemic psychology' (Strong, 1990), which has amplified weight-related stigma and moralising action, there are antecedents. For instance, in 1952 the Director of the National Institutes of Health claimed obesity was 'the number one nutritional problem in the United States' (cited by Gaesser, 2002: 44). Similar concerns were expressed in Canada, related, in part, to national anxieties generated during the Cold War (McPhail, 2017).

Calls to tackle 'excess' weight/fatness/obesity persist in national and inter-national contexts (e.g. DHSC, 2019, 2020; OECD, 2017; WHO, 2021), despite mounting critique (Chapter 2). Definitions of population weight (gain) as a 'big' problem requiring urgent solutions appear irresistible when obesity is conflated with overweight, alongside downward revisions of BMI thresholds that render most people 'too heavy' (Oliver, 2006). Calls to combat weight/fatness 'feed off' normative cultural values about self-control, care, responsibility and body malleability. Of course, the world war on obesity – or 'globesity' (WHO, 2021) as it has been called – is not uniform in its embodied effects and affects. This is because 'health discourses flow across territories and national boundaries' thus entering different 'socio-political systems' with varying degrees of inequal-ity and 'status differentials' (Evans and Davies, 2020: 739). Nonetheless, the aforementioned healthist values are shared across many neoliberal nations, meaning the imperatives of obesity discourse, whilst unpredictable, often resonate. Thille (2019: 892), in an article on anti-fat stigma in primary healthcare, writes: 'In the US, Canada, Australia, New Zealand, and Britain, people commonly assert weight and body composition are highly malleable and under individual control through eating and exercise practices'. Such tenets underpin public health pedagogies that target 'risk behaviours' and presumed ignorance via technologies such as the BMI, tape measure (Dukelow, 2017; Lupton, 2014, 2018) and social media (OECD, 2017), with the normatively healthy body symbolising 'morally worthy' citizenship (LeBesco, 2011: 154). Embedded in globally circulating pedagogic systems of symbolic and economic control, which invite obsessive comparison and competition in policy fields (Evans and Davies, 2020; Chapter 3), such citizens are ideally self-disciplined and motivated to resist an 'obesogenic environment' wherein 'toxic' overconsumption and sedentary living are deemed endemic (Schorb, 2013: 5; Chapter 2).

Gard (2011) professed a decade ago that the end of the obesity epidemic was nigh due to a levelling of rates in the West and increasing life expectancy. Yet, events scuttled that bold prediction. Thereafter life expectancy declined or stalled in high-income nations (Marmot et al., 2020a), attributable to suicide, drug overdose (Ho and Hendi, 2018), austerity policies and social vulnerability (especially for women and the elderly) (Annandale, 2022). Moreover, many enterprising actors continued or reinvigorated the war on obesity. These actors are variously described as '"anti-obesity proponents" (Saguy & Riley, 2005), "obesity alliances" (Strategies to Overcome and Prevent [STOP] Obesity Alliance), "obesity crusaders" (Basham & Luik, 2008), or "obesity alarmists" (Gard, 2011)' (O'Hara and Taylor, 2018: 2). Drawing from classic and contemporary social theory, including interactionist writings on 'the moral entrepreneur' (Becker, 1963) and Foucauldian-inspired scholarship on the new public health (Petersen and Lupton, 1996), Monaghan et al. (2010) refer to these actors as 'obesity epidemic entrepreneurs'. They include: scientists, journalists, policymakers, drug companies, charities, celebrities, clinicians, weight-loss consultants and dieters. Interests and practices include: establishing rationalised benchmarks (e.g. the BMI), dramatising the epidemic, campaigning for legislation, launching taskforces, writing reports, devising policy, 'educating' the public, profiteering and displaying moral worth. Drawing from Monaghan et al.'s typology of obesity epidemic entrepreneurs, O'Hara and Taylor (2018: 4) describe these as 'promulgators of the WCHP' and a crucial element of its *context*.

These enterprising types, or continually refashioned modes of entrepreneurship, have been busily reproducing the obesity epidemic as a national and/or global problem. For instance, the WOF launched World Obesity Day in 2015, with subsequent events dedicated to calling on governments to invest in treatment, end childhood obesity and weight stigma. The WOF is the rebranded name for the International Association for the Study of Obesity, criticised in the *British Medical Journal* given its ties to the pharmaceutical industry and for proposing to expand potentially harmful definitions of childhood obesity (Moynihan, 2006a, 2006b). The WOF, in asserting its credentials or 'symbolic capital' (Saguy, 2013), reportedly 'represents professional members of the scientific, medical and research communities from over 50 regional and national obesity associations' (WOF, 2019). In 2016, its president, Professor Ian Caterson, called for strategic action because: 'The obesity epidemic has reached virtually every country in the world, and overweight and obesity levels are continuing to rise in most places' (cited by Boseley, 2016a). Such concerns were subsequently crystallised with 'the first unified World Obesity Day' on the 4 March 2020, signalling a more integrated approach from an expansive coalition of organisations from around the world. The campaign website, dedicated to 'the root causes of obesity', stated: 'Obesity is a global crisis that affects 650 million people worldwide' and 'by working together on a unified day, the power and reach of our activities can be multiplied' (World Obesity Day, 2020; for a related report pertaining to 200 countries, see Lobstein and Brinsden, 2020). The WOF is also part of *The Lancet* Commission on Obesity (Swinburn et al., 2019), which, as noted earlier, frames the putative problem as a 'global syndemic' entwined with climate change and undernutrition.

The UK's Obesity Health Alliance has also been advancing a public health crisis narrative at the national level. Established in 2015, this 'coalition of 45 leading health charities and medical royal colleges' (Bauld et al., 2021) campaigns for ministers to take tough action to fight obesity and counter alleged 'government inertia' (on the UK policy context, see also Boswell, 2016). The Alliance's latest report, *Turning the Tide: A 10-Year Healthy Weight Strategy* (2021), claims to offer 'a far more nuanced' approach to 'the complexities' of weight by invoking issues such as the obesogenic environment and the problem of COVID-19 'for those living with obesity' (p. 8). Alliance members have also proven to be active independent producers of the obesity crisis narrative in recent years. For example, the Academy of Medical Royal Colleges' (2013) widely publicised report declared fatness is 'a problem of epidemic proportions' that 'must now be tackled urgently' (p. 7). Fiscal concerns and unfavourable comparisons with Europe apparently bolstered their claims, reported by news media under headlines such as 'Obesity crisis risks making Britain "fat man of Europe"' (Dixon, 2013). Such declarations have political effects, with the UK Government subsequently revising its policy response, especially for childhood obesity (DHSC, 2019; Chapters 3 and 5) and, thereafter, for children and adults (DHSC, 2020). Responding to obesity and COVID-19, the latter report enacts earlier policy concerns and proposed solutions that drift towards lifestyles (Popay et al., 2010; Chapters 3 and 8), belying assurances that 'less emphasis' is currently being placed on 'individual responsibility' for obesity (Obesity Health Alliance, 2021: 8).

Other governments have similarly renewed their anti-obesity offensive in recent years. The Irish Government is a case in point, evidenced in *Healthy Weight for Ireland: Obesity Policy and Action Plan 2016-2025* (DOH, 2016). That document extends concerns expressed in an earlier report, which claimed 'body weight is now the most prevalent childhood disease' [*sic*] (The Report of the National Taskforce on Obesity,

2005: 6). The Irish Government's subsequent plan attracted a flurry of media attention. National newspapers featured headlines such as: 'government launches 10-year war on obesity' (Hallissey, 2016), 'new strategy aims to tackle Irish obesity levels' (Cullen, 2016) and 'revealed: new plan to stop Ireland becoming the fattest country in Europe' (O'Regan, 2016). The state television and radio broadcaster, RTÉ, joined this cacophony. Quoting the Minister for Health, the RTÉ website reported that 'obesity is a ticking time bomb which has already to some extent exploded as 60% of adults and 1-in-4 children in Ireland are either overweight or obese'. The Minister of State at the Department of Health is also quoted, announcing that 'Ireland is "becoming the fattest nation in Europe" and the new strategy aims to get people to a healthy weight "as a norm"' (RTÉ, 2016; also Quinlan, 2018). Furthermore, there appeared to be public support for harsh penalties on the grounds that 'irresponsible' parents are to blame for rearing fat kids. Reporting on the new state strategy, one newspaper headline presented opinion poll results as such: '25% back prosecuting parents of obese children' (Baker, 2016). Because mothers traditionally take primary responsibility for childcare and are often blamed for 'the broken society' (Jensen, 2018), the implication is clear. Reflecting on the moralisation of health in the USA, LeBesco (2010: 74) states mothers of fat children 'are framed as the scourges of civilization' (cited by Quirke, 2016: 140). Yet, in Ireland, as elsewhere, it seems to matter little that epidemiological data contradicted claims about escalating childhood obesity (Share and Share, 2017).

We have already mentioned the US context and several decades of obesity alarmism. US health agencies continue to recycle obesity discourse. Kwan and Graves (2013) describe the US Centers for Disease Control and Prevention (CDC) as a leading producer of the 'health frame' that defines 'fat as fatal' (though there are internal contradictions, with the CDC publishing reports that destabilise this frame and weight-loss recommendations; see Rothblum, 2018; Saguy, 2013). After surveying the CDC website and citing a report titled *Obesity and Severe Obesity Forecasts through 2030* (Finkelstein et al., 2012), Kwan and Graves (2013: 138) state 'from a public health standpoint, the problem has not subsided'. More recently, the CDC (2020) lists obesity among several 'underlying medical conditions' that render 'people of any age … at increased risk for severe illness from COVID-19' (though see Chapter 2). The definition of obesity as a serious and protracted problem that demands solutions has also been advanced in a report by the US Department of Health and Human Services, *Healthy People 2020* (US DHHS, 2014). This 'bible' of American public health lists numerous objectives, including: increasing the proportion of adults at a healthy weight; reducing the number of children, adolescents and adults considered obese; and preventing inappropriate weight gain in youth and adults. Interestingly, a subsequent report on the CDC website states: 'No significant changes were seen in either adult or childhood obesity prevalence in the United States between 2003–2004 and 2011–2012' (Ogden et al., 2015: 1). However, citing data for 2011 to 2014, it still defines obesity as a big problem: 'The prevalence of obesity among U.S. adults [crude estimate of 36.5%] remains higher than the Healthy People 2020 goal of 30.5%' (p. 1). Thereafter, US researchers predicted 'that by 2030 nearly 1 in 2 adults will have obesity … and the prevalence will be higher than 50% in 29 states and not below 35% in any state' (Ward et al., 2019: 2440). Most recently, *Healthy People 2030* (US DHHS, 2020) continues to buttress the WCHP by seeking to '[r]educe overweight and obesity by helping people eat healthy (*sic*) and get physical activity' – the reiteration of lifestyle prescriptions.

We could also refer to many nations outside of the Anglophone sphere. For example, obesity is defined as a big public health problem in China, not least given population size and concerns about the Westernisation of lifestyles (Greenhalgh, 2019). We have also drawn attention, in our introduction, to the OECD's 2017 obesity report which cites campaigns in its member states (e.g. Turkey's *Move for Health* and *Reducing Portion Sizes*) (p. 12). Spain, ranked the healthiest country in the world on the 2019 Bloomberg Global Health Index (Miller and Lu, 2019), is also projected to have problems. Drawing uncritically from public health research, the media warn '80% of men and 55% of women in Spain will be overweight by 2030 […] which will mean an additional cost to the health system of €3 billion' (Quintáns, 2019). Obesity discourse also circulates in high-income nations such as Japan (Borovoy and Roberto, 2015; Castro-Vázquez, 2019), France (Saguy, 2013; Saguy et al., 2010), Germany (Mata and Hertwig, 2018; Schorb, 2013), Norway (Grønning et al., 2012), Finland (Gailey and Harjunen, 2019; Setälä and Väliverronen, 2014) and, increasingly, middle- and low-income nations in the Global South (Brewis et al., 2018). However, rather than referring to an expansive list of countries, we will contextualise our discussion by briefly referring to two additional Anglophone nations with which we are most familiar: Canada and Australia.

The Canadian Medical Association has continued to pontificate about the country's 'growing problem' (McPhail, 2017), using national and international data to declare obesity a 'costly pandemic' and 'an expanding threat' (Wisniewski, 2013: 358). Such concerns were further legitimated by the Parliament of Canada's (2016) report, *Obesity in Canada: A Whole-of-Society Approach to a Healthier Canada*. Highlights from the report, published on the parliamentary website, begin as such: 'There is an obesity crisis in this country. Canadians are paying for it with their wallets — and with their lives' (though see Ellison et al., 2016; Medvedyuk et al., 2018). The report generated media commentary lamenting the apparently dire nature of the nation's health and the need to revise Canada's Food Guide (Harris, 2016; Kirkup, 2016), or arguing against a proposed sugar-sweetened beverage tax (Riediger, 2016; see also Riediger and Bombak, 2018). Concerns about childhood overweight and obesity also feature heavily in Canadian public health policy (Medvedyuk et al., 2018), alongside representations of its Indigenous population as a problem (McPhail, 2013, 2017).

Finally, obesity remains a 'symbolically violent' policy concern in Australia (Warin, 2020; Warin and Zivkovic, 2019), following government aspirations to become the healthiest country by 2020 (National Preventative Health Taskforce, 2009). As well as targeting tobacco and alcohol consumption, the Australian Government Taskforce aimed to '[h]alt and reverse the rise in overweight and obesity' (p. 7) through a phased approach comprising, for example, community-based intervention trials that seek to '[e]mbed physical activity and healthy eating in everyday life' (p. 13). The Australian Institute of Health and Welfare subsequently released two reports in 2017 that defined obesity as a major problem that was most pronounced among youth and Indigenous people (Australian Government, 2017a, 2017b). Finances again figure in these reports, with a cost of $8.6 billion attributed to obesity in 2011–2012 (2017a: vii). The nation's media have also amplified obesity concerns, with false claims that 'Australia is the "fattest nation" in the world' (Holland et al., 2011: 31; Chapter 2). Drawing from Cain et al.'s (2017) research on Australian (and US) online news reports (from 2013 to late 2015), Lupton (2018: 100–1) flags *continued* media reference to 'an obesity epidemic … that requires interventions on the part of government, urban designers, the food industry and individuals themselves'. Highlighting themes that we will discuss in subsequent chapters, Lupton adds that news reports have continued to emphasise personal responsibility and the importance of behavioural change, though 'the social and economic determinants of eating behaviour' have also garnered attention alongside the problem of 'fat-shaming' (p. 101).

In summary, despite evidence of stabilisation of obesity prevalence rates in various nations (Ogden et al., 2015; O'Hara and Taylor, 2018; Share and Share, 2017), the world reportedly remains in the grip of a costly public health crisis or epidemic requiring various interventions. Proponents of 'the anti-obesity perspective' have even coined 'the neologism "globesity", to denote the spread of the epidemic around the world' (Lupton, 2013: 15), with youths often emerging as a focus of concern (WHO, 2016). Rather than witnessing 'the end of the obesity epidemic' (Gard, 2011), or its decline on the policy agenda (Boswell, 2016), there is evidence of re-emergent, recycled and reinvigorated calls to wage worldwide war on 'excess' flesh. Indeed, millions of people continue to be targeted by an anti-obesity offensive amidst a flurry of government and media reports in various nations, most recently compounded by problematic responses to COVID-19 (Chapters 2, 6 and 8). This metaphorical war equates weight-loss and slenderness with virtuous healthiness, fitness, pandemic preparedness and actively supporting, rather than needlessly burdening, the economy and state. Arguably, these shared concerns are reflective of the highly competitive dynamics of a world-capitalist system facing an unresolved global crisis (Wallerstein, 2011). This is an unstable, exploitative and wasteful system based on the endless accumulation of capital wherein much anxiety surrounds productivity, consumption and the relative standing of nation-states. In such a context, obesity is a pre-eminent vehicle, symbol and metaphor for widespread societal dis-ease.

A matter of perspective or frames? From public health to social justice

Whether viewed as frames, discourses or narratives (Boswell, 2016; Evans et al., 2008; Kwan and Graves, 2013), the alarmist picture outlined above has dominated global public health debates, thinking and action for over 20 years (WHO, 1998). The basic and ubiquitous formulae, especially in Western culture, is that 'fatness = unhealthy = bad' (LeBesco, 2011: 155). A more insidious rendition, noted by Evans et al. (2008: 2) with reference to socially divided Britain, is that 'fat equals working-class failure, thin equals virtue and middle-class success'. Accordingly, in order to avoid being 'framed' as slovenly and greedy 'weight deviants' (Monaghan et al., 2010: 65) who are subordinated, marginalised and socially immobile, every-one everywhere is urged to combat obesity and achieve a better life.

Frames or perspectives *contesting* obesity discourse are also identifiable and have been analysed by sociologists for over two decades (e.g. Saguy, 2013; Saguy and Riley, 2005). However, before we outline these alternatives below and expand upon critical perspectives in subsequent chapters we will tease out 'the signa-ture elements' or 'rhetorical devices used to describe representations' (Kwan and Graves, 2013: 13) of 'the obesity problem'. These signature elements include the following 'constellation of ideas' (Boswell, 2016: 39), all of which may be conten-tious: fat is a killer; it has expanded relentlessly and is costly; this is an epidemic primarily caused by poor diet and/or lack of physical activity in an obesogenic environment replete with 'junk food' and energy-saving devices; the problem must be urgently combated with the assistance of weight-loss industries, their staff and wares (e.g. personal trainers and group fitness instructors, specialised foodstuffs, weighing scales, mobile tracking devices and other technologies), gov-ernments, the mass media (e.g. newspapers and reality television shows promis-ing solutions), celebrities (e.g. chefs such as Jamie Oliver), the pharmaceutical industry, clinicians (e.g. bariatric surgeons and dieticians), public health work-ers, schoolteachers and other educators. Corrective and preventative action is essential since obesity is a leading public health issue, possibly eclipsing tobacco and alcohol, which governments can ill afford (Sturm, 2002). As explained by Boswell (2016: 39), actors offering particular narratives in policy-relevant settings may not recount all of these ideas 'in full', but they form a discourse that serves to 'order people's perspectives on understanding of political issues, sometimes at a distance from or beyond their own apprehension' (see also Chapter 3, where we offer a pedagogical reading of anti-obesity public health policy).

The *vulnerability* of childhood, an idea-element evinced in many nations, is also a key signature element in the above discourse or 'problem frame' (Backstrom, 2020; Quirke, 2016; Saguy, 2013). Entwined with patriarchal ideology, which reasserts traditional gender norms under the rubric of 'mother blame' (Bombak et al., 2016; Friedman, 2015), publics are told that children, if they are to avoid becoming obese adults, require healthy 'parental' (*sic*) nurturance from con-ception onwards. Children symbolise the future, which needs to be secured through anticipatory medicine and a pre-emptive war on obesity (Evans and Colls, 2011). Whilst developments in scientific research on the foetal origins of disease have implications for how women's reproductive bodies are imagined and framed, for instance, as 'smoking guns' for childhood obesity (Warin et al., 2012), one can also discern here echoes from the past. Child-saving crusades and the demonisation of typically working-class mothers were observed in England during the Industrial Revolution amidst middle-class anxieties about a broken nation (Evans et al., 2008). Whilst the contents of health crusades differ (e.g. the emphasis on drunkenness rather than fatness in the eighteenth century), contemporary state interventions and sanctions proceed on the hardly original grounds that we must safeguard children's future and the future of society (Evans and Colls, 2011; Jensen, 2018; LeBesco, 2010, 2011). Indeed, following a highly cited US medical report on a potential decline in life expectancy (Olshansky et al., 2005), it has even been predicted that children could die at an earlier age than their parents if urgent action is not taken to fight obesity (Saguy, 2013).

The scientific veracity of the above framing is questionable (Gard, 2016; Gibbs, 2005; Chapter 2), but it has real effects. If we stick with childhood obesity or 'fat kids' for the moment – a relatively neglected topic within fat studies (Boero and Thomas, 2016) – multiple strategies have been mobilised. Whilst Boero and Thomas immediately refer to the US *Let's Move!* campaign (see also Backstrom, 2020), other nations also seek to fight childhood obesity on various fronts. Strategies in the UK, for instance, include: food industry regulations, such as calls to eliminate television advertisements for 'junk food' at times when children are most likely to be watching; taxation (e.g. on sugar-sweetened beverages, see Wise, 2016); mass surveillance (e.g. regularly measuring and tracking schoolchildren's BMI; see Evans and Colls, 2009, 2011); removal of 'morbidly obese' children from their families (Johnson, 2014) and regional initiatives (e.g. encouraging young people to embrace physical activity and sound nutritional practices). The community, regional and national dimensions of governing childhood obesity have been critically explored by sociologists with reference to reality television (e.g. Rich, 2011; Warin, 2010) and young people (e.g. Evans et al., 2013; Monaghan, 2014a). Ultimately, though, as part of the ubiquitous personal responsibility 'blame frame' (Saguy, 2013), individuals and families must exercise 'healthy choices' – a key motif in various governments' public health anti-obesity 'educational' policies and campaigns (e.g. Mulderrig, 2017, 2019; Chapter 3). To the extent that children are unable or unwilling to control their weight, responsibility falls on parents (mothers), and, failing that, a broader 'obesity assemblage' (Rich, 2010) comprising state agencies such as schools, child welfare and even the criminal justice system (Bell et al., 2009; Boero, 2009; Herndon, 2014; LeBesco, 2011; for recent research on how children in Poland are deemed 'individually responsible' for obesity, see Boni, 2020).

The above signature elements and practices characterise the dominant understanding of 'excess' weight/fatness as a massive public health problem that demands urgent solutions. For Rail et al. (2010: 261), this discourse constitutes a Foucauldian 'regime of truth' that is constructed by 'state-science' without acknowledging that it is ideological (also Bombak, 2014b; Gard and Wright, 2005; Medvedyuk et al., 2018). This regime has also been defined as a commercially 'manipulated' field of science and policy, spanning the globe from the USA to China, wherein corporations provide considerable research funding (which may exceed state funding) (Greenhalgh, 2019). In Chapter 2 we will bring together insights from a range of critical perspectives on obesity discourse whilst remaining reflexive about complex relations of power and inequality. In building on this, Chapter 3 critiques the 'lifestyle drift' (Popay et al., 2010) or behaviourism that dominates many public health interventions. We do this with specific reference to state-backed anti-obesity policies and social marketing campaigns, which draw from private sector principles for public ends (Mulderrig, 2017). However, our aim in the remainder of this section is to outline how sociologists apply 'frame analysis' to this terrain, a common approach when studying 'social problems'. In so doing, we will be better placed to scrutinise different, overlapping and conflicting interpretations on an uneven field of power.

Employing frame analysis in this problem field

> Framing is an unavoidable part of life. The world is too complex to be perceived in all its intricacy. If we did not frame our experiences of phenomena we encounter, we would be overwhelmed by the sheer mass of information.
> *(Saguy, 2013: 5)*

Frame analysis, a form of 'content analysis' applied to cultural messages and artefacts (Kwan and Graves, 2013: 13), is often traced to Goffman's (1974) work on the social organisation of experience. In the realm of social problems, framing is employed by claims-makers who offer versions of reality and seek resonance with their audiences. Kwan and Graves (2013) and Saguy (2013) offer two useful texts that analyse framing in the contentious 'fat field', that is, 'a semiautonomous' domain of practice '[o]rganized around a topic, rather than a single institution' comprising 'its own rules and forms of relevant capital' (p. 31). Both texts elucidate shared and alternative ways of defining 'the problem' and mobilising action. The first book (Kwan and Graves, 2013) is based on US research, whilst the second text (Saguy, 2013) includes both America and France. One insight is that with 'different national cultural lenses' (Saguy, 2013: 105), there are different points of emphasis and orientations to policy. For instance, US media compared to French media tend to emphasise 'individual blame' for obesity, whilst the latter are more likely to discuss possible 'policy solutions, which may be related to greater support for state intervention' (pp. 103–4). Yet, what is common across both national contexts, and evidenced in other research in countries such as Norway, with a still relatively generous welfare state, is that obesity is defined as a *problem* that connotes moral 'badness' and it demands solutions (Grønning et al., 2012).

Building on some of her earlier co-authored work on 'framing contests over obesity' (Saguy and Riley, 2005), Saguy (2013) begins with a vignette depicting a girl tearfully asking, 'Mommy, why am I fat?' alongside parental dilemmas. Focusing instead on media and scientific studies, Kwan and Graves (2013) immediately cite contradictory statements on weight, the fat body and life expectancy.

What can be taken from both books, however, is that frame analysis offers a means of getting to grips with this complex, contradictory and emotionally charged field wherein actors/organisations 'possessing' different 'volumes' of capital (economic and symbolic) engage in 'credibility struggles' (Saguy, 2013: 29). For Kwan and Graves (2013), relevant questions include: what does a frame say about an issue, how is it said, what is not said, what are the similarities and differences within and across frames? They acknowledge that reality is more complex than implied by their study but stress that framing analysis offers a useful *heuristic*. This is an important point. Even authoritative bodies, such as the CDC, comprise different groups of scientists who have produced wildly contrasting reports on deaths associated with 'excess' weight (Saguy, 2013).

Readers not attuned to such controversy could be forgiven for thinking that in a field dominated by biomedicine, frame analysis is redundant. Guthman (2009: 119), for example, reveals how some undergraduates taking a course that she co-taught on the politics of obesity 'were particularly taken aback by challenges to medical representations and the notion that the obesity epidemic was in any sense socially constructed' (see also Cameron and Russell, 2016). However, as noted in our introduction with reference to Saguy (2013: 5, emphasis in original), whilst 'the term *obesity* implies a medical frame' there are 'competing frames' pertaining to health, beauty and civil rights. Kwan and Graves (2013) agree, subjecting four main frames to systematic analysis: (1) an aesthetic or 'fat as frightful' frame, (2) a 'health' or 'fat as fatal' frame, (3) 'a choice and responsibility frame' and (4) 'a social justice frame'. They analyse each frame with reference to documents, public statements and other artefacts (e.g. media reports, advertisements, books, statistics and images) produced respectively by: the fashion and beauty industries, the CDC, the Center for Consumer Freedom (CCF, a financially powerful group tied to the food industry) and the National Association to Advance Fat Acceptance (NAAFA) (a 'civil rights organization dedicated to "protecting the rights and improving the quality of life for fat people"' (cited by Kwan and Graves, 2013: 95). We will outline each frame below, citing other literature and related themes where appropriate.

The aesthetic frame, often critiqued by feminist scholars when challenging gendered power and the regulation of women's bodies (Bordo, 2003; Saguy, 2013; Tischner and Malson, 2011), is manufactured by an amorphous fashion-beauty complex. This complex advertises and sells products promising 'bodily perfection' and an attendant good life in 'consumer culture' (Featherstone, 1991), peddling what have also been called 'perfection codes' within pedagogic systems of 'symbolic and economic control' (Evans and Davies, 2020: 737–8). This conventionally attractive body – although challenged in popular culture by, for example, Dove's 'Real Beauty' campaign (Saguy, 2013: 32) – is slim, toned and highly prized. This normative body is the antithesis of the 'grossly obese' body that is stigmatised within and across different nations (Brewis et al., 2018; Gailey and Harjunen, 2019). Although fat is framed as 'frightful' (Kwan and Graves, 2013) and a symbol of 'personal failure' (subordination on gendered, racial and class hierarchies), it is also deemed 'fixable' within a neoliberal rationality via marke-tised lifestyle choices, such as gym and diet group membership (O'Toole, 2019) and surgery (Throsby, 2012). Men and boys deemed fat/obese are not immune to these aestheticised and commercialised imperatives (Monaghan, 2008, 2014a, 2015; Chapter 2). However, insofar as women and girls tend to be judged more harshly on their physical appearance and perceived fatness (Fikkan and Rothblum, 2012; Tischner, 2013), the costs of body non-conformity (e.g. stigma, isolation and loneliness) remain highly gendered (Kwan and Graves, 2013; see also Part 2 of *Rethinking Obesity*).

Insofar as the aesthetic frame inscribes the slender and toned body as a personal accomplishment, it accords with a 'postfeminist sensibility' that embodies neolib-eral values (Gill, 2016; Chapter 5). This is a sexy and desirable 'looking-glass body' (Waskul and Vannini, 2006) that looks and feels good; a 'body project' (Shilling, 2012) proffering hope for a better life that 'consumers/citizens' must simply 'choose' (Lupton, 2018: 34). Such incitements are challenged by fat activist groups, such as NAAFA, which lack Dove's economic and symbolic capital (Saguy, 2013) but are committed to advancing alternative definitions of beauty. The aesthetic frame is also repudiated by critics who observe fat is seldom 'fixable' through diets or weight-loss programmes (Mann et al., 2007; Rothblum, 2018). Indeed, serious doubts have been cast on the validity of claims made in weight management research (Aphramor, 2010), and there is much to indicate that weight-loss is 'ill-fated' (Kassirer and Angell, 1998; O'Hara and Taylor, 2018; Chapters 4 and 7).

Our discussion has already included much on the *'health' or 'fat as fatal' frame* (Kwan and Graves, 2013), a dominant variant of the 'problem frame' (Saguy, 2013). To reiterate, within the health frame, 'excess' weight can be life-threatening and is an expensive crisis that must be urgently tackled. Attributing frames to specific cultural producers, Kwan and Graves (2013) explain that the CDC substitute mor-tality risk for appearance when constructing the obesity problem. Other 'allied' organisations advancing this frame, and which also exhibit high levels of symbolic capital, include the WHO and the US National Institutes of Health (Saguy, 2013). According to Kwan and Graves (2013) the CDC, when making claims about the causal roots of obesity, acknowledge complexity, including structural elements such as socio-economic factors (see Chapters 2 and 3 on the obesogenic environment). However, individualistic logics prevail in line with 'the Energy Balance Equation' (p. 46) that infuses obesity discourse as enacted in various national and regional policy reports (Medvedyuk et al., 2018). This equation attributes fatness to an excess of calories consumed relative to those expended, resulting in an emphasis on 'the big two' (diet and exercise) despite many other possible contributors (Keith et al., 2006; O'Hara and Taylor, 2018; Chapter 2). There is, then, overlap between the aesthetic and health frames regarding some core assumptions about weight/fat as a problem, its aetiology and proposed solutions:

> [T]he CDC addresses structural factors primarily as barriers to behav-ioural (that is, individual-level) outcomes. In other words, the CDC engages

structural factors insofar as they make personal changes in lifestyle difficult to accomplish. The indictment of personal behavior appears to be central. As the surgeon general asserts: 'Change starts with the individual choices we as Americans make each day for ourselves and those around us'.

(Kwan and Graves, 2013: 45)

The above reference to making choices for others also has to be interpreted in the context of the CDC's emphasis on mothers' perceived role in America's obesity crisis. Elsewhere, as Maher et al. (2010) and Backstrom (2020) observe, where parental responsibility for children's health and weight is raised in public and policy discourse, mothers are often located as the key actor/agent. Again, the operation of gendered power is not only manifest in beauty ideals and the aggressive militaristic metaphors used in the war on obesity (Monaghan, 2008), but also the implication that mothers are culpable and should rectify this in crisis times.

Kwan and Graves (2013) describe alternative frames as reactions to the health and aesthetic frames. Those advocating *'the choice and responsibility frame'* reject the idea that fatness is necessarily a social problem to be fixed by external agencies. Lupton (2018: 18–9) makes the same point with reference to 'Libertarian sceptics'. For Kwan and Graves (2013: 71, emphasis in original), the CCF is noteworthy because it is *'especially* vocal about obesity' and has financial clout. Presenting itself as a defender of truth and consumer choice, the CCF refutes what it terms 'obesity myths' as propagated by the CDC, 'food cops' and 'radicals' (pp. 76–7). Such rhetoric, which is similar to that expressed by various actors 'performing the Nanny State narrative' in UK and Australian policy-relevant contexts (Boswell, 2016: 91), might be interpreted as an understandable reaction to the media's 'intense coverage' of the obesity epidemic. According to Cohen et al. (2005: 154), US media reports of obesity increased almost fourfold between 1999 and 2005 (see also Chapter 2 on media and 'fat panic'). Whilst the CCF cite scientific reports in an attempt to establish credibility, this organisation cannot extricate itself from the profit motive because it receives significant funding from large food corporations – a problem also noted by Greenhalgh (2019) with reference to the global soda industry. Such connections mean that organisations like the CCF may have economic capital but, unlike the CDC, they lack symbolic capital (Saguy, 2013).

Similar to the health frame, individualistic logics pertaining to bodies and behaviours pervade the above 'choice and responsibility frame', though, in the case of children, parental responsibility is again emphasised (Kwan and Graves, 2013). As lobbyists for the food industry, the CCF unsurprisingly blame weight gain on lack of physical activity. This, like diet, is framed as a personal choice that has nothing to do with 'big government' (p. 78). Similar sentiments were hinted at above with reference to reactions to the Canadian Government's proposed sugar tax. Yet, such regulations appear inescapable: in March 2015, Berkeley, California, became the first US city to introduce a sugar-sweetened beverage tax amidst concerns about obesity (Boseley, 2017). Over 40 countries and cities have since followed suit, enacting WHO policy recommendations to reduce sugar consumption via taxation (Bridge et al., 2020). Governments have also introduced increased taxes on food (e.g. chocolate, sweets) in an attempt to combine both fiscal and health benefits (Sarlio-Lähteenkorva and Winkler, 2015). This taxation approach to encouraging reduced consumption has been widely used for decades in relation to alcohol and tobacco. Amidst increased food regulation and vilification of the global food and drink industry, Kwan and Graves (2013: 79) note that the CCF 'fires back with its neoliberal rhetoric' that stresses the role of supply and demand in regulating a 'free market' wherein 'consumers [can] make their own choices' without state interference. As an aside, the invocation of 'free markets' is an old strategy in the USA and the UK as the political right enact 'strategic ignorance' for their own ends (McGoey, 2019).

Finally, what Kwan and Graves (2013) call *'the social justice frame'* is deemed reactionary and subversive (though, as we will suggest, it could be considered compatible with, rather than subversive of, neoliberal relations and logics; see also Aphramor, 2016, 2018). Instead of pathologising fatness, the central claim is that 'weight-based discrimination' or oppression is the problem (Solovay, 2000). Such a view has been expressed in the USA over several decades by NAAFA, with an advisory board including 'scientific, medical and legal leaders from all over the country' (Kwan and Graves, 2013: 95). As a caveat, NAAFA cannot simply be treated as a proxy for fat activism, itself a complex social movement (Cooper, 2016a). Even so, it is through a review of NAAFA documents and related material that Kwan and Graves (2013) seek to highlight how the social justice frame opposes discrimination in contexts ranging from employment and physical activity to education and healthcare. NAAFA cite research in order to bolster their claims regarding, for instance, the relationship between stigma and poor health. Unfair treatment, which seriously compromises 'psychological, social, and physical well-being' (p. 98), is attributed to assumptions that 'fat people' are blameworthy. Regarding causality, some advocates claim fatness is a product of biological inheritance, whilst environmental factors are downplayed. Others maintain that searching for a cause is unnecessary since it implies fatness is a problem requiring a solution, rather than a product of 'natural bodily diversity' (also Saguy and Riley, 2005).

The social justice frame prioritises civil rights, an objective to be advanced through education, letter-writing campaigns (or their online equivalents), calls for size-related legislation and other forms of activism. As noted in our introduction, the word 'fat' is also reclaimed in order to extol positive appropriations of language, ways of thinking about fatness and 'fat identity' (Wann, 1998). Other solutions include calling for state regulation of the weight-loss industry and embracing HAES (Chapter 7). This is a weight-inclusive health movement, advanced by the Association for Size Diversity and Health (ASDAH) that reportedly enjoys more symbolic capital than NAAFA (Saguy, 2013). Yet, whilst size-based discrimination or stigma are problematic and have reportedly increased (Puhl and Heuer, 2010; Chapter 2), various scholars have critiqued fat activism with reference to embodied subjectivity and emotions (Lupton, 2018; Murray, 2005a). Furthermore, Kwan and Graves (2013) suggest that the social justice frame does not easily resonate with the public. Boswell (2016) makes a similar argument regarding *the marginal status of what he calls 'the Moral Panic narrative'* in Australian and UK policy contexts, wherein critical attention is directed at those defining obesity as a massive problem rather than the behaviours and bodies of people labelled obese. If such a depiction is accepted (much may depend on which publics and contexts are being referred to) then the deeply ingrained nature of anti-fat prejudice plus the relative distribution of (and search for) economic and symbolic capital could partially explain this. What may also matter is the degree to which size discrimination correlates with other subordinated and intersecting identities, such as being a woman and poor. 'Race' cannot be ignored here either. 'To the extent that fat people are also poor minority women', writes Saguy (2013: 19) in the US context, 'discussions of irresponsible "fatties" shore up prejudices against women of colour'. The same point might also apply to policy concerns about Indigenous people, a so-called 'problem population' (*sic*) in nations such as Canada (McPhail, 2013).

In their conclusion, Kwan and Graves (2013) underscore the issue of resonance and implications for causal attribution and policy. They explain that the aesthetic and health frames are hegemonic and demand conformity in line with common assumptions about bodies, lifestyles and weight (gain). Given 'the internationalization of the "obesity epidemic" narrative' (Schorb, 2013: 3), their argument corresponds with fat studies and other analyses of anti-obesity policies and campaigns outside of the USA (e.g. Boswell, 2016; Lupton, 2018). Amidst (bio)medicalisation and other processes that demand rational forethought (Gibson and Malcolm, 2020; Monaghan, 2014a), it is unsurprising that bodies labelled fat or obese are pathologised. Such bodies are not only deemed unattractive but also more or less blameworthy for (possible) health problems that extend to childhood obesity, especially via a focus on poor and/or racialised mothers (LeBesco, 2010; Quirke, 2016). Saguy (2013: 70–1) complements this discussion, citing 'deep seated U.S. political and cultural traditions of self-reliance and the increasingly powerful political-economic ideology of neoliberalism, in which costs are shifted from the state to individuals and their families'. The global reach of neoliberalism as an ideology and practice is uneven and contested (Bell and Green, 2016), but it cannot be underestimated (Harvey, 2005), particularly after the 2008 Great Financial Crisis and deep cuts to social safety nets. Indeed, the implications of such events have been critically explored with reference to reinvigorated weight-related stigma and scapegoating in nations such as Britain (Monaghan, 2017). Yet, despite possible constraints on alternative ways of thinking and acting, 'frame dialogues' and 'interframe connections' (Kwan and Graves, 2013: 21) are conceivable. For instance, proponents of the biomedical frame could learn from the social justice frame, which incorporates a multidimensional view of health. We endorse this possibility and return to it in Part 3, with *critical* reference to HAES and alternative approaches. Before that, however, we will discuss research, policy and barriers to rethinking obesity within a broader cosmology that does not simply equate the sacred with religion (Bernstein, 2000; Moore, 2013), and which extends to health matters (Evans et al., 2008; Monaghan, 2008).

In sum, literature on framing usefully explores how definitions of weight/fatness are socially constructed and responded to. Even so, there exists a much larger and only partially understood reality outside of frames, meanings and discourses (Williams, 2003), throwing into relief the possibility of rationally evaluating different ways of knowing, being and intervening in a stratified world that has ontological depth (Bhaskar, 1989; Scambler, 2020a). Kwan and Graves (2013) are cognisant of related political and economic concerns insofar as they expose the 'corporate underpinnings' (p. 132) of the aesthetic and choice and responsibility frames. Similar to Saguy (2013), Kwan and Graves (2013) also critique neoliberal ideology, which includes a pervasive emphasis on personal responsibility and a 'laissez-faire rhetoric' that can lead to a 'patronizing' public health model and victim-blaming, especially in 'trying economic times' (p. 6). Arguably, though, when rethinking obesity and an attendant lifestyle drift within public health pedagogy, much more needs to be written. We focus on that task in Chapter 3. For now, in the interests of laying some further foundations for our critique (to be expanded upon in Chapter 2 with reference to science, media, stigma and meta-critique), we will underscore embodied political matters.

Embodying politics (power): from definitional practices to body materiality

Whether referring to fat activists who challenge discrimination, or governments lamenting the alleged costs of obesity on the national coffers (e.g. DHSC, 2019), politics saturate the health field. Politics entail the exercise of power relations and the regulation of life, incorporating consequential practices such as performing policy knowledges (Boswell, 2016; Ulijaszek and McLennan, 2016) and health education as public pedagogy (Evans et al., 2008, 2013; Fitzpatrick and Tinning, 2014). These and other readings on the politics of health (e.g. Banks and Purdy, 2001; Metzl and Kirkland, 2010; Popay et al., 2010; Rail et al., 2010) dissect matters such as: ideology and policy (e.g. how shifts in ideas about state welfare impact collectivist healthcare provision via institutions such as the NHS that are founded on the principle of social justice), social stratification and growing inequalities, experiences of health and illness, health fascism as a form of micro-political power, and health as a new morality. Recent literature on community health also underscores how socio-political domination, stigma and scapegoating (a divide-and-rule strategy used by the wealthy and powerful), impact public health (Friedman et al., 2022; see also O'Flynn et al., 2014). Some clinicians also scrutinise the politics of health (care); for instance, when critical dieticians discuss the gendered history of their profession and advocate 'for more social, political, and economic understandings of health in our practice' (Gingras et al., 2014: 3). Such scholarship includes calls for dieticians to consider how their strict adherence to the biomedical view of obesity has unfortunate 'practice implications' when working with stigmatised groups (Joy and Numer, 2018: 54; see also Chapter 2).

Insofar as bodies are the source, location and medium of society (Shilling, 2005), politics are inescapably embodied. Collective anxieties about possible war in historical context serve as an obvious example, where healthy bodies are equated with national fitness and preparedness (McPhail, 2017; Shilling, 2012). The same point extends to preparedness for further 'waves' of COVID-19, as expressed by UK health authorities during the summer of 2020 (Chapter 8). Because human bodies are located, categorised, surveyed, regulated, measured, (de)valued, disciplined and punished in social space, they are at the heart of politicised or 'biopolitical' concerns (Foucault, 2008; Guthman, 2009). Scholarship on biopolitics attends to 'the governance and regulation of individuals and populations through practices associated with the body' (Wright, 2009: 1). Whilst body concerns pertaining to warfare have long influenced national policies, current corporeal preoccupations (e.g. associated with a demographic transition and chronic illness, techno-science, viral infection and risk) have led sociologists to define contemporary society as a 'somatic society' wherein 'major political and personal problems are both problematized in the body and expressed through it' (Turner, 1996: 1; for related discussion on the Indian Government's early response to COVID-19, see Rahman, 2020). Drawing from Turner (1992), Shilling (2012: 1) observes that 'the body in modern social systems has become "the principal field of political and cultural activity"'. Yet, appreciating that embodiment is constituted within and constitutive of a larger body politic can also lead to very different conclusions. Note, for example, how health researchers use the same concepts (such as neoliberalism) in contradictory ways as part of a social justice agenda that seeks to tackle inequity or 'how politics makes us sick' (Schrecker and Bambra, 2015; for critiques, see Monaghan et al., 2018; Schorb, 2021). Simply recognising that obesity and health are embodied political concerns is not enough. Rather, there is a need to be reflexive about how predefined political agenda may foster blind spots, limit critique and (unintentionally) sustain an oppressive 'stigma system' (Friedman et al., 2022).

Before focusing specifically on fat politics and explaining how we approach weight-related matters in subsequent chapters, we will elaborate on the general issue of body politics and related concepts pertaining to education, subjectivity, citizenship and agency. Responding to the supposed 'naturalness' of human bodies, social scientists usefully explore the politicisation of somatic existence in a broader context, critically elucidating, for example, governmental concerns about 'maximizing our human capital', productivity and ensuring national fitness (Dukelow, 2017: 89). Rail (2012: 229, emphasis in original) points towards such concerns with reference to 'the moral regulation of *bios*, or life', incorporating discourses on population risk, disciplinary techniques and lifestyles. Whether discussing particular bodily matters such as hygiene, new reproductive technologies, abortion, euthanasia and genetic engineering – or, more generally, what is deemed 'normal' (Meleo-Erwin, 2012) – the social sciences demonstrate that human bodies are entangled in consequential power relations. As we will elaborate in Chapter 2, when exploring science, popular media and stigma, these processes socially construct (de)valued bodies and embodied subjectivities. Sociologists of the body and physical education conceptualise such processes as 'body pedagogies' (Evans et al., 2008), evident, for instance, in school curricula, but also unfolding within larger society comprising 'general forms of body pedagogics' (e.g. idealised notions of healthy embodiment) (Shilling, 2010; also, B. Evans et al., 2011a). Importantly, theorising these processes need not be equated with a conception of humans as cultural dopes devoid of agency. Evans et al. (2013: 324) maintain that health education policy may 'frame and regulate', but it does not determine thought and action (see also Evans and Davies, 2020).

Other scholars have similarly explored the pedagogical operations of key institutions, such as: governments, schools, family, medicine and healthcare. Wright (2009) draws analytical attention to the imbrications of human corporeality and institutional knowledge/power with reference to education, media and biopower. Wright calls these ubiquitous biopolitical instructions 'biopedagogies' that frame and regulate what people should consume, their physical (in)activity, relations to biomedicine and basically how to live (see also Mulderrig, 2019). In that respect, politics and the regulation of life are connected to the 'biomedicalization' (Clarke et al., 2003, 2010) of bodies in a moral and political economy wherein failure and the promises of technoscience are pervasive themes (Boero, 2010). Research on public health anti-obesity campaigns is noteworthy here. As reported in Dukelow's (2017) Foucauldian analysis of neoliberal governmentality, public health incites responsible, self-monitoring citizens to overcome their possible 'denial' about their fat bodies and comply with 'expert' modes of subjectification. At the same time, it is understandable why people may resist or reject these ethically suspect pedagogies of fear and disgust (see also Lupton, 2015, 2018). Indeed, as seen in UK-based research, even when public health biopedagogies deploy 'soft' forms of power (e.g. nudging), they position subordinated groups and cultures as irrational (Mulderrig, 2019). We return to this in Chapter 3 when critiquing anti-obesity public health policies and campaigns wherein, as explained by Ulijaszek and McLennan (2016), ideology and values apparently matter more than evidence.

Understanding bodies as sites of intervention, contestation, regulation, struggle, negotiated interests and emotions underpins the sociology of embodiment (e.g. Nettleton and Watson, 1998; Shilling, 2008, 2012; Waskul and Vannini, 2006; Williams and Bendelow, 1998). This flourishing subfield is irreducible to Foucault's popularised notions of biopower, biopolitics, governmentality and the regulation of bodies in social space (Turner, 1992). Similar to interactionists of the body/embodiment (Waskul and Vannini, 2006), Shilling (2008) teases out the significance of well-established pragmatist philosophy for contemporary body studies (see Chapter 4). Additionally, as Nettleton and Watson (1998) observe, there are, inter alia, important antecedents to the study of embodiment and body politics in feminist scholarship (see Chapter 5, which utilises feminist theory). Citing women's efforts to reclaim their bodies from a 'male dominated medical profession', Nettleton and Watson credit feminist scholars who have 'revealed the political status of the body and demonstrated how it was a medium through which women have been exploited by men' (p. 4). The politicisation of the body is also integral to disability activism, which contests social oppression and disablism, and fat activism which centres the politics of size (e.g. Cooper, 1997, 2010).

Fat politics are crucial when rethinking obesity, with politicisation extending to the use of language to describe bodies. As explained in the introduction to *Rethinking Obesity*, fat activists and allied social scientists substitute 'fat' for biomedical labels because the latter pathologise bodies (defining them as risky, unhealthy and diseased). The politicisation of fatness, and, in particular, women's fatness, has been an organising principle in fat activist groups from the late 1960s onwards. On that note, Cooper (2016a) gives more credence to The Fat Underground than NAAFA, which was initially established by fat feminists and radical therapists rather than men with a sexual preference for fat women. Cooper explains that The Fat Underground was the first group 'to theorise fat oppression, a major contribution of the movement' (p. 119) that has benefitted subsequent generations of fat activists and fat studies scholars (Rothblum and Solovay, 2009). The politicisation of fatness has also informed HAES (Chapter 7), a movement that appeals, albeit in a qualified sense, to those writing on the politics of obesity (LeBesco, 2010). Politicised approaches that challenge fat oppression are needed, especially in the twenty-first century, insofar as obesity discourse fuels a bellicose rhetoric that 'dehumanises fat people' and constructs them as 'passive or pitiful sites for intervention' (Cooper, 2011: 164). Using British mass media to advance her cause, Cooper (2016b) states that being a fat activist means 'I think fat is a political subject'. She adds:

> Fat is typically framed as a health problem but health is not apolitical, as bodies of work in the social sciences have come to reveal. Debates about the NHS, and fat people being held responsible for funding crises, are just one area in which fat is a political subject. The social hatred and scapegoating of fat people can also be seen as political.

The politicisation of fatness – including the politics of managing 'spoiled identity' (Goffman, 1968 [1963]; Monaghan, 2017) – is important and we will return to this throughout our book. As reported in qualitative research undertaken by Andrea among women identifying as obese (Chapter 4), her contacts also vocalised politicised concerns about size discrimination and discussed their (sometimes ambivalent) relationship with HAES. However, our approach to fat politics, whilst partly indebted to and largely sympathetic with fat activism, is not simply predicated on the task of trying to make life less demeaning for a subgroup of 'fat people' who suffer from fat oppression. After all, a central tenet of obesity epidemic discourse is that most people are 'weight deviants' (Monaghan et al., 2010: 65), with 'everyone everywhere' (Gard and Wright, 2005: 19) medically defined on the BMI as overweight, obese or at risk of becoming so. Evolving obesity science and concerns about obesogenic social networks also mean that 'the current waist sizes and body shape of the majority of the population' are labelled abnormal within public health campaigns (Dukelow, 2017: 88). Whether these publics can be defined as or identify as 'fat people' is, nonetheless, an entirely different matter and it is debated elsewhere. Meleo-Erwin (2012: 389) suggests that those engaged in fat politics 'must look carefully at the tactics and strategies we choose precisely because the movement is helping to produce "Fat" as a mode of subjectification, identification and collectivity'. Critiquing identify-based politics, Meleo-Erwin argues that 'fat politics may be better framed in terms of *what we desire* rather than *who we are*' (2012: 389, emphasis in original). In doing so, she states the core of fat politics should involve arguing for a more complex, inclusive framing and troubling of 'normal' ideas and ideals of health (also Nash and Warin, 2017).

There is another way in which our approach to fat politics might differ from (some) strands of fat activism, itself a personally challenging or potentially unsatisfactory movement (Murray, 2005a) comprising conflicting politics, thorny relations and the acrimonious ending of specific groups (Cooper, 2016a). As mentioned already, some size acceptance activists tend to be personally invested in the idea that fatness is a product of 'natural bodily diversity' (Saguy and Riley, 2005) or genetic inheritance (as a likely means of repudiating narratives of gluttony and sloth that spoil their identities) (Cooper, 1998; LeBesco, 2004). HAES practitioners, who are 'wise' or sensitive to the plight of the stigmatised (Goffman, 1968 [1963]; see also Monaghan and Hardey, 2011), support such a view. For example, Burgard (2009) asserts that human bodies are naturally diverse and are comparable to different breeds of dog, so that whilst some people's build could be compared to the greyhound others are more like the St. Bernard. However, there are problems here, ranging from the performance of 'the good fatty' (Pausé, 2015) who is blameless, to the erasure of ontological matters. Aside from the fact that pedigree dogs are the product of potentially harmful human practices (selective breeding is associated with many health problems), we remain open to possible and likely complex body-society imbrications that render the idea of a 'natural' or 'naturalistic body' (Shilling, 2012) questionable, if not politically naive and debilitating. We must at least be open to the idea that the reciprocal body–society relationship could result in unwanted adiposity (an inescapably value-laden judgement). Furthermore, this possibility may have real consequences for people's health (practices), identities and relations not only across their own lifecourse but also across generations (Yoshizawa, 2012).

Whilst such matters warrant further discussion, our main point here is that the social sciences should cautiously engage with biology and body materiality in a non-reductionist manner (Williams et al., 2003). The need to rethink biology has recently been echoed in critical obesity studies with reference to material feminism and maternal nutrition (Warin, 2015), a potential minefield given common discourses of 'mother blame' identified above and elsewhere (Bombak et al., 2016). Such calls open up the possibility of posing, if not fully addressing, important questions. For example, what about the impact of poverty on pregnant women's nutritional status and foetal development? What does this mean for birthweight, distribution of adiposity and future health outcomes, especially when families migrate from low- to high-income nations (Aphramor, 2005)? Other questions, which similarly point to the need to reclaim the ontology of the body and for transdisciplinarity (Yoshizawa, 2012), might include: What about the possible relationship between weight-related stigma (including that reproduced through public health policy), eating and the pathophysiology of obesity (Tomiyama, 2014)? What about possible contributors to secular trends in obesity, such as side effects from medicines and endocrine disruptors in the environment (O'Hara and Taylor, 2018; Keith et al., 2006), which also cast a different hue on lifestyle prescriptions to exercise more and eat less (Chapters 2 and 3)? As implied by such questions, an embodied approach takes us beyond identity politics, frame analysis and discursive critique. More ambitiously, the aim here is to incorporate the body politic, its potentially deleterious effects on 'lived bodies' across the weight spectrum and efforts to rethink obesity, health and society more generally.

Summary and preliminary reflections

According to various authoritative and well-publicised claims, it would seem that there is no scientific, philosophical or moral controversy in this field: overweight and obesity constitute a crisis which, despite some evidence of stabilisation, demands urgent action. Yet, the world war on obesity has generated a backlash and a burgeoning field of critical scholarship which, in varying degrees, draws from and extends fat activists' and feminists' politicised concerns for social justice. Within this broader discursive context, it is reasonable to ask: is weight/fatness really the problem of the type, scale and prevalence reported in obesity discourse or is this alarming/alarmist picture something to be problematised? Restated, and in drawing from Kwan and Graves (2013) and Saguy (2013): should medical and public health crisis frames be taken at face value or should we draw from other frames and approaches that render the very idea of an obesity crisis problematic? Insofar as sociology teaches us that 'things are not what they seem' (Berger, 1963: 34), our approach entails exercising critical judgement when confronted with the WCHP and navigating a course that is widely informed and defensible.

In paving the way for such an undertaking, this chapter outlined overlapping and competing constructions of the putative obesity crisis. For Kwan and Graves (2013), the 'fat as fatal' frame is hegemonic, not least given the resources and credibility of agencies such as the CDC in the USA, or the WHO internationally. Other cultural producers and definitions include the fashion-beauty complex and the aesthetic frame that construct fat as frightful. The claim that fatness is a problem – that it is ugly, unhealthy and costly for individuals and populations – has cultural resonance in high-income nations. However, alternative responses include an emphasis on consumers' rights to make their own choices without state interference or framing the problem as one centred on oppression and the struggle for civil rights. In the latter frame, challenging size discrimination takes priority as seen in fat activism and fat studies.

Insofar as fat activism and the idea of an obesity epidemic emerged in the USA (Saguy, 2013), it is perhaps unsurprising that elements of neoliberal ideology (e.g. the rhetoric of choice, personal responsibility, individual freedom and deference to the market) emerge to some degree and with different emphases in all of the surveyed frames. Often taken as 'common sense' (to be differentiated from 'good sense' that critiques misleading, obfuscating and prejudicial thinking) (Harvey, 2005: 39), neoliberal ideology is powerful, pervasive and tacit. Indeed, its influence is not always recognised even in critical public health scholarship that is somewhat contradictory when invoking this concept (Bell and Green, 2016). However, whilst neoliberalism is incoherent, messy, subject to different interpretations and never complete, its primary effects are observable in terms of the reproduction and reinvigoration of class as a social structure, driving growing inequalities in wealth and health (Scambler, 2012, 2018). Neoliberalism also implicates gender through, for instance, a 'postfeminist sensibility' (Gill, 2016) that emphasises, inter alia, personal choice, empowerment and a makeover paradigm. This sensibility shapes girls' and young women's embodied subjectivities as self-responsible, depoliticised individuals who must maximise their own successes in life. Consider, then, how different fat frames hardly disrupt this class, gendered and racialised project, feed it even, or further stigmatise people most vulnerable to health inequalities (Rich et al., 2015).

We would apply the previous point to the four frames referenced above. Just as proponents of the choice and personal responsibility frame, such as the CCF, lambast what they consider unnecessary government interference in the 'free market', the health and aesthetic frames largely define fatness as an individualised behavioural problem (Kwan and Graves, 2013). Accordingly, the obesity problem is to be prevented or fixed by responsible citizens qua consumers who are favourably disposed to the market, which, as we will explore in Chapter 2, is saturated with digital media through which people (especially youths) are incited to monitor and discipline their flesh. 'Empowered' techno-bodies are receptive to public body pedagogies (Evans et al., 2008), which further stigmatise fatness and set weight-loss or management as crucial 'body projects' (Shilling, 2012). Even if not beautiful bodies, these 'civilised' (Elias, 2000 [1939]) bodies (seek to) pass as acceptable rather than abject (Monaghan, 2014a). Advocates of the social justice or 'fat rights' frame (Saguy, 2013) also paint a picture with a neoliberal hue wherein 'fat people' are positioned as individuals or groups of individuals whose freedoms are being unfairly curtailed. According to this frame, fat folk are routinely barred from everyday freedoms (e.g. to make one's own decisions without social censure, to be happy and loved) or enjoying 'the good life' routinely marketed in consumer culture. Arguably, a frame that draws from the individualistic rights-based discourse that works through neoliberalism can only ever be an exercise in damage limitation, in a broader marketplace of ideas and therapies for alienated and oppressed groups. Again, relatively enduring power structures – such as intersecting class and gender relations that (dis)credit bodies – remain unscathed. Efforts to frame fatness simply (defensively or innocently) as natural bodily diversity are similarly limiting, arguably impeding a nuanced reading of the body and society.

These are complex embodied issues and themes, entwined with body politics and the political economy. It is difficult doing justice to such an extensive range of concerns. Indeed, we have merely scratched the surface. Nonetheless, our aim in this chapter has been to provide context and a basis for ensuing chapters, including, but also going beyond those presented in Part 1. Whether referring to public health accounts that prioritise the obesogenic environment, the macro-social structural underpinnings of weight-related stigma, the everyday frustrations of dieting or the promises and pitfalls of alternative interventions, our goal in this chapter has been to provide some orientation to a large, potentially confusing and contested field.

As suggested by Aphramor (2005: 317) well over a decade ago: 'A first step in getting to grips with fatness may be to dismantle the old ordinances and draw up new maps'. We are of the view that whilst important inroads have been made by scholars who challenge the WCHP, there is a need to survey, evaluate and selectively draw from existing critical literature in order to move forward. Our aim is to devise a map that could assist in this shared journey across a complex, changing and obstacle strewn terrain. We further that task in Chapter 2 by offering an extensive review of critical perspectives, research and meta-critique.

2

CRITICAL PERSPECTIVES

Key themes and meta-critique

The previous chapter explained that health and aesthetic frames define fatness as fatal and frightful (Kwan and Graves, 2013). The dominant rendition, well-rehearsed internationally, is that 'fat bodies' not only look and feel bad, but they also die sooner and suffer more illnesses than their 'normal weight' counterparts. 'Excess' weight or fatness, medically defined as overweight and obesity, must therefore be urgently combated. The salience of biomedical health cannot be underestimated when problematising weight/fatness as overweight and obesity. Appeals to health rationalise the aesthetic, evoking far weightier issues than the 'superficial' (feminised) preoccupations of the fashion-beauty complex. The wealth and security of the nation are also underscored in this 'problem frame' (Saguy, 2013), alongside the health of 'our' children who symbolise and embody the future.

The certainty and authority of alarming claims about an obesity crisis belie the controversy and contestation at the heart of this field (O'Hara and Taylor, 2018). As highlighted in our book's introduction, burgeoning literature invites readers to take a critical perspective on the anti-obesity offensive and WCHP. Whilst critical perspectives have antecedents in fat activist writings and are mushrooming within the interdisciplinary field of fat studies (Lupton, 2018; Rothblum and Solovay, 2009), critical contributions have also emerged from within the health sciences, for example: exercise physiology, dietetics, medicine, nursing, epidemiology and public health (e.g. Allison et al., 2016; Bacon and Aphramor, 2011; Casazza et al., 2013; Cohen et al., 2005; Doehner et al., 2015; Flegal et al., 2013; Gaesser, 2009; Kassirer and Angell, 1998; Kuk et al., 2018; Rogge et al., 2004). Hence, contrary to certain depictions, it is inaccurate and misleading to present this field as one wherein fat activists, and their 'friends' in the social sciences and humanities, lock horns with 'enemies' from the health sciences (Gard, 2009a).

DOI: 10.4324/9781315658087-4

This chapter reviews four key themes in this critical literature. First, we note that whilst Gard and Wright (2005) offered a seminal critique of 'the obesity epidemic', epidemiological and scientific understandings have evolved. Building on Bombak (2014b), we offer an updated critique of these understandings. Second, because mass media play a crucial role in dramatising and amplifying the sense of crisis, we will review critical literature on media, 'fat panic' and body pedagogies. Third, we outline research on weight-related stigma. Fourth, we broach the issue of meta-critique, or how critical perspectives are also open to critical interrogation, inviting further responses and counter-responses. In practice these areas overlap. For instance, science and medicine are inseparable from cultural values in a mediated social environment populated by lived bodies. Hence, our approach is intended as a heuristic, providing readers with a detailed, though by no means exhaustive, map for orienting to an ever-expanding and complex field. As part of this endeavour, we will also tease out some of the nuances within 'critical perspectives', thus avoiding the simple polarisation of protagonists versus antagonists.

Evolving obesity science and epidemiology: updating the critique

Published in 2005, Gard and Wright' pivotal book, *The Obesity Epidemic: Science, Morality and Ideology*, is widely cited by scholars who are critical or sceptical of the WCHP. Gard and Wright review the portrayal of obesity in scientific literature, mass media and popular non-fiction books. They observe that science is invariably presented as the remedy for the obesity epidemic. Within science the body is conceptualised as a machine and obesity causation is explained through an energy imbalance model, i.e. excessive caloric intake and/or insufficient caloric expenditure. However, Gard and Wright observe that despite years of research, no consensus has emerged on the actual components of this energy imbalance. Regardless, science persists as the only recognised means of rectifying the epidemic and is routinely presented as being exempt from doubt, contradictory evidence or uncertainties.

Although Gard and Wright expose the contradictions and uncertainties in the primary scientific research field, obesity science has progressed. This, in turn, has added further complexities and evidence challenging the WCHP. For example, when revising the definition of 'metabolically healthy obesity' to include people with zero metabolic risk factors (e.g. elevated blood pressure, glucose or lipids), Kuk et al. (2018) state obesity does not appear to be independently associated with increased risk of dying early. However, elevations in metabolic risk factors are strongly associated with mortality risk, even for 'healthy weight' individuals. Recent scientific sources, discussed further below, also increasingly reference environmental contributors to obesity, low sustained weight-loss levels and limitations of measures such as the BMI. At the same time a weight-centric discourse persists and as seen in the UK, for instance, continues to frame public health policy in individualistic terms despite evidence of socio-economic factors (Ulijaszek and McLennan, 2016; Chapter 3). Accordingly, critics must engage with recent science if they are to scrutinise biomedical, public health, government and media attachment to the WCHP and the belief that obesity is a modifiable, self-imposed risk (Bombak, 2014b).

In providing a basis for such work this section broaches the following themes: early reflections on COVID-19 and obesity; increased caution and reflexivity among some obesity scientists; problems attributing type 2 diabetes mellitus to obesity; questions about putative causes, which extend to the obesogenic environment; the ineffectiveness and harms of weight-loss interventions; the limitations of measurements of overweight and obesity; flawed reasoning as a basis for apocalyptic predictions and debate about the 'obesity-survival paradox'.

Early reflections on COVID-19 and obesity

Pausé et al. (2021) critique early claims and measures that 'problematise fatness in COVID-19'. Calling for health justice, Pausé et al. resist the dominance of the WCHP that reproduces individualised understandings of health (risk) alongside tendencies to scapegoat 'fat people' for governments' inadequate preparedness for disaster and crisis. We concur, albeit with our eyes on how obesity discourse frames most people as weight deviants who need to take greater personal responsibility for their health (similarly, see O'Connell et al., 2021). Writing in June 2020, some obesity researchers admitted that data on SARS-CoV-2 (the virus that causes COVID-19) and obesity were 'limited' (Rychter et al., 2020: 1). Nonetheless, during this period British medical authorities and policymakers still prescribed weight-loss in the community as a putative protective measure *for practically everybody* in accord with a WCHP that conflates various chronic illnesses with obesity (DHSC, 2020; see also Chapter 8).

Amidst much uncertainty, such prescriptions might have seemed prudent as a precautionary measure. Thereafter, accumulated evidence suggested 'severe obesity' might be a 'risk factor' for increased mortality following viral infection (Ioannidis, 2020a; Tartof et al., 2020). Yet, we would also note Dingwall's (2020a) advice on 'injecting some sense of proportion into the risks represented by SARS-CoV-2'. Admittedly, such words could cause consternation given 'the moralization of COVID-19 health response' and its elevation to 'a sacred value' (Graso et al., 2021). However, in an account that scrutinises the imprecise nature of death certification, Armstrong (2021) states that COVID-related mortality is not high relative to past epidemics that disrupted social order. Biomedical literature, which acknowledges the difficulties in disentangling deaths from COVID-19 and 'harmful response measures', is also salutary. Towards the end of 2020, Ioannidis (2020a) inferred from 82 seroprevalence study estimates (mainly from locations hardest hit by the pandemic) that the 'global infection fatality rate' was 0.15 to 0.2 per cent (0.03 to 0.04 per cent for those under 70 years of age). Furthermore, whilst there was a reported '1.5- to 5-fold' increase in mortality risk for various conditions, including 'severe obesity', there 'was no increased risk' for 'mild obesity' (p. 3).

Besides age and gradations of obesity, other considerations include healthcare, sex and time. As reported in a US state with relatively equal healthcare, weight/ fatness only appeared to elevate the risk of death from COVID-19 among male (not female) patients with 'severe obesity' (BMI ≥40 kg/m^2) and mortality risk declined with age and calendar time (Tartof et al., 2020). Whilst that publication reported on a single healthcare organisation and observations from <7,000 patients, the association between male sex, increasing BMI and mortality was not confirmed in a subsequent systematic review and meta-analysis of observational studies of adults admitted to intensive care in 2020 (58 studies, >44,000 patients) (Taylor et al., 2021). Variables that did appear to elevate the risk of death from COVID-19 in that review included increasing age, smoking, diabetes, renal disease and hypertension, among others.

In our view many questions demand attention in a scientific field that is rapidly changing, subject to revision, possible errors (Speakman, 2021) and misunderstandings (Popkin et al., 2021). For instance, even if obesity is unequivocally linked to the risk of infection and worse COVID-19 outcomes (for some groups) why are ineffective and potentially harmful weight-loss prescriptions repeatedly endorsed (Rothblum, 2018; Chapter 7)? And, when positing a link, are researchers controlling for confounding variables – in addition to those flagged above with reference to Tartof et al. (2020) and Taylor et al. (2021) – such as: social class and/or status, racism, stigma, metabolic and cardiorespiratory fitness, a history of weight fluctuation and diet drug use (Campos, 2011; Ernsberger, 2009; O'Hara and Taylor, 2018)? Our reading of the literature, including other meta-analyses (e.g. Popkin et al., 2020), would suggest that such variables are largely ignored. Caution would therefore appear to be prudent when forming conclusions and proffering evidence-based policy recommendations, especially in view of findings from studies of an earlier pandemic. For instance, reviewing studies of the H1N1 influenza pandemic between 2009 and 2011, Sun et al. (2016) observe that associations between obesity and poor outcomes disappeared after adjusting for early antiviral treatment.

The enduring tendency to problematise weight or fatness in the time of COVID-19 is disconcerting not least when respected social epidemiologists, who are attuned to socio-economic inequality, reproduce obesity discourse based on slim and speculative evidence (Marmot et al., 2020b). One might add to this mix concerns about various biases, mistakes and exaggerated claims in early communications about COVID-19 more generally (Brown, 2020; Caduff, 2020; Ioannidis, 2020b), themes to which we will return in Part 3 when critically discussing what we term 'the dual crisis frame' of COVID-19 and obesity.

Reflexivity, 'diabesity' and 'the big two'

Given the scant progress produced by the ongoing focus on energy imbalance and the innovation stifling-effect of the presumption of obesity's causal role in disease, some obesity researchers have been developing a more reflexive tone over the past decade (e.g. Casazza et al., 2013; Hebert et al., 2013). Hebert et al. (2013) maintain that 'solutions' to what they regard as a major public health problem are mired by a lack of 'clear understanding', with impediments such as 'lax application of scientific standards of review, tenuous assumption making, flawed measurement and other methods, [and] constrained discourse limiting examination of alternative explanations of cause' (p. 593). Similarly writing for a medical audience, Casazza et al. (2013: 446) review the scientific field and offer the following words:

> Many beliefs about obesity persist in the absence of supporting scientific evidence (presumptions). Some persist despite contradicting evidence (myths). The promulgation of unsupported beliefs may yield poorly informed policy decisions, inaccurate clinical and public health recommendations, and an unproductive allocation of research resources and may divert attention away from useful, evidence-based information.

Slack standards and the glossing over of uncertainty have been explored with reference to diabetes research. Type 2 diabetes mellitus is often conflated with obesity as one dreaded, burdensome disease brought on by unrestrained eating and physical inactivity. McNaughton (2013) critiques this conflation with reference to Australian public health concerns about so-called diabesity. She underscores the complexities, contradictions and uncertainties surrounding knowledge of diabetes, noting: diabetes can occur at multiple body sizes, weight gain as a possible *symptom* rather than *cause* of diabetes, age, family history and genetics. Yet, public health largely elides such considerations, ignoring concerns from within dietetics about the validity of the claim that weight-loss or management prevents diabetes (Aphramor, 2010). More recent critical analyses of diabetes intervention literature reveal that despite 'surprising', mixed and misleadingly reported results, researchers continue to posit an indelible linkage between diabetes and weight in a variety of forms (as risk factor, lifestyle change, intervention or trial outcome) (Bombak et al., 2020; Riediger et al., 2018).

Arguably, the general reluctance among proponents of diabesity to revise their thinking could be attributed to the 'paradigm effect' and 'paradigm paralysis' whereby conflicting data are difficult to recognise (Barker, 1993, cited by O'Hara and Taylor, 2018: 15). Others might see this as a case of 'strategic ignorance' (McGoey, 2019), which is protective of elite interests. Although not using the concept of strategic ignorance, Cyr and Riediger (2021) provide an illustration of what we have in mind when critically discussing 'weight, diabetes and health' among 'Indigenous populations' (weight was a poor predictor of risk). Challenging conventional public health in Canada, which is arguably complicit in propagating 'colonial violence', they suggest that 'returning stolen lands' would likely be a better policy to reduce health inequalities than banal advice to eat 'traditional, land-based food' (pp. 494–5).

Difficulties in 'recognising' conflicting evidence extend to putative causes of the obesity epidemic. Keith et al. (2006) assert that evidence of possible contributors to secular trends in obesity is equivocal and there are many puta-tive factors beyond diet and physical inactivity, or 'the big two' (e.g. smoking cessation, sleep debt, endocrine disruptors in the environment). Yet, their work returns to the big two, which is perhaps unsurprising given the appeal of simplis-tic behavioural explanations, prescriptions and entrepreneurial interests in profit-ing from a reductionist and corrective focus on lifestyles (Monaghan et al., 2010; Chapter 3). O'Hara and Taylor (2018) summarise evidence on myriad possible contributing factors, ranging from polycystic ovarian syndrome (which affects up to 1 in 15 women) to the effects of maternal famine, whether real or induced through dieting. Weight-gain among young women has also been linked to 'key life events' (e.g. marriage, attending university, motherhood, bereavement) (Pegington et al., 2020). Even if age-old habits of mind return to the body as machine – or calories in/out – the scientifically questionable yet routine empha-sis on diet and physical inactivity is asymmetrical. As reported in the USA and China, greater scientific and policy attention is directed at physical inactivity than diet. Greenhalgh (2019) attributes this to 'manipulation' by the soda indus-try, highlighting the corporate underpinnings and influence of the 'choice and responsibility frame' (Kwan and Graves, 2013), outlined in Chapter 1.

Other scientific work, although marginalised or ignored in policy debates (Boswell, 2016), seeks to go beyond behavioural causes. Recently, several novel determinants of obesity, which could provide a more nuanced biomedicalised perspective on a simplistic energy imbalance model, have been gathering cre-dence. For example, the role of gut bacteria or the gut microbiome – the com-position of which is linked to lifestyle, environment, antibiotic exposure and genetics – is growing in prominence as a more variegated perspective on obesity development (Compare et al., 2016; Dehghan et al., 2020; John and Mullin, 2016; Miller et al., 2018; Rasmussen et al., 2018; Saad et al., 2016). Obesogens, chemicals that may disrupt hormonal action and increase likelihood of fatness in humans, particularly if exposure occurs during developmental stages, have also been presented as a potential contributor to the obesity epidemic (Heindel et al., 2015; Janesick and Blumberg, 2016). And, chronic exposure to ambient air pollution has been associated with obesity among older adults (N. Zhang et al., 2019a). As we will see in Chapter 3 on pedagogising obesity knowledges, such evidence tends to be ignored or negated within public health policymaking via an empha-sis on healthy lifestyles/behaviours/choices. Even then, such factors are, as hinted at above with reference to Pegington et al. (2020), also embedded in broader systems rather than 'free floating'.

Appeals to the obesogenic environment: a more socially mindful account?

The obesogenic environment, or modern system comprising 'toxic' living condi-tions leading to sedentary behaviours and overconsumption, has become a com-mon framing device for obesity (Bombak, 2014b; Colls and Evans, 2014; Schorb, 2013).

Citing an influential UK report on obesity, Colls and Evans (2014: 734) explain that this ecological or environmental account is 'defined in policy terms as "the whole range of social, cultural and infrastructural conditions that influence an individual's ability to adopt a healthy lifestyle" (Foresight, 2007: 52)'. Despite this problematic emphasis on lifestyles (Popay et al., 2010), the obesogenic account is viewed by Gard (2009b, 2013) as a structurally minded and, by extension, more compassionate approach within the new public health. Whether this 'environmental frame' reduces individual blame is an empirical question, though Saguy and Almeling (2008) previously expressed scepticism with reference to literature on smoking and attributions of personal responsibility for disease. Indeed, as we will discuss in Chapter 3 – and building on insights from popular media and stigma research reviewed below – seemingly helpful representations in anti-obesity policies and campaigns are ethically suspect. Indeed, they tend to be entwined with pedagogies of fear and disgust (Dukelow, 2017; Lupton, 2018).

The recontextualisation of the obesogenic environment account has proven influential, mobilising European health policy (Schorb, 2013). However, evidence supporting a simple link between environmental factors and obesity remains slim (Bombak, 2014c). The evidence for a link between physical environments and adult weight is weak, with the exception of urban sprawl and land mix use in North America (Mackenbach et al., 2014). Similarly weak evidence is produced when focusing on psychosocial environments and adult weight (Glonti et al., 2016). A recent development in obesogenic environment research is a linking with neurobiological accounts of eating (Sinha, 2018). Such accounts present obesogenic environments as contributing to the stress–induced overeating of accessible 'highly palatable' foodstuffs. This construction basically invokes two primary accounts of obesity aetiology: it is caused by the modern environment, but it is also due to fat/obese persons' addictive natures and/or stressful, adverse and even traumatic circumstances that contribute to weak willpower or pathological eating patterns (McPhail, 2010; McPhail and Bombak, 2015). Arguably, this construction illustrates how obesogenic framing continues to thrust the onus of change onto 'deficient' individuals, even when ostensibly concentrating on environmental reform (Bombak, 2014d; Kirkland, 2011). What is also telling in terms of the social values that 'inform' science is that even a recent meta-analysis, detailing the possible impact of 'long working hours on adverse weight-related outcomes' (Zhu et al., 2020: 12), does not frame formal employment and demanding working conditions as part of the obesogenic environment.

Whilst working long hours, historically associated with male-coded public life and the formal economy, is not classed as an obesogenic environment by Zhu et al. (2020), others conceptualise the family home and women's wombs in these terms (Hajj et al., 2014; Reid et al., 2015; Schrempft et al., 2015; Sookoian et al., 2013). This framing throws into relief how the obesogenic environment discourse continues to reinforce an individualistic and potentially sexist health focus, despite its nominal reference to structural factors. Indeed, defining homes as 'obesogenic' is likely to exacerbate 'mother blame' for children's weight (Warin et al., 2012). Moreover, evidence to support the claim that family home life is obesogenic may be just as scanty as labelling external environments obesogenic. So-called obesogenic home environments were not associated with English pre-schoolers' BMI, despite an association with diet, television viewing and physical activity measures (Schrempft et al., 2015). Referring to several studies, these authors also note how 'lower socioeconomic status groups and some ethnic minority groups may live in more obesogenic home environments' adding they 'may be heavier than other demographic groups' (pp. 12–7). Such words illustrate how obesogenic environment discourse can further marginalise already oppressed groups. Overall, whilst presumably offering a more humane account of obesity aetiology, obesogenic environment framing perpetuates a depoliticising, if not stigmatising, behavioural focus and simplistic understanding of energy balance that has now comingled with other accounts, such as 'food addiction'. There is, of course, nothing unique about this; the concept of 'addiction' is often marshalled to pathologise 'unwanted behaviour' and justify questionable policies (Schorb, 2013: 4) that might be deemed meddlesome (Edgley and Brissett, 1999).

From weight-loss interventions to 'the obesity-survival paradox' (paradigm)

Scientific wisdom regarding the effectiveness and safety of weight-loss interventions has come under increasing scrutiny (Bacon and Aphramor, 2011; Rothblum, 2018). We elaborate upon this in Chapter 7 before critically discussing alternatives, notably HAES, but it is worth flagging here that intentional weight-loss cannot be regarded as a panacea for the putative obesity crisis. Indeed, efforts to lose weight have been found to produce profound physiological effects on thermogenesis (caloric expenditure), subjective hunger, fat oxidation, appetite-related hormones and other involuntary impetuses that stimulate weight regain (Greenway, 2015; MacLean et al., 2011; Rosenbaum et al., 2008; Rosenbaum and Leibel, 2016; Schwartz et al., 2017; Sumithran et al., 2011). In short, weight does not appear to be as malleable and subject to personal control as suggested by advocates of the WCHP.

A notable example of the above physiological processes is provided by research on reality television weight-loss competitors, whose fame is premised on their massive and highly visible physical transformation. Research on former contestants from *The Biggest Loser* demonstrates that most regained substantial weight and experienced extreme metabolic slowing (Fothergill et al., 2016). The authors write: 'Mean RMR [resting metabolic rate] after 6 years was ~500 kcal/day lower than expected based on the measured body composition changes and the increased age of the subjects' (p. 1617). Still, rather than critiquing the war on obesity, the authors conclude 'long-term weight loss requires vigilant combat against persistent metabolic adaptation that acts to proportionally counter ongoing efforts to reduce body weight' (p. 1618). Other commentators acknowledge the unrealistic and inaccurate portrayals of larger persons on such programmes and appear to call for lower weight-loss targets and more tolerance of body diversity (Ravussin and

Ryan, 2016; Tremblay, 2016). Yet, such inaccuracies prevail, fuelling erroneous assumptions and stigma.

Biomedical researchers are also demonstrating greater reflexivity about the limitations of measurements of overweight and obesity, particularly the BMI (Bosy-Westphal and Müller, 2021; Hebert et al., 2013). There are calls for more precise measurements that would facilitate biomedical understandings of the diversity of health and embodiment represented by such daunting characterisations as: metabolically healthy phenotypes, metabolically obese normal weights, and the so-called obesity-survival paradox (Bosello et al., 2016). Obesity scientists call for more research amidst uncertainty and speculation, though two recent publications further complicate the idea that fatness simply equals badness independent of specifying, among other things, type of adiposity and overall body composition. First, Becher et al. (2021) provide interesting observations from over 50,000 patients who had received a tomography scan following the diagnosis, treatment or surveillance of cancer. Their study indicates that 'thermogenic' brown adiposity (which dissipates, rather than stores, energy) 'is associated with cardiometabolic health' and 'beneficial effects' among the overweight or obese 'were more pronounced' (p. 1). Second, Bosy-Westphal and Müller (2021) review evidence that casts doubt on 'traditional understandings of the pathophysiology of obesity' that centre 'fat mass' (p. 1). Challenging the 'adipocentric paradigm of obesity' they conclude: 'the definition and diagnosis of obesity based on "adiposity/overfat" and characterized by BMI does not represent a meaningful outcome' amidst a range of 'body composition phenotypes' (p. 5). This does not mean they simply view fatness as always and necessarily benign or protective; rather, the picture is complex. Other considerations include stage in the lifecourse, sex, health status, the distribution of and capacity to store body fat, and, moreover, the relationship between fat-free mass and fat mass when 'diagnosing obesity-related risk' (p. 4).

Arguably, such calls are important given the well-worn practice of conflating size or fatness with health or disease and a dire future – definitional practices that are recontextualised and sensationalised in mass media (see the next section). For instance, whilst endlessly reiterated, the contention 'that obesity will lead to a significant decline in life expectancy' (Gard, 2016: 245) and related claims that children will die before their parents misrepresent a study comprising a 'back-of-the-envelope calculation' (Saguy, 2013: 4; see also Gibbs, 2005). What the paper in question (Olshansky et al., 2005) actually determined was that if obesity rates continued as projected (an assumption that proved erroneous), and all obese persons' mortality could be attributed to obesity (a fundamentally flawed assumption), then children may die at an age several months younger than their parents. Despite such flaws, and consistent epidemiological findings that question moderate obesity's association with heightened mortality risk (Flegal et al., 2013), claims about children dying before their parents continue to circulate like some shocking 'urban legend' (Fine, 1980). That parents' 'worst nightmare' might be realised, with them burying their kids, has even been graphically portrayed in a US public health campaign (see Saguy, 2013: 158–9).

Most revealingly, the findings contradicting the 'obesity canon' (Moss and Petherick, 2016) have been termed 'obesity paradoxes' (Lavie and Loberg, 2014; Liu et al., 2020; McAuley and Blair, 2011). Observations include: individuals deemed obese and with particular health conditions surviving longer than their normal weight counterparts, overweight status being protective of mortality risk compared to normal weight, cardiorespiratory fitness eliminating the heightened mortality risk associated with obesity, and the large component of overweight and obese populations who are metabolically healthy (Bacon and Aphramor, 2011; Flegal et al., 2013; Lavie et al., 2015; McAuley and Blair, 2011; Tomiyama et al., 2016; Wildman et al., 2008). These 'paradoxes' are not exclusive to studies using the BMI to measure obesity and thus they cannot be dismissed as an artefact of this flawed measure (Hebert et al., 2013). Interestingly, after reporting on the *consistent finding* that higher bodyweight is associated with lower mortality among people with a broad spectrum of cardiovascular diseases and conditions, an editorial in the *European Heart Journal* called for a move away from the term obesity 'paradoxes' (implying an unexpected or contradictory situation) in favour of the more constructive term 'paradigm' (Doehner et al., 2015). Even then, the authors' concern about inappropriate terminology is belied by their continued use of 'obgobbing' (Aphramor, 2018).

The question of whether fatness constitutes a 'legitimate' form of mortality protection in some contexts has generated considerable debate, with some authors suggesting this could be merely an artefact of existing methods (Braun et al., 2015). Bosy-Westphal and Müller (2021) stress the need to better understand how different body composition phenotypes, such as 'sarcopenic obesity' (low lean mass at a high fat mass), may not enjoy the same benefits as heavier individuals whose bodies comprise high levels of fat but also lean mass. Amidst ethical concerns in a context of uncertainty, some recommend a greater focus on maximising fitness and quality nutrition, as optimal weights may exist for different ages and disease populations, outside the narrow bands suggested by the BMI (Dixon et al., 2015). However, Stevens et al. (2015) are concerned that 'confusing messages' could ensue from so-called obesity paradoxes and undermine public health. They advocate that findings contradicting the received canon must not displace encouraging weight-loss, obesity prevention and the ongoing use of the BMI. Peeters (2018) even suggests a halt to publications on 'obesity paradox' research that are not clinical trials focused on survival outcomes, to mitigate methodological bias.

In short, despite the increasingly shaky scientific foundations of the war on obesity, advocates continue to justify their position. This entrenchment cannot simply be attributed to recent (questionable) concerns about COVID-19 and obesity. In a time of austerity, 'fiscally prudent' governments have also legitimated 'the science' that would render us all conscientious weight watchers. However, a final point worth making in view of what we have described above and to echo Gard and Wright (2005) is that the 'true' financial costs of 'the obesity epidemic' cannot be stated with precision and certainty. Moreover, claiming obesity will bankrupt health systems is dubious. According to Gard (2016: 247), 'the more

well-documented drivers' of increasing healthcare expenditure tend to be ageing populations and 'advancing technologies'. Other considerations within the
capitalist world-system might include the profit motive, or rapacious greed, of the
Biomedical TechnoService Complex Inc.

Media, 'fat panic' and body pedagogies

Obesity is typically framed as a big problem, with mass media widely circulating defiling content and 'melodrama' that can be 'told and *sold*' (Raisborough,
2016: 63, emphasis in original). Boero (2012), Campos et al. (2006) and others
(see Fraser et al., 2010), describe the mass media as purveyors of a 'moral panic'
(Cohen, 2002 [1972]), or 'fat panic' (LeBesco, 2010). For Saguy and Almeling
(2005: 19), 'heightened public concern over obesity cannot be attributed to perceived medical risks alone'; rather, it 'is largely a response to the perception of
threats to social values and public morality'. This section outlines critical perspectives on such matters. We also introduce nascent scholarship that analyses new
media (digital) formats (Lupton, 2017) and related popular 'body pedagogies' that
'tend to frame our thinking about our bodies and health' by constantly instructing us that overweight/obesity/fatness are 'bad things' (Evans et al., 2008: 4–6).
Such analyses are important because defiling representations of fatness influence
beliefs, prejudice and policies (Boero, 2013; Frederick et al., 2016; Saguy et al.,
2014; Stanford et al., 2018). Following Evans and Davies (2020: 747), who are
concerned about such outcomes in relation to young people, we will foreground
'assemblages of meaning around health' which form, via sites of practice, 'the
body pedagogies that regulate consciousness'.

Divided into two, this section first introduces literature that critiques negative
representations of fatness/obesity in various media. The second part explicitly
focuses on reality television and digital media as public or body pedagogies. Our
discussion is not exhaustive. For instance, we reserve discussion on social marketing public health campaigns for Chapter 3.

Introducing critical media studies of fatness/obesity: from movies to scientific news reports

Fat studies scholars have usefully contributed to media analyses (Evans and
Cooper, 2016). Part IV of *The Fat Studies Reader* (Rothblum and Solovay, 2009),
for instance, explores 'size-ism' in movies (e.g. *The Nutty Professor* and *Shallow
Hal*) (Mendoza, 2009) and televised celebrity culture (Bernstein and St. John,
2009) wherein fat suits, damaging stereotypes, cheap laughs and self-hatred prevail. Such literature complements LeBesco's (2004) framing analysis of representations of obesity as disability in popular media (movies, talk shows, animation),
representations that occasionally challenge 'fat oppression' but which 'ultimately
capitulate' (p. 82) to dominant readings of fat as abject. Concerns about the stigmatising effects of so-called fattertainment (popular media replete with sizist

stereotypes) (Heuer, 2010) have, without any sense of contradiction, also been advanced by The Obesity Action Coalition, who frame fatness as obesity. In so doing they partially co-opt fat activists' objections about unfair treatment and bias whilst nonetheless medicalising and thus pathologising fatness.

Social scientists have devoted much attention to typically alarmist news coverage in this field, including how obesity is framed as a social problem, how media report on the science of obesity and its relation to social policy (Boero, 2013). On framing, Raisborough (2016: 5) states that 'fact-based alarmist claims ("fat bomb" statistics, for example) have become commonplace in this genre', prompting sustained social scientific interrogation. Boero (2012) offers one such example, drawing from 751 articles in *The New York Times*. She states the newspaper has tended to construct a chaotic scene wherein ideas of individual responsibility for health prevail and pre-existing beliefs about fat people are confirmed. Also concerned about the potential mechanisms propelling weight-based stigmatisation and discrimination, Glenn et al. (2013) analyse print media coverage of weight-loss surgery in Canada. Themes include the dissemination of 'a strong fairy-tale narrative' (p. 633). Here heroic doctors and biomedical discourse reinforce neo-liberal ideals of responsible individuals who seek surgery so that they are better able to control their choices and behaviour and avoid becoming a costly burden.

Other considerations include national context, audience responses and space for alternative frames. First, Ries et al. (2011) suggest that whilst major newspapers in the USA, Canada and the UK similarly frame obesity as a 'lifestyle' problem, 'attitudes' towards policy prescriptions vary in terms of the emphasis given to the shared role of individuals, government and industry 'in addressing modern environments to promote healthier choices' (p. 73). Also, Saguy et al.'s (2010) international research suggests that US media is less likely to emphasise socio-structural factors than French media (though there was no difference in the reporting of weight-based discrimination). For Boero (2013), such observations indicate a need for more comparative research, an important point especially in view of subsequent work indicating newspapers play a key role in communicating science and mediating 'biological citizenship' in Nordic countries (Setälä and Väliverronen, 2014). Second, audiences, including those discredited by stigmatising stereotypes, are neither homogenous nor passive. Holland et al.'s (2015) research with Australians defined as obese reveals various viewpoints, including those challenging news media reporting that is typically derogatory and reflective of journalists' tendency to uncritically rely on pre-packaged information. Third, even traditional media and their online counterparts sometimes include alternative perspectives, aesthetics and 'paradoxical' scientific evidence (see Monaghan et al., 2019). Yet, this should not detract from the fact that amidst 'the growing social prominence of health and well-being as a driver of risk language' in news media, journalists tend to 'reproduce and amplify expert risk assessment yet also create limited opportunities for counter definitions to emerge' (Gabe, 2022: 163).

Understandably, then, critical social scientific literature often refers to how media proliferate obesity epidemic rhetoric, peddling negative judgements and stigma via appeals to health and normality (Fraser et al., 2010). Whether referring to British print media that equates women's obesity with terrorism (Borland, 2015), Canadian coverage articulating fairy-tale narratives of weight-loss surgery (Glenn et al., 2013), or Australian journalists who erroneously claim theirs is the fattest nation on earth (see below), critics often flag dramatising news stories. This way of introducing the topic is salutary. Rhetoric about 'killer fat' (Boero, 2012) and disgrace (inflected by ideologies of gender, social class, age, etc.) is ubiquitous. For example, De Brún et al. (2013) analyse 346 Irish newspaper articles on obesity from six major publications. They observe mothers were often blamed 'for childhood obesity and media messages aimed to shame and disgrace parents of obese children through use of emotive and evocative language' (p. 17).

Such pedagogies also reproduce class divisions and disdain. In the UK, Evans et al. (2008), who critique body pedagogies for propelling some young women into disordered eating, immediately refer to a *Daily Mail* story about an 'overweight 8 year old, weighing 218 pounds' who risked 'being placed on the childcare register' (p. 1). They state this story 'carried tropes' that are 'now familiar' in UK media 'reporting of "obesity" issues' (e.g. parental and working-class irresponsibility, inadequacy and the problems of poor diets and laziness). Comparable US news reporting has been critiqued with reference to *racial* stereotypes and inequalities (LeBesco, 2011; Saguy and Gruys, 2010). Indeed, detailed US media research suggests that such degradation is likely to disproportionately impact African American women and girls (Saguy and Gruys, 2010; though, for discussion on how weight-focused television discredits the poor *and* White in Britain, see Raisborough, 2016).

Classic literature informs critical media analyses in this field. Indebted to Cohen's (2002 [1972]) study of Mods and Rockers, Saguy and Almeling (2005) are just some of the authors who conceptualise heightened public concern about obesity as a moral panic. Analysing over 200 media articles reporting on scientific studies of obesity, Saguy and Almeling maintain that this 'panic' comprises exaggerated portrayals of obese people as 'folk devils' who putatively violate social norms and values (see also Mannion and Small, 2019; Saguy and Almeling, 2008). 'Fat panic' also includes a surge of alarmist media attention that is disproportionate to the increase in obesity rates (Cohen et al., 2005). Accordingly, Saguy and Almeling (2005) challenge the assumption that the media simply report on objective facts about public health in tandem with the reductionist foci of biomedicine and obesity science. Campos et al. (2006) offer a similar argument with reference to contested epidemiology, social change, increased media attention, cultural anxieties and 'an exaggeration or fabrication of risks' that are projected onto already stigmatised groups (p. 58).

Holland et al. (2011) have researched intersections between science and the media with reference to coverage of a scientific report, *Australia's Future 'Fat Bomb'*. This report, from a leading national medical institute, lent a new sense of urgency to the issue, supporting journalists' interest in seeking a 'novel' angle on an already well-rehearsed story. Similar to Boero's (2012, 2013) and Saguy and Almeling's (2008) observations on science and US newspaper reporting, Australian journalists largely failed to exercise critical judgement when reporting 'the facts' voiced by a professor qua spokesperson for the *'Fat Bomb'*. Australian media also took at face value the professor's unsubstantiated claims regarding the nation's status as a world leader in obesity league tables, or an imagined fat Olympics (salient during the run-up to the Beijing Games). Newspapers drew from a repertoire of familiar tropes when using the report as a platform to denigrate the overweight and obese. One columnist, for instance, compared fat Australians to pigs with their snouts in the trough, culpable for draining the health system and failing to heed multimillion-dollar government campaigns to promote healthier lifestyles (see Chapter 3). What is clear from this and similar media analyses is that fatness is routinely discredited. And, whilst news media might take a more dramatising and moralising tone than scientists, the latter are not exempt from this.

When typifying the media as moralisers and amplifiers of the obesity epidemic, Monaghan et al. (2010) note that obesity scientists also magnify the crisis through, for example, emotive language and downward revisions of the BMI. However, crucially, the media disseminate news to a larger audience and create 'conditions for further stereotyping, myth-making and labelling' (p. 51). This mode of entrepreneurship is located within a broader assemblage of practices and interests, including but not limited to those of governments, the pharmaceutical industry, healthcare providers and the person in the weight-loss club qua 'entrepreneurial self' (Petersen and Lupton, 1996). Monaghan et al. (2010) qualify their approach to moral panic theory, thus distancing themselves from critics who might 'adopt the conspiratorial aspect of this concept rather too easily' (p. 44), but they stress that media practices are crucial in 'drawing public attention to and typifying a particular social problem over time, thus increasing and reinforcing their significance' (p. 50). Similar to US-based research, critical reference is also made to disproportionality; for example, in the UK at the turn of this century the percentage increase in articles on obesity in two years exceeded the total percentage rise in obesity that had reportedly occurred in the previous 20 years. Other points include how the media further 'sensationalise' obesity 'through the melodramatic use of terms like "epidemic", "time bomb" or "war on obesity", or what Cohen (2002 [1972]: xx) terms the 'metaphors we discriminate by'''. Mention is also made to images, graphs and 'shock' headlines which are 'the archetypal carriers of moral panics' (Cohen, 2002 [1972]: xii; see also Chapter 8 on COVID-19).

Finally, it is worth pointing to analyses of news media and their online equivalents at a time when governments have reinvigorated concerns about the 'costly' obesity crisis (Chapter 1). Farrell et al. (2016) address such concerns via an analysis of articles and reader comments on an Australian news and current affairs website (for further discussion on digital media and production, see below). Their research explores 'how popular anxieties about the "obesity crisis" and vitriol directed at obese individuals circulate alongside understandings of the appropriate role of government to legitimise regulatory reform to address obesity' (p. 543).

Underscoring the complex role of emotions via an approach that does not regard these as antithetical to reason (a complaint levelled at moral panic theory: see Fraser et al., 2010; Raisborough, 2016), Farrell et al. (2016: 543) write: 'obesity regulations achieve popular support within affective economies oriented to neo-liberal and individualist constructions of obesity'. Furthermore, these economies 'preclude constructions of obesity as a structural problem in popular discourse; instead positioning anti-obesity regulations as a government-endorsed vehicle for discrimination directed at obese people' (p. 543).

New forms of health media as instructional: from reality television to digital media

Social historians explain that the media have long fashioned understandings of the body, weight and fatness (Schwartz, 1986; Stearns, 2002). However, the discernible advent of 'the obesity epidemic' as a discursive truth from the 1990s onwards has provided grist for new media that visualise, target, monitor and fight the spectacle of 'aberrant' flesh. The emergence of new forms of media indicates a shift towards the more 'surveillant' (Andrejevic, 2002a) and instructional format of health media (Rich, 2011). What we have in mind here relates, first, to reality television and, second, digital media that provide opportunities for resistances but also transform today's body into something akin to 'a walking sensor platform' (Smith, 2016: 108). We will discuss each of these in turn.

Weight-loss, diet and fitness have increasingly become the focus of multiple 'reality science' (Cohen, 2005) and 'reality television' productions, involving 'first person programming' (Wood and Skeggs, 2008) and the public. Scrutinising media centred on cosmetic surgery (including weight-loss), such as *Extreme Makeover* (US and UK editions), Heyes (2007: 17) suggests that such representations 'have contributed to the evolution of a contemporary discourse in which one's body must be made to represent one's character'. Raisborough (2016), Raisborough et al. (2019), Rich (2011) and Warin (2010) analyse various popular weight-focused television shows within this genre, exploring what these 'achieve' in societies wherein fatness is commonly framed as the consequence of '*lifestyle crimes*' (Raisborough, 2016: 6, emphasis in original). Often articulated through 'the spectacle of celebrity concern' (Vander Schee and Kline, 2013) and critiqued for side-lining 'the more complex, structural causes of overweight and obesity' (p. 575) in favour of 'bad' behaviour (e.g. neglectful parenting, laziness and ignorance), the lessons emanating from such programmes are clear. Indeed, these authors demonstrate the *constitutive* role of television in popular understandings and experiences of obesity, including how weight-focused shows (e.g. *Too Fat to Work*) form a broader genre of 'poverty porn' that centres the 'failings' of predominantly poor White people who depend upon social welfare. Accordingly, bodies denigrated as fat, bad, sickly and sad become embroiled in larger class antagonisms, sensibilities, scapegoating and abjection in austerity Britain (Raisborough, 2016). Raisborough et al. (2019) add to this critique, explaining how ostensibly educational reality television shows, which frame fat characters as deviant, 'are put to the work of securing public consent for a post-welfare society in the UK' (p. 279).

Emphasising public pedagogy, Rich (2011) undertakes a critical reading of obesity television shows as cultural texts, but also reveals how such texts function as instructional devices. Focusing on *Honey We're Killing the Kids* and *Jamie's Ministry of Food*, Rich reveals the 'complexities of how surveillance associated with these health imperatives circulates relationally and affectively as public pedagogy' (p. 6). Framed as 'factual' reality-style programmes, these media draw on instructional narratives of self-improvement. The growth in this type of reality media reflects broader changes in the way in which learning about health is undertaken in sites beyond formal schooling (Evans et al., 2008; Miah and Rich, 2008; Rich, 2011; Sandlin et al., 2011). Whilst an approach that focuses on dominant discourses or frames provides some valuable insight, Rich and Miah (2014: 307, emphasis in original) caution against focusing only on 'the *content* of pedagogy rather than its *relational* derivation'. They explain that learning is shaped by affective relations between different elements of this assemblage.

In line with this affective turn, scholars emphasise how fear, guilt, shame and humiliation emerge in 'reality' weight-focused television shows about 'ordinary people' (Lupton, 2018: 51). Inthorn and Boyce (2010), after analysing 28 prime-time British television programmes about obesity, explain that shame, rather than knowledge, prevails when instructing the public to take control of their weight. This pedagogy is part of a related media genre that denigrates celebrities for gaining weight/fat, with magazines and websites reproducing the 'aesthetic frame' (Chapter 1; Kwan and Graves, 2013). Regardless of whether the targets of these body pedagogies are the public, or celebrities, such media fuel disgust (see Lupton, 2013: 52–5).

Second, there is an emergent literature on *digital media*, surveillance, body pedagogies (Goodyear et al., 2019; Lupton, 2017; Rich and Miah, 2014, 2017; Smith, 2016) and public pedagogies (Rich, 2018). Reflecting the shift from Web 1.0 through Web 2.0 and 3.0, over the last decade new media have been radically altered by the expansion of digital practices that permeate people's lives and enable them to *produce* and not simply consume text, images and other data about and on the body. Attuned to public pedagogy, Rich and Miah (2014: 301) write: 'it is necessary to recognise how [digital] technology is inextricable from the manner in which people learn about health'. Digital mobile and wearable media promote search learning, which could be scrutinised with reference to the social rules (including 'the evaluative rules') of a 'pedagogic device' (field of forces) that is implicated in consciousness and 'symbolic control' (Bernstein, 1996, 2000, 2001; Evans and Davies, 2020; Chapter 3). Some of these technologies are not only instrumental in framing (and challenging) obesity as an individualised, behavioural problem; they are also used to predict, diagnose, monitor and regulate various health issues whilst, paradoxically, possibly leading to 'embodied exhaustion' (Smith, 2016).

The ubiquity and design of mobile and wearable digital devices provide *opportunities* as well as peer-based *expectations* (especially among young people) to upload and share 'data' via multiple, interconnected social media platforms. Common digital platforms, implicated in the potentially tiresome 'work of being watched' (Andrejevic, 2002b; Smith, 2016), include: apps, social media, blogs and websites. In her editorial of a special issue of *Fat Studies* on 'digital media and body weight', Lupton (2017: 129) brings together fat studies and critical social analyses of digital media to examine the 'representations, practices and performances' in and with these technologies. Lupton highlights the myriad voices and images present within digital media and the tensions between them, including: fat activism, body positivism, fat shaming and stigmatisation, pro-anorexia, thinspiration and fitspiration. Whilst it is difficult doing justice to the richness of such work here, this emerging literature suggests that the advent of digital platforms has facilitated the representation of diverse perspectives on bodies, weight, size and shape. Lupton cites, inter alia, examples of digital media used by fat activists to promote fat acceptance and admiration (including eroticisation) via 'the Fatosphere' (p. 122). 'Rad fatties' offer a particularly interesting display of recalcitrance, subverting the idea that they should be apologetic (Pausé, 2015), whilst other body positivity sites (focusing on themes such as exercise, fashion and sex) invite visitors to 'feel' comfortable in their bodies via an emphasis on affect (Hynnä and Kyrölä, 2019). However, despite these and earlier attempts to challenge fat stigma online (Monaghan, 2005b), negative constructions persist. Hamera (2019) offers a recent analysis with reference to online US-right wing populist media, highlighting the contradictions of anti-feminist invective aimed at fat women and fat studies.

A nascent literature highlights the dominance of individual-level frames within social media communications about obesity and the presence of derogatory and misogynist sentiment (Chou et al., 2014). In a content analysis of 120 obesity-related messages on the social media platform Twitter, So et al. (2016) found the tweets that were emotionally evocative, humorous and invoked individual-level causes for obesity were more frequently retweeted than their counterparts. Yet, whilst negative (often humiliating) portrayals of fatness and fat people are dominant in digital media (Lupton, 2017; see also Chapter 6 in the context of the declared COVID-19 pandemic), such environments are also being harnessed in ways that might be considered supportive rather than oppressive, both for people who wish to lose weight and for those resisting this imperative.

Regarding the first point, Atanasova's (2018) research on obesity blogs demonstrates the importance of a metaphor of 'Journey' rather than 'War' that 'can be seen as affirmation of the potential of blogs to offer a space where alternative to the mainstream narratives can surface' (p. 8; for a critique of the 'Journey' metaphor, see Lupton, 2017). Regarding the second point, and in underscoring further the relevance of the Fatosphere, or 'online fat acceptance community' (Dickins et al., 2011: 1679), digital environments enable users to resist weight-based oppression (Rich, 2016). Indeed, fat blogs, social media, e-zines and other digital spaces are often utilised as part of the assemblages of more critical practices such as those endorsed by HAES (Burgard, 2009; Robison, 2005). Instagram and 'digital media activism' also enable advocates of HAES to challenge 'mainstream media' representations of the normative yoga body (Webb et al., 2019: 156). The micro-blogging platform Twitter has been used by the HAES community through the hash tag #HAES. Hence, social media can provide a counter-institutional space for reframing and learning about weight (loss), fat, physical activity and health in ways that challenge, circumvent and resist dominant narratives and metaphors. Further work is needed to address the pedagogical influence (Rich and Miah, 2014) of these digital technologies in an age of risk, uncertainty, mistrust, mass surveillance and 'datafication' (Smith, 2016). Such work would seem ever more urgent in light of 'the problematisation of fatness in COVID-19', with various media entrenching but also challenging anti-fat attitudes and discrimination (including that encountered by multiple oppressed groups in triage policy) (Pausé et al., 2021). Such research could identify what people are learning about health, well-being, weight and obesity/fatness within and through complex digital assemblages.

Finally, many of the studies described above examine particular media in isolate. As new media forms continue to emerge, researchers will need to consider how these interrelate. An example is offered by Hass (2017), who examines television makeover narratives, revealing how they extend beyond their traditional boundaries into digital media. Indeed, the capacity for viewers to actively comment live on media through accompanying social media (e.g. hashtags associated with television shows) further complicates assumed boundaries between media producer and consumer. Based on their analysis, Hass suggests that digital media offer 'affective spaces' for challenging 'officially sanctioned' accounts via communications 'between viewer and performer', incorporating 'direct exchanges in comments threads on Facebook' (p. 1489). Elsewhere, Cain et al.'s (2017: 184) study of digital news media also reveals that 'attempts to disrupt the dominant anti- "obesity" rhetoric are indeed making their way into the public discourse, albeit primarily through the more informal channels afforded by comments sections of digital media'. Yet, it should be stressed that the socio-technical infrastructure of digital media, as explained by Brooker et al. (2018) with reference to online news, may help perpetuate weight stigma. More also needs to be learnt about the salience of political divisions and big money's influence within nation-states and how such matters intersect with the declared COVID-19 pandemic. We will return to such matters in Part 2 of our book with an analysis of an online media platform (Chapter 6).

Weight-related stigma: the embodied effects and affects of obesity discourse

'The machinery of inequality' (Tyler, 2020) works in and through bodies that are stigmatised, or risk being discredited. As a concept, stigma refers to a social process or 'complex' (Pescosolido and Martin, 2015) wherein individuals and groups are marked as outsiders, immoral, apathetic, inferior, undesirably different, etc. (Goffman, 1968 [1963]). Weight-related stigma – incorporating negative attitudes, stereotypes, discrimination and oppression – has been defined as a 'truly global/ized' and 'emotionally damaging' phenomenon (Hackman et al., 2016: 58–9). Although thinness is stigmatised in certain contexts, 'excess' weight or fatness is framed as the archetypal physical stigma in somatic society. Stanford et al. (2018) flag this when discussing the media and obesity. Citing literature on the social, psychological, physiological and behavioural consequences of *negative attitudes* towards heavier people (defined as 'weight bias') and *humiliating treatment* (defined as 'fat shaming') (p. 186), these authors highlight themes such as: stigma and its relation to binge eating, exercise avoidance and metabolic health (e.g. blood pressure, cortisol levels); weight bias among health professionals and avoidance of doctors by patients who anticipate weight-related comments. Yet, it should also be reiterated that obesity discourse does not simply target 'fat people'. Wann (2009: xv) suggests 'people all along the weight spectrum may experience fat oppression', whilst Raisborough (2016: 7), drawing from Levay (2014), states 'a "fear of fat" works to pull all women, and increasingly men, into "constant micro-practices of self-monitoring"'.

Other literature points towards possible anxiety, social isolation, depression, disordered eating and poor body image (Friedman et al., 2005; Pearl and Puhl, 2018; Strauss and Pollack, 2003). In a systematic review of studies on 'weight bias internalization' or 'self-directed weight stigma', Pearl and Puhl (2018: 1141) write: 'Results showed strong, negative relationships between weight bias internalization and mental health outcomes'. They state such evidence has been accumulating over the past decade and especially during the last one to two years prior to their publication (p. 1159). Whilst we would not dispute the validity of these empirical findings, they emerge in an official journal of the WOF, which, as noted in Chapter 1, is a global proponent of the problematic WCHP.

The previous point is important in terms of how we conceptualise, represent and respond to weight-related stigma. Sociologically, rather than such stigma being a property of the self or being 'self-directed' by the obese, it is traceable to the broader society, *including* the operations of (bio)medicalised and widely circulating public health narratives (see also Brewis and Wutich, 2019). For Murray (2005b: 111): 'the persuasive power and dominance of medical narratives in generating a moral panic about the "obesity epidemic" have further pathologised fatness in the public consciousness, effectively legitimizing and sanctioning prejudice and discrimination against fat bodies'. Similarly, Tischner (2013) states that public health promotion fuels stigma amidst assumptions that weight is malleable and claims that it is costly for health services and the nation. Such arguments might be read alongside more recent literature on how a broader 'stigma system', comprising socio-political domination and scapegoating, shapes public health in ways that serve the wealthy and powerful (Friedman et al., 2022). Clinicians and public health workers *might* grapple with tensions here, remaining sympathetic to the 'psychological harm' of weight-related stigma or bias and the need to condemn, for example, popular mass media, yet also remain convinced of the need to address obesity (Cain et al., 2017; Flint et al., 2018). This view is partly rationalised on the basis that 'obesity stigma' is not considered as seri-ous or afforded the same recognition as other forms of stigma, prejudice or bias (Cain and Donaghue, 2018). Thus, tackling 'the global epidemic' (WHO, 1998, 2021) is considered a greater public good. However, not only are stigmatising approaches unethical, they may also be ineffective and iatrogenic (Meadows and Bombak, 2019). We would remind readers here of O'Hara and Taylor's (2018: 14) point, noted in our introduction, that the WCHP contributes to 'an enhanced adipophobicogenic environment'.

Our position is that the growing problem of weight-related stigma or bias (Pearl and Puhl, 2018; Puhl and Heuer, 2010), which disproportionately impacts women and children (Brewis, 2014; Fikkan and Rothblum, 2012; Herndon, 2014; Tischner and Malson, 2011), should be challenged without endorsing the war on obesity. With that in mind, we will outline burgeoning literature that attends to the harm-ful *embodied* effects and psychosocial affects of obesity discourse (Evans et al., 2013), incorporating 'the weight of expectation' in contexts of 'uncertainty and morality' (Williams and Annandale, 2020: 421). This literature draws on a range of perspec-tives on 'the body in culture' (e.g. Evans et al., 2008), foregrounding the impact of obesity discourse on the 'lived experience of fat embodiment: how it feels to be fat in a fat-phobic society' (Lupton, 2018: 2), or the fear of becoming fat. Reviewing such work through an embodied sociological lens is important not least given psychologists' tendency to emphasise cognitive rather than carnal dimensions in 'obesity stigma' research (Williams and Annandale, 2019). We cannot fully explore such literature here, including reflections on racial hierarchies (slim, White bodies as civilised bodies) (Farrell, 2011) and disability theory (Aphramor, 2009; Cooper, 1997), or the contradictions that emerge when obesity epidemic entrepreneurs lament and seek to end weight bias and stigma (WHO, 2017; WOF, 2018). More could also be presented on gendered and class-based resistances, which are not spe-cific to fat activism, and how types of social theory illuminate such processes (e.g. Warin et al., 2008). Rather, we document the impact and negotiation of weight-related stigma among predominantly cis gendered adults in various social con-texts before identifying studies of young people, especially in schools. Taken in the round, such work speaks not only to the (potential) intersection between biology and culture but also to how obesity discourse is shaped across various sites, between bodies and in ways that (re)produce difference, subjectivity and identities. To this end, we again draw attention to 'what inequalities are being formed and reformed' (McLeod and Yates, 2006: 3).

Research on adults and weight-related stigma

Social scientific research demonstrates the impact of weight-related stigma in var-ious contexts, including healthcare wherein size-ism, like racism, may be enacted without individual conscious intent (cf. Porter, 1993). Whilst most research focuses on cis gendered adults, some recent literature underscores how weight-related stigma and fatphobia intersect with trans- or non-gender conforming identities, sexualities and healthcare. Even in clinical settings geared to supporting marginalised groups, such as LGBTQ healthcare in the USA, there is evidence of intersecting stigma and weight bias undermining ethical patient-centred care (Paine, 2021). Elsewhere, commenting upon research on fat cis women's unsatisfactory experiences of reproductive healthcare (Ward and McPhail, 2019), Sojka and Sanchez (2019) underscore the need to also heed trans masculine and intersex patients' voices and advocate for 'trans inclusion in fat studies' given the intense stigma experienced by such people.

Research on cis gendered women and motherhood in Canada also paints a disconcerting picture. It reveals how those of higher weight felt wrong or disgusting due to the pathologising or derogatory language they encountered in reproductive contexts in which their pregnancies were deemed 'high risk' (Bombak et al., 2016; McPhail et al., 2016). This risk often pertained to the alleged severe consequences of the women's weight on foetal outcomes, but these risks were largely unspecified and poorly delineated. For *some* participants, this 'mother blame' could result in outright refusal of fertility care, or access to midwifery services. These authors also discuss internalised blame, which relates to whether or not women deemed obese 'deserve' to have children. Whilst we acknowledge embodied critiques of internalisation discourse (Williams and Annandale, 2019), the impact of what psychologists term 'internalised weight stigma' is noteworthy. This problem is said to occur when people adopt and personally endorse negative weight-related stereotypes. Studies indicate that such stigma also moderates the efficacy of weight-inclusive health interventions (e.g. HAES) that might otherwise improve multiple health indicators (Mensinger et al., 2016; Mensinger and Meadows, 2017; Chapter 7).

Elsewhere, Lewis et al. (2011) document the weight-based stigma experienced mostly by women labelled obese in Australia. The researchers describe the different types of obesity stigma participants faced (direct, environmental and indirect), how they responded and the impact on their health and well-being. Participants reported using extreme weight-loss techniques to avoid stigma, avoiding taking part in activities that might improve physical health and well-being, and becoming socially disconnected because of indirect stigma. The researchers also observed that self-blame was common, concluding that initiatives intended to challenge obesity stigma will 'likely' have to 'be more complex' than those for other 'health conditions' because 'weight bias is everywhere and is inherent in the contemporary "war on obesity" (Gard & Wright, 2005)' (Lewis et al., 2011: 1354; see also Lee and Pausé, 2016).

Following Lewis et al. (2011) and others (e.g. Grønning et al., 2012; O'Toole, 2019; Williams and Annandale, 2020), imputations of blame for obesity, and even self-blame for experiencing stigma, evidently pervade the global war on fat. Whilst there is a need for more *cross-cultural* research, existing literature is suggestive of a 'shared experience of being fat' (Gailey and Harjunen, 2019: 374) in the Global North (see also Puhl et al., 2015) and, increasingly, the Global South as governments 'roll out large scale and costly anti-obesity efforts' (Brewis et al., 2018: 2). It is under such conditions that weight-loss becomes an apparently 'logical choice' (obligation) for people with the necessary resources, i.e. time, energy, money, access to medicalised technologies and procedures. Yet, even here, stigma gets 'under the skin' (Williams and Annandale, 2019) and 'spoils identities' (Goffman, 1968 [1963]). Given the focus on individual responsibility within neoliberal thinking in general (Harvey, 2005), and obesity discourse in particular (Glenn et al., 2013; Monaghan et al., 2018), there are moral implications for people who appear to have reneged on the duty to exercise self-care even when publicly seeking (and paying for) redemption. O'Toole (2019) explores morality and accountability among women attending a commercial weight-loss club in Ireland, wherein the 'quest' to achieve 'a "better" body' (p. 15) unfolded in a setting that 'crafted weight stigma'. Indeed, the stigmatisation of fatness was overt; for instance, club posters informed members that 'A Flabby Body is a Flabby Mind' (p. 18). O'Toole's ethnography also describes narratives of self-blame, lack of personal control and 'the insatiable nature of women's appetites' (p. 17).

Adults hoping to slim down are presented with numerous 'options' within a biomedicalised marketplace of products and services, rendering 'excess' weight/ fatness apparently inexcusable. Throsby's (2009) UK-based qualitative research reveals the discursive work taking place when participants (again, mostly women) are unable to lose weight using pharmaceuticals and decide to undergo weight-loss surgery in a hierarchy of interventions. Throsby argues that 'failure' to lose weight, by whatever means, can lead to

> not only a burden of bodily labour in the form of repeated efforts to lose weight via escalating levels of intervention, but also a burden of discursive labour in order to pre-empt and rebut the negative moral evaluations of others for having 'failed' and for 'not trying hard enough'.
>
> *(p. 202; see also Throsby, 2008a, 2008b)*

Other research on weight-loss surgery, which again underscores moral dimensions and stigma, is also noteworthy. Recent examples include Meleo-Erwin's (2019) research on blog posts by bariatric patients and Vogel's (2018) study on patients who are 'entangled in webs of emotional, moral and sensorial relations' (p. 519). The former article reveals how personal responsibility is reproduced online, whilst the latter challenges the idea that people make individual free choices (the ideology of the self-contained liberal subject).

Insofar as fatness and weight-loss interventions tend to be associated with femininity, men labelled obese must negotiate certain contradictions that could spoil their identities: the idea that their physicality is effete yet efforts to lose weight may also carry feminine/feminising connotations (e.g. when joining a commercial weight-loss club populated by women). As described in Monaghan's (2008) ethnography, medicalisation is implicated in the masculinisation of dieting, i.e. it promises men the opportunity, even if illusory and ill-fated, to take control of their health and reduce risk. This vision was especially attractive to middle-aged men, including those who had taken public health campaigns and alarmist media reports to heart.

Subsequent studies have provided further critical insights on men and weight-related issues, which are useful given the usual research focus on women and girls in feminist (Bell and McNaughton, 2007) and fat activist literature (Cooper, 2016a). Whilst Bell and McNaughton (2007) bemoan the invisibility of 'the fat man' with reference to feminist scholarship, there is a growing literature on male bodies, weight/fatness, stigma and related body projects among diverse groups (e.g. Groven et al., 2018; Joy and Numer, 2018; Lozano-Sufrategui et al., 2016; Monaghan, 2015; Monaghan and Hardey, 2011; Newhook et al., 2015; Whitesel, 2014). Indeed, such work contradicts the recent claim in a leading obesity journal that 'studies of weight stigma within men have been primarily absent from the literature' (Himmelstein et al., 2019: 1598). Groven et al. (2018), for instance, describe the long-term experiences of men receiving weight-loss surgery in Norway. Exploring narratives about pre- and post-operative lives, these researchers address: men's anxieties about their employability, being ignored when fat, distress associated with repeatedly failed diets, emotional eating and public stories of success post-surgery despite ongoing struggles with food and potentially fatal side effects. Groven et al. problematise men's tendency to silence their suffering. Here, 'doing' gender is challenged for 'reinforcing stigma, lack of support, pain (physical, social and psychological), and self-blame' (p. 8).

Research is also accumulating on the social situation of gay men identifying as fat and the cultural emphasis on 'the ideal body' (e.g. Joy and Numer, 2018; Whitesel, 2014). Joy and Numer (2018) review accumulating scholarship and highlight implications for dieticians. Referencing, inter alia, ethnographies, psychological surveys and studies of (digital) gay media, they foreground themes such as denigration, rejection, isolation and body dissatisfaction. Whilst such problems may be compounded by the dietetic profession subscribing to the medical model of obesity, they note that gay men also engage in meaningful resistances or 'lines of flight' (p. 54) by entering size positive spaces. Similarly, Whitesel (2014) documents the politics of stigma in his ethnography of the US Girth and Mirth gay subculture. Both studies cite Monaghan's (2005b) virtual ethnography of fat male embodiment, size admiration and sexuality. Such research shows that 'fat men' with diverse, including marginalised, sexual orientations may subvert stigmatised identities along with supportive others. Bears and Chubbies are two such groups where fat gay men seek validation and manage 'spoiled identity' (Goffman, 1968 [1963]). Yet, there are limits. Subsequent research among Taiwanese gay men furthers understanding of Bears, specifically, differentiations according to size and how men typified as 'too fat' are insulted as 'Pigs' (Tan, 2016: 852).

Elsewhere, Monaghan and Hardey (2011) explore 'vocabularies of the discredited male body' and attendant sensibilities among British working-class men mainly identifying as heterosexual. They present ethnographic data on various orientations to the dominant cultural aesthetic, which equates men's fatness with deviance (e.g. the possibility of becoming a proud 'fat bastard' rather than a passive victim of the prejudiced). Whilst such literature complicates the idea that it is only women and girls who must negotiate stigmatising body norms (also

Roehling, 2012), none of this is antithetical to feminist concerns for gender justice. For example, Monaghan and Malson (2013) describe how 'big fellas', who encountered stigma and sought to lose weight, defined women and girls as most likely to suffer from weight-related 'troubles' in visually oriented culture, even if they were not fat. This seems to align with Rich and Evans' (2013) research on the impact of obesity discourse on young women's subjectivities vis-à-vis what they imagined their future lives and choices would be like if they were fat. Their study foregrounds the prominence of narrative and storying the future in relation to 'becoming fat'. Reflecting the broader culture of stigma, participants storied obesity with reference to fears of social isolation and bullying. These fears are understandable in view of evidence that fat is a feminist issue, including harsher penalties for women in contexts ranging from employment and healthcare to dating and education (Fikkan and Rothblum, 2012; Saguy, 2012).

Young people, obesity discourse and schooling

Obesity discourse has impacted schools' policies and practices, potentially stigmatising young people. Weight-based oppression has even been described as 'rampant in educational settings' (Cameron and Russell, 2016: 5). Of course, schools, and particularly Physical Education (PE), have long been positioned as sites intended to militate against disease (Fitzpatrick and Tinning, 2014), but obesity discourse has intensified and directed such concerns to bodily appearance and behaviours. A growing international literature examines the relationship between obesity discourses and the policies, curricula, pedagogies and practices of formal education (Burrows and Wright, 2004; Burrows et al., 2002; Cale and Harris, 2013; Cliff and Wright, 2010; Cameron et al., 2014; Evans et al., 2008; Evans and Colls, 2011; Gard and Pluim, 2014; Harwood and Wright, 2012; Leahy, 2009; Monaghan, 2014a; Powell and Fitzpatrick, 2015; Rich, 2010; Sykes and McPhail, 2008). This literature reveals the extent to which body pedagogies centred on obesity prevention have resulted in heightened surveillance, significantly impacting young people's embodiment and well-being.

Numerous scholars describe the above in terms of the impact of 'new health imperatives' (Harwood and Wright, 2012). In schools, these imperatives prescribe the 'lifestyle choices' young people should make in relation to physical activity, the regulation of their bodies and diets. Evidence, even from researchers who fail to problematise the 'existence' and 'urgency surrounding "childhood obesity"' (Boero and Thomas, 2016: 91), suggests that weight-centric health imperatives are highly corrosive. Among children and adolescents, exposure to weight stigma, harassment and bullying may have profound effects on physical and mental health, fitness, body dissatisfaction, eating behaviours, healthcare avoidance, psychosocial stress, adverse coping mechanisms, social well-being and educational performance (Greenleaf et al., 2014; Jendrzyca and Warschburger, 2016; Larkin and Rice, 2005; Puhl, 2011; Puhl et al., 2011, 2013; Weinstock and Krehbiel, 2009). Stigma and weight bias among children and adolescents are pervasive, strong and have increased over time (Puhl, 2011; Puhl et al., 2011). Young people labelled overweight and subject to weight bias may find that their peers are disinclined to help them (Patel and Holub, 2012; Puhl et al., 2013). Weight-related teasing is the most common form of teasing among students, and weight bias is also present among teachers and pre-service teachers (Puhl, 2011; Puhl et al., 2013; Russell-Mayhew et al., 2015). Whilst teachers' weight-related attitudes, expectations and attributions may disadvantage heavier students (Peterson et al., 2012), researchers have found pre-service teachers fear fat, dislike higher weight persons, have poor body image, high levels of implicit weight bias and anti-fat attitudes, and low self-efficacy for dealing with weight-related issues (Glock et al., 2016; Russell-Mayhew et al., 2015). Hence, schools are potentially unsafe environments for many students typified as fat. Indeed, they are 'common targets for bullying', defined as repeated aggressive acts perpetrated by more powerful people or groups (Weinstock and Krehbiel, 2009).

At this juncture, we draw caution towards simply reading bodies as being acted upon or assaulted by global obesity discourse, as if without resistance or struggle. These discourses are articulated and experienced in multiple ways; indeed, research by J. Evans et al. (2011b) indicates that whilst many young people are deeply troubled by the weight-centric health imperatives in British schools, others are emboldened or privileged (see also Evans and Davies, 2020). In Ireland, obesity discourse enabled young people with a common chronic illness (asthma) to define themselves as 'healthy looking bodies' in contrast to 'fat bodies'; the narrators' discreditable (unobtrusive) stigma was eclipsed by reference to visibly 'inferior' (usually female) bodies against whom they evaluated themselves and asserted their moral worth (Monaghan and Gabe, 2016). Other research on children's health, schooling, parenting and ethnicity in the USA reveals that given 'ever-present media reports' on how Black women and their children are at an elevated risk of obesity, Black parents understandably 'chose to distance themselves from perceived obesity-related lifestyle choices, avoiding yet another level of stigmatization' (Parsons et al., 2016: 611). Further work is needed to understand the complexities of fat embodiment through intersections of class, gender, ethnicity, nationality, age, sexuality, disability, culture and relations of shame and blame, etc. For example, how do different girls and young women invest in, negotiate and/or resist (postfeminist) discourses of health/obesity (Atencio and Wright, 2009; Rich and Evans, 2013; Gailey and Harjunen, 2019; Haugue, 2009; Skeggs, 1997; Youdell, 2005; Zannettino, 2008)? What about boys' bodies and embodied experiences, especially given the documented problem of bullying (Atkinson, 2014; Kehler and Atkinson, 2010; Monaghan, 2014a)? And, how might insights on the structures underlying (weight-related) stigma and its 'weaponising in neoliberalism' (Scambler, 2018) inform empirical research and interventions (Lewis et al., 2011; Monaghan, 2017)? Emerging research and perspectives on weight/fatness will likely need to draw from a range of theoretical concepts and recognise myriad resistances, or, alternatively, 'pragmatic enactments that make sense within specific social contexts' (Monaghan, 2015: 260). Indeed, as

Walkerdine (2009: 201) suggests, we need to be cautious about invoking a simple 'relation between the effectivity of biopower and the subject working on the self, or resisting'. This is not to downplay the important contributions already made to the study of pedagogies of weight/obesity but rather to understand complex relationalities in broader contexts. We explore these contexts elsewhere in our book with reference to anti-obesity policy, for example, in Chapter 3.

Meta-critique

Presumably the above literature could prompt a general rethink of the anti-obesity offensive. Furthermore, given the 'humanitarian' impulse to improve public health within the anti-obesity camp, one might anticipate there would be a receptive audience for research on the harms of obesity discourse, or what others term 'fallout' and 'collateral damage' from the war on obesity (Herndon, 2005; O'Connell et al., 2021). Yet, such a view is idealistic, if not naive, in a politicised field wherein obesity is, among other things, equated with domestic terrorism and 'emotional gratification' may be derived from holding beliefs congruent with neoliberal tenets (Gibson and Malcolm, 2020). Rail et al. (2010: 261) explain that the 'regime of truth' promulgated by obesity science largely 'ostracizes those with contradictory, and hence "deviant", forms of knowledge'. Of course, in a fraught world that is full of (metaphorical) battles, this reaction is not peculiar to the obesity wars (see, for example, Latour, 2004).

Besides ignoring critical perspectives, obesity epidemic entrepreneurs have rubbished some of the material cited above. Consider, for example, reactions to Flegal et al.'s (2013) meta-analysis of epidemiological research that contradicted the usual narrative about 'excess' weight and mortality. Even though the study was published in a leading medical journal it was publicly lambasted by a prominent researcher. The Chair of the Harvard School of Public Health's nutrition department, Willett, described the research on US National Public Radio as 'a pile of rubbish, and nobody should waste their time reading it' (cited by Hughes, 2013: 428). Willet then organised a symposium to explain why Flegal et al.'s (2013) study 'was absolutely wrong' (Hughes, 2013: 428). As reported by Hughes, Willet also 'attacked' earlier work lead by Flegal, though she offered a robust counter-response and additional epidemiological evidence to support her team's conclusions. This example might seem peculiar – after all, Flegal et al. (2013) were reporting data that could reassure millions of people who are medically classed as overweight – but such caustic responses are not, unfortunately, unusual.

'Attacking' seems to be the name of the game even when researchers simply *question* obesity orthodoxy. Referring to higher education in New Zealand, Burrows (2016: 102) describes how 'two international experts who raised questions about the veracity of "obesity" science were accused of sullying the university's reputation' and their reasoning was 'cast as "mad," "crazy," "unscientific," and/or embarrassing'. Cameron's (2016) international research with critical obesity scholars in higher education points to similar reactions, which, as might be anticipated, could negatively impact academic careers. Such admonishment is also problematic in terms of advancing the knowledge base. The science of obesity, nutrition and energetics is littered with errors that have been proven to be highly unresponsive to correction (Allison et al., 2016). In such an environment it is disconcerting that critical social science perspectives are also misrepresented and possibly undermined by fellow critics of obesity alarmism. When offering reflections on how some of our own work has been attacked an immediate caveat is in order: we are not claiming that alternative perspectives and apparently disconfirming evidence should not be subjected to critical inspection, revision and perhaps rejection. Questioning Campos et al.'s (2006) reproduction of gendered dichotomies and the denigration of emotions when invoking moral panic is a case in point (Fraser et al., 2010). Scholarship that destabilises obesity discourse must be well informed, systematically researched, reflexive about uncertainty and open to debate in a shared community of learning (Rich et al., 2011). Our point extends to alternative interventions such as HAES, a sentiment also evidenced in an online exchange between practitioners and critics (Lupton, 2012; Chapter 7). However, our argument here is that not all criticisms directed at critical work can be taken at face value.

We will draw this section to a close with some reflections on critical scholarship, within the social sciences, which scrutinises critical weight studies and fat activism. Drawing from Lee's experiences, we comment on how rethinking obesity entails meta-critique, or how critical perspectives beget critical responses that invite further interrogation. Lee has previously offered sociological explanations for some of the antagonistic responses he has encountered, including media misrepresentations of his approach, when entering 'the obesity debate' (*sic*) (see Monaghan, 2008: 13–21). Thereafter he describes how objections may even come from 'unexpected quarters' (2013: 87), a fellow critic of obesity epidemic rhetoric. Specifically, Monaghan challenges Gard's (2009b) review of *Men and the War on Obesity* (Monaghan, 2008). According to Gard (2009b), Monaghan (2008) apparently criticises doctors for harbouring hatred towards 'obese people'. He is also apparently unaware of the new public health, which, for Gard (2009b: 236), seeks to avoid 'victim blaming' with its focus on 'obesogenic environments' (though, see our earlier discussion *and* Monaghan, 2008: 42).

In response, Monaghan (2013) explains that he *does not* berate individual medical doctors (or others committed to fighting fat, notably slimming club employees who are thanked early in his ethnography). Certainly, when reporting empirical data, Monaghan (2008) cites men who were critical of clinicians, though their views varied. One interviewee, for instance, stated that his general practitioner was 'fantastic' in a section of the book where Lee writes: 'Some clinicians are sensitive to the needs of larger people' (p. 85). And, contrary to Gard's (2009b) claim that Monaghan (2008) seems unaware of modern public health and its focus on obesogenic environments, he discusses these matters with reference to Petersen and Lupton's (1996) *The New Public Health*. Mindful of the symbolic violence enacted in this field, Monaghan (2013) conceptualises Gard's (2009b) reading as a case of 'misrecognition' (Bourdieu, 2001). That is, 'cognitions, sentiments and actions (typically embodied within the white, bourgeois, masculine habitus), which legitimate relations of dominance (claims to distinction and so on) over subordinated groups who are not granted full recognition' (Monaghan, 2013: 87–8). To be sure, there are legitimate (unacknowledged) debates to be had here, notably regarding aspects of Bourdieu's theorising on 'the field' rather than 'world' where many people are doing various things together, beyond seeking to dominate (Becker and Pessin, 2006). However, Bourdieu's concept, 'misrecognition', seemed apt here not least because Gard (2009a) also depicts fat activism in a way that belies the complexities of this heterogeneous movement – for instance, activists are not necessarily seeking to mitigate culpability for fatness through 'the will to innocence' (LeBesco, 2004: 111).

After Monaghan (2013) flagged these and other problems, Gard (2013) offered *some* concessions. For instance, he acknowledged that his approach to social constructionism was 'unhelpful, vague and sloppy' (p. 108). However, his response is titled 'disagreement not misrecognition' and the overall tenor is one of defensive retrenchment in a piece containing questionable counter-responses and the eliding of mistakes that should be beyond debate or disagreement. For example, because Monaghan (2008) explicitly refers to 'the obesogenic environment' and the new public health, it is wrong to claim otherwise. Rather than acknowledge this, Gard (2013) suggests to Monaghan (2013) that medicine's use of militarised metaphors 'has been part and parcel of medical discourse in numerous fields of enquiry throughout medical history' (Gard, 2013: 113). Yet, the introduction to Monaghan (2008: 1, emphasis added) states: 'Medicine's military metaphor, as explained by Sontag when discussing the war on cancer, *first became popular in the 1800s*'. Our concern here is that there are already enough constraints on the uptake of critical scholarship (subsequently amplified in the time of COVID-19; see Chapter 6 and our epilogue) without the sort of 'friendly' review offered by a fellow critic who, on other occasions, has contributed valuable work. Arguably, challenging 'misrecognition' within the 'fat field' (Saguy, 2013: 31) is vital today given (global and national) public health authorities' 'esurient' (Dew, 2014: 141) tendencies to constrain our everyday embodied, affective, spatial and intellectual life worlds.

One last example underscores the need for defensible or revisable (meta-)critique. Responding to Gard's (2009a) apparent adoption of what could be called a 'statesman' role, where he recounts and evaluates the work of other critical scholars, Monaghan (2013: 87) writes:

> I do not think this move is necessarily bad, even among 'like-minded' critics who might be considered 'friends' rather than 'enemies'. Those who scrutinise obesity orthodoxy will encounter opposition, even from unexpected quarters. Hence, while the uptake of critical scholarship will always be unpredictable, it remains a truism that we must offer intellectually robust and defensible work, or at least be prepared to modify our always partial analyses not least if we aim to present credible studies that have real world relevance (Monaghan et al. 2011). As with science more generally, critical weight studies are corrigible.

Yet, when 'disagreeing' with Monaghan (2013), Gard (2013: 106) immediately writes: 'I argue that while groups of scholars and activists may share broad social and political commitments, this does not mean that they should never challenge each others (*sic*) points of view'. Given the above excerpt and other points raised in this section, Gard is evidently disagreeing with a straw man. Gard's framing unfortunately sets the tone for the remainder of his reply, incorporating problematic references to assumed invitations, alliances, interpretations of science and HAES. More could be written but we will simply refer readers directly to Monaghan (2013) and Gard (2013) for further points and counterpoints and leave it to others to make up their own minds on the merits or otherwise of each contributor's case.

Conclusion: moving the debate forward

The above section is a stark reminder that we cannot assume homogeneity or predictability when critiquing obesity discourse and the WCHP. For such very good reasons we are implored to consider the nature of knowledge and critique amidst broader sociological and philosophical reflections on 'matters of concern' (Latour, 2004). As evinced above, the war on obesity can be examined through various critical perspectives. There are nuances and differences across this critical work. This remains a complex assemblage of discourses, affects and interests; hence, in the remaining chapters we aim to capture the complexity of science, policy and people's embodied experiences as we engage with a range of critical work, theoretical perspectives and empirical research. In all of this, there is a need to challenge health inequalities and the harms of obesity discourse. However, we also reflect on the political utility of our own and others' work if participants fail to engage in ethical and respectful debate across communities, professions and disciplines. Drawing from Giroux (1992, 2004), for instance, Mansfield and Rich (2003) explore how this form of 'border crossing' within assemblages might lead to new perspectives/understandings of health and physical activity. This is a salutary point, possibly urging contributors away from disciplinary silos and what might be read as disagreeable positions and antagonisms that stymie 'meaningful social change' (p. 357).

The work of this chapter is done. We addressed four main areas when reviewing critical perspectives on the obesity crisis: (i) critique of epidemiology and evolving obesity science; (ii) analyses of media, 'fat panic' and body pedagogies; (iii) empirical studies of stigma and (iv) meta-critique. Our aim has been to assist readers, who may not necessarily be familiar with this literature, to orientate to a potentially difficult and conflictual terrain rather than 'adding more ruins to the ruins, adding even more smoke to the smoke' (Latour, 2004: 228). In so doing, we have provided some 'insider' understandings that might be useful for those seeking to make their own way through and perhaps go on to help (re-)shape a changing and *open* landscape, itself 'a consequence of being "peopled" by actors and agents who possess critical reflexivity and creativity towards the world in which they live' (Williams, 2003: 59).

In taking a different tack to politics, the next chapter analyses the pedagogising of obesity knowledges and the recontextualisation of policy. In so doing, we provide a means of scrutinising the 'sacred' status of state-sanctioned obesity discourse and the WCHP, as enacted in public health policies and campaigns. As will be seen, such communication strategies not only drift towards lifestyles when ostensibly tackling the social determinants of health; they are also potentially stigmatising. Hence, they are ripe for ethically informed critique which could, in turn, pave the way for a different approach.

3

PEDAGOGISING OBESITY KNOWLEDGES AND THE RECONTEXTUALISATION OF POLICY

In previous chapters we revealed how an abundance of critical literature has examined the discursive shifts through which 'obesity knowledges and matters of fat' (Land, 2018) have been 'framed' (Kwan and Graves, 2013; Saguy, 2013). Some of this work has begun to trace policy developments and implementation (e.g. in schools via measurement programs and state-funded multi-media public health campaigns), often using Foucauldian analyses to do so (e.g. Dukelow, 2017; Mannion and Small, 2019; Wright and Harwood, 2009). These approaches have offered interesting analytical and empirical insights on biopedagogies, not least in terms of revealing the powerful expressions of neoliberalism which come to frame weight and/or fatness as obesity and its precursor, overweight. However, we also recognise the risk of conceptualising neoliberalism as an omnipresent force shaping public health knowledge(s) and policy (analysis) (Bell and Green, 2016; Monaghan et al., 2018; Williams and Fullagar, 2019) without providing a detailed exploration of the processes and mechanics of the production and communication of these policies. Such considerations matter because, as Maguire et al. (2015: 485) argue, policy enactment is a far more 'fragile and unstable process than is sometimes documented in policy analysis and implementation studies'.

This chapter takes a modest step in advancing a pedagogical reading of the rule-bound social processes that 'legitimate' obesity as a public health problem requiring policy solutions (see Monaghan et al., 2010: 53–5), or 'prescriptions' (Warin and Zivkovic, 2019: 212). In so doing, we will utilise an eclectic range of literature, including pedagogy scholarship (e.g. Bernstein, 2000), in order to critique how 'received wisdoms or "sacred" health knowledge' (Evans et al., 2008: 19) are produced and communicated via anti-obesity policymaking and practice. Accordingly, we will extend pedagogy scholarship that 'rest[s] on a particular view of policy as process not object, inherently social in its making, implementation and purpose, inevitably value laden and loaded with cognitive and affective intent' (Evans et al., 2013: 333).

DOI: 10.4324/9781315658087-5

The materials informing this chapter emerge from existing international literature on anti-obesity public health policy and interventions (e.g. Backstrom, 2020; Dukelow, 2017; Lupton, 2015, 2018; Ulijaszek, 2014; Warin and Zivkovic, 2019). When analysing the globalising and pedagogising of policy we draw from scholars who have critically surveyed specific national policy fields in addition to foregrounding the role of ideology and values in an ostensibly rational and unbiased process (e.g. Ulijaszek and McLennan, 2016). Just as we recognise that the biomedical concept of obesity denotes a multifaceted and contested field (Chapters 1 and 2) that cannot be divorced from particular places, actions and corporeal matters, we are also mindful of Ulijaszek's (2014) reference to complexity when describing types of policy within *and* outside of government organisations in just one jurisdiction and time period. Described as a 'confusing' landscape, Ulijaszek refers, among other things, to competing interpretations, the diversity of disciplines involved and 'the increasing sophistication of different policy positions' (p. 126). Hence, it is not our aim to identify and dissect key policy reports, strategy documents and recommendations since the advent of 'globesity' (Chapter 1). Such a task, even if limited to obesity agenda setting over the past decade, would likely require a book, if not several volumes. Rather, in critiquing this field as affective (as distinct from effective) and embodied public pedagogy, we proffer a theoretically informed reading of what currently pass as *ethically* justifiable public health policies and campaigns. We take it as axiomatic that 'pedagogy always implies a relationship that is driven by intentions and desires for particular kinds of shifts in subjectivity', thereby necessitating 'the case for the articulation of an ethical imperative that is always the premise of any discussion about pedagogy' (Gaztambide-Fernández and Arráiz Matute, 2014: 52–3).

This ethical imperative is evidenced in other social scientific literature in the fat field. As explained by Lupton (2015) when dissecting 'pedagogies of disgust', ethical concerns trump claims about effectiveness in public health – a pertinent point that does not depend upon, but is worth making with reference to, the general *ineffectiveness* of health policy (Evans et al., 2013; Kelly and Barker, 2016). Kelly and Barker, for instance, state the reason why changing health-related behaviour is so difficult is because 'policy makers make it so. They do this by seeking simple non-scientific answers to complex problems' (p. 109; see also Kelly and Russo, 2018). In addition to philosophical and human rights matters (O'Hara and Taylor, 2018), ethical concerns prompt us to ask various questions when discussing anti-obesity policy processes or 'enactments' (Maguire et al., 2015); for example: What does it mean to frame obesity as socially determined in public health policies inspired by epidemiology, psychology and economics; why are behavioural responses to a putative environmental problem ultimately preferred by state-backed policymakers and administrators; and what are the 'affects' of policy prescriptions that drift towards lifestyles and/or appearance as a presumed index of poor (unhealthy) choices, parental practices and national fitness?

This chapter is divided into three main sections. First, we outline our conceptual approach when scrutinising the pedagogising of obesity knowledges and their reshaping and enactment through policy. A pedagogical approach is apt given the relatively recent emphasis within high-income nations on 'communication policies' to 'tackle obesity' (OECD, 2017: 1). Our analysis synthesises Bernstein's (1990, 1996, 2000, 2001) theorising on 'recontextualisation' and 'the pedagogic device' with literature on health education, policy, campaigning (e.g. Dukelow, 2017; Evans et al., 2008, 2013; Popay et al., 2010; Sandlin et al., 2011) and obesity epidemic entrepreneurs (Monaghan et al., 2010). This synthesis informs our discussion on the production and pedagogic communication of various policies and interventions within a broader political economy of health (Evans and Davies, 2020; Scambler, 2018). In the second section, organised into three subsections, we revisit and build on work that has informed some of our earlier critique of obesity policy (Evans et al., 2008). Specifically, we deploy Bernstein's concepts as part of a 'three rules approach' to delineate dominant government-sponsored responses to obesity. In so doing, we aim to render visible that which may otherwise remain tacit and accepted, such as marketised ideology, values, power and the hidden injuries of class. As part of that analysis we will draw from Popay et al.'s (2010: 148) commentary on 'lifestyle drift' or 'the tendency for policy to start off recognizing the need for action on upstream social determinants of health inequalities only to drift downstream to focus largely on individual lifestyle factors'. We also deploy Bernstein's (1996) concepts of 'evaluative rules' and 'symbolic control' when drilling down into the bases of 'social marketing' (Mulderrig, 2017) anti-obesity campaigns, critiquing the (unintentionally) stigmatising pedagogical modalities utilised by policymakers and recontextualising agents as they attempt to 'positively' influence or 'nudge' (groups of) individuals towards making 'better' (healthier) choices. In the final section we reflect on the value of a Bernsteinian approach when explicating pedagogical processes and practices and what such theorising might offer critics hoping to interrupt ethically dubious public health policies.

Theorising anti-obesity policy as pedagogy: the focus on communication

Lest we are immediately accused of being 'overly theoretical', consider the representation of policy responses in an authoritative international report (OECD, 2017). That document is not unusual in its points of emphasis, as might be inferred from recent critical commentary on *The Lancet* EAT Commission's (2019) report that 'frames premature death as primarily a consequence of individual dietary and lifestyle choices, repeating the term "healthy diets" nearly 100 times' (The Nutrire CoLab, 2020). In its update on efforts to tackle obesity, the OECD (2017) prioritise what are termed 'communication policies that promote healthy diets by improving health literacy and empowering consumers, or by regulating marketing of potentially unhealthy products' (p. 8). The report continues by noting member states have recently been utilising various 'new technologies' such as 'social media' or 'have revised the arrangements for more traditional communication policies such as food labelling or regulation of marketing, in order to tackle the problem of obesity' (p. 8). In our view, this framing of the matter as a need to 'communicate' with and 'sensitise' (p. 1) consumers (with much reference made in that report to the less-educated) invites a theoretically informed reading of policy as pedagogy and its modalities of enactment within various arenas. In so doing, we learn that the policy process, structured by various principles and ideology, is less stable than implied by the OECD and is open to contestation.

Importantly, whilst the framing of obesity as a public health crisis has remained a consistent theme within health policy across Western societies for over two decades (Saguy, 2013; Schorb, 2013; Ulijaszek, 2014), arguably there is a lack of consensus over responsibility for, definition of and responses to a so-called wicked problem that is highly complex and intractable (Boswell, 2016; Warin and Zivkovic, 2019). We would add that efforts to tackle obesity through policy (prescriptions) are challenging given the complexity of such processes as '*emplaced, enacted* and *embodied*' (Evans et al., 2013: 320, emphasis in original). Whist Evans and Davies (2020) unpack what each of these terms means in some detail and what underlies them, the crux of their argument is that mediated policy is ongoing and contingent rather than definitive and causal given the myriad contexts, actors and processes (social, biological, psychic) involved therein. Furthermore, even within nation-states, there are innumerable policy documents from different departments and national public bodies that point towards different causes and solutions to the obesity crisis. Consequently, in the UK at least, there have been calls for more joined-up approaches across government departments (DHSC, 2019). Amidst such complexity and the ways in which different policies 'call up different forms of enactments' (Maguire et al., 2015: 485), our task is to advance a theoretically informed reading of policy matters as pedagogy. Rather than undertaking an empirical analysis of policy documents, or enactments of those policies by actors 'on the ground' (p. 485), we present a conceptually rich means of scrutinising messy and multilayered processes of policymaking. In so doing, we interrupt claims that 'communication policies to tackle obesity are advancing' (OECD, 2017: 8) and the implications of such assertions for ongoing public health interventions.

Our argument is premised on the sociologically informed view that one cannot adequately understand the pedagogising processes of policy – their instructional, regulative, educative and affective dimensions – without acknowledging their relationship with other discourses, values, ethics, histories, organisations and actors. Such considerations sensitise us to how, for example, tensions emerge between approaches emphasising individual responsibility and behaviour change and those lamenting health inequalities. Other medical sociologists and social theorists of health also recognise such tensions in broader political context. Note, for example, recent critiques of lifestyle drift (Kirkland and Raphael, 2018; Williams and Fullagar, 2019), a policy process entwined with the problem of 'short-termism' in central government and its deleterious effect on democratic engagement (Popay et al., 2010: 148).

Elsewhere, as Rizvi and Lingard (2010, 2011) suggest in their work on social equity and higher education, what is also of interest is how pedagogical matters are 'performed' in public policy and linked to other values; or to draw on Bernstein (1996), with reference to *who* is involved in knowledge distribution. If we synthesise such thinking with Monaghan et al.'s (2010) typification of obesity epidemic entrepreneurs, these actors include those legitimating obesity science as a governmental concern via policymaking and those who campaign and/ or administer (or even enforce) the state-sponsored war on obesity in various settings (e.g. the school and clinic) (see also O'Hara and Taylor, 2018). If such prescriptions or pedagogies are to be accepted, however, they must also align or mesh with the 'embodied dispositions' of those whom Monaghan et al. (2010: 44), following Petersen and Lupton (1996), term '"the entrepreneurial self", i.e. the person who actively, reflexively and responsibly works on their body as part of the new public health'.

We are not the first to seek a more nuanced reading of policy. For instance, the concept of 'assemblage' has been used in policy research (e.g. Rizvi and Lingard, 2011), but less so in relation to weight-centric public health policy and campaigns (though, for exceptions, see: Evans and Davies, 2020; Lupton, 2015; Monaghan et al., 2010; Rich, 2010). Drawing from scholarship on normalising/regulating body pedagogies, Monaghan et al. (2010: 41) explain this 'assemblage' comprises 'a matrix of interactions, measurements and interventionist approaches' that are multi-sited and potentially harmful (e.g. with reference to size-ism and stigma). Citing Evans et al. (2008: 13), they add: 'such processes should not be seen as the product of "conspiracy on the part of science or expression of political mischief or health educators' malicious intent" but rather larger social historical processes (e.g. changes in conceptions of health in the 20th century, regulation of populations, consumerism)' (Monaghan et al., 2010: 41). This caveat is important considering the misrecognition of critique discussed in Chapter 2 and mounting barriers following the outbreak of COVID-19 (see also Part 3).

When looking towards pedagogy scholarship to advance our reading of policy and the arenas within which it operates, Bernstein's theories and concepts are promising (e.g. Bernstein, 1990, 1996, 2000, 2001; see also Evans et al., 2008; Loughland and Sriprakash, 2016; Moore, 2013). To be sure, Bernstein needs to be re-read in a corporeal light. For instance, Evans et al. (2008: 96) explain that Bernstein 'was not particularly concerned to interrogate how social relations were "embodied"' (see also Evans and Davies, 2020). Nonetheless, his toolbox of ideas, originally applied to 'educational knowledge' in schools, could be extended to other forms of knowledge development and, we would add, bodywork. For instance, amidst growing concerns about obesity and metabolic syndrome, Castro-Vázquez (2019) draws from Bernstein when referring to state-backed nutritional education and media reports in Japan. The responsible entrepreneurial self is defined here as a 'totally pedagogised self' who uses knowledge and acquired experiences to become a 'healthy self'. Additionally, whilst sociologists of education use Bernstein's work to examine the politics of curricula in class-divided societies, his concepts can be utilised and extended to examine policy itself (see Loughland and Sriprakash, 2016; Singh et al., 2013).

Some of Bernstein's concepts, which we will employ, include 'recontextualisation' (comprising an 'official recontextualising field' or ORF and a 'pedagogic recontextualising field' or PRF), and 'the pedagogic device' with its three inter-related rules: 'the distributive rules', 'the recontextualising rules' and 'the evaluative rules' (Bernstein, 1990, 2000). We consider these key concepts to analyse the complex relationalities between a range of elements that operate throughout, or flow through, totally pedagogised (micro) societies 'where health education is everywhere and everyone's concern' (Evans et al., 2008: 6). Such rule-bound pedagogical mechanisms incorporate not only everyday actions and prescriptions but also organisational (meso-social) and globalising (macro-social) political economic processes. We lack space to fully explicate these concepts with reference to Bernstein's oeuvre and its antecedents in British social anthropology, linguistics and classic French sociology (Moore, 2013). However, our discussion below should provide enough orientation when scrutinising policy as pedagogy – a social process entwined with a broader moral order, or cosmology, where there are enduring regulative concerns pertaining to the sacred and profane. On the latter point, note how anti-obesity policies foreground quasi-religious moralising about 'gluttony or sloth' (Evans, 2006), or how 'new wave public health' constructs 'folk devils' (Mannion and Small, 2019). None of this, we will stress, can be divorced from class/command (Scambler, 2018), or what Dingwall (2020b), in the context of COVID-19, calls 'patrician policymaking' that reflects circumscribed, individualised, elite interests that are indifferent to the plight of the poor. Recently reflecting on their use of Bernstein when researching embodied policy concepts and the political economy of health, Evans and Davies (2020: 741) remind us that 'the sacred (valuable, important, high status)' is elevated above the 'profane' and therefore helps to 'perpetuate social class and cultural hierarchies and differences'.

For Bernstein (2000), recontextualisation entails the selective appropriation of knowledge from one place, such as a specific scientific discipline, and its translation in another, such as a textbook that has pedagogic functions. To the extent that knowledge is moved from one place to another – it is delocated, relocated and refocused – there is space for the play of ideology and other social dimensions that are amenable to critique. Chapter 2, when reviewing literature on media as popular pedagogy, noted how learning goes beyond the classroom as obesity science is selectively recontextualised – and typically dramatised – in news reports and other sources, with ethically dubious affects/effects. Recontextualisation in the fat field could also refer to how epidemiological knowledge provides the basis for (early) health interventions in schools once such knowledge is translated or filtered 'through the ideologies and policies of neo-liberalism and free market economics' (Evans et al., 2008: 14). Similarly, public health social marketing campaigns recontextualise ideas assembled in one discursive terrain, biomedicine, and reproduce them elsewhere as part of a social process that is inseparable from values, culture, economics, power, bodies, subjectivity, affect, etc.

Recontextualisation comprises an ORF and PRF. The former is 'created and dominated by the state and its selected agents and ministries' (Bernstein, 2000: 33), whereas the latter consists of pedagogues who may be more or less aligned with the ORF that has colonising tendencies, as seen in UK curriculum policy since the 1980s (Evans et al., 2008) and elsewhere (Loughland and Sriprakash, 2016). As explained further below, various interrelated rules structure the ORF of obesity where knowledge is distributed through specialised actors and agencies associated with health, biomedicine and knowledge creation (for discussion on 'creators' as a mode of obesity epidemic entrepreneurship, see Monaghan et al., 2010: 47–50). More generally, the ORF is entwined with and influenced by marketised logics in capitalist societies (see Scambler, 2018), and it gives 'legitimacy' (Monaghan et al., 2010) through symbolic means to the war on obesity. Additionally, Bernstein (2000) draws attention to what he terms the PRF, which may be relatively autonomous, though, for Evans et al. (2008: 155), this 'has been weakened by extension and growth of the [ORF]'. The PRF is analytically significant because policymaking involves 'negotiation, contestation or struggle between different groups who may lie outside the formal machinery of official policy-making' (Ozga, 2000: 13, cited in Maguire et al., 2015: 486). In the case of obesity policymaking, the PRF includes organisations and agents who operate within health education fields – Monaghan et al.'s (2010) 'administrators/enforcers' – and those with a special motivate, or moralised investment, in the anti-obesity campaign (e.g. celebrity chefs, who have also influenced policy on school meals provision; see Chapter 1).

The pedagogic device, a concept related to recontextualisation, refers to the 'social grammar' of educational knowledge. This device 'has internal rules which regulate the pedagogic communication which the device makes possible' (Bernstein, 2000: 27). This device is not a thing per se but a field of forces that has observable effects that are political (relating to power and control) and ideological (requiring legitimation) (Moore, 2013). The concept can be used to examine how particular discourses are appropriated, regulated and resisted. Drawing from Bernstein, Evans et al. (2008: 19) explain, 'the pedagogic device' refers to 'a grammar for producing specialised messages, realizations, a grammar which regulates what it processes: a grammar which orders and positions and yet contains the potential of its own transformation'. Such thinking helps to make sense of how policies are 'pedagogised', i.e. how particular discourses, which are 'not neutral' (Bernstein, 2000: 27), become legitimised forms of knowledge and thus what becomes intelligible, creditable and doable amidst possible contestation in democratic societies (Moore, 2013).

For Bernstein, the pedagogic device acts through three interrelated rules: the distributive rules, the recontextualising rules and the evaluative rules. These rules provide the 'intrinsic grammar of pedagogic discourse', thus setting out the conditions of (re)production and transformation of culture (Bernstein, 1990: 80):

> These rules are themselves hierarchically related in the sense that the nature of the distributive rules regulates the recontextualizing rules, which in

turn, regulate the rules of evaluation. These distributive rules regulate the fundamental relation between power, social groups, forms of consciousness and practice, and their reproductions and productions. The recontextualizing rules regulate the constitution of specific pedagogic discourse. The rules of evaluation are constituted in pedagogic practice.

Our analytical focus is on how these rules interrelate in and through anti-obesity policymaking and pedagogic practice. Such rules guide our analysis towards the role of particular social groups, power and their capacity to construct legitimate health knowledges and communicative practices. This conceptualising also appeals to us because, rather than analysing these rules in isolation, we can explore their interplay and how they 'give rise to three respective arenas containing agents with positions/practices seeking domination' (Bernstein, 2000: 202). This approach provides a useful organising framework to understand processes of anti-obesity policymaking and how symbolic control of 'lived bodies' (Williams and Bendelow, 1998) materialises through the pedagogising of policy.

Substantively, we will focus on recent developments that have come to impact major anti-obesity policies and initiatives across many high-income nations (Chapter 1) and, in turn, what it means to be evaluated and symbolically marked as an (un)healthy body. We highlight how neoliberal (Harvey, 2005; Scott-Samuel et al., 2014), or 'advanced liberal' (Williams and Fullagar, 2019), discourses of individualism and healthism have come to reshape anti-obesity policy through 'new forms of standardization, comparison and commensurability' (Loughland and Sriprakash, 2016: 232), but which have also been recontextualised in ways that develop novel relationships with discourse about the environmental influence on obesity (Colls and Evans, 2014). Similar to but also extending contemporary Bernsteinian analyses, we consider the mechanics through which policies are 'employed, gain traction' (Loughland and Sriprakash, 2016: 231) and are communicated with embodied affects in a broader symbolic universe. Guided by and adapting Bernsteinian thinking to weight-related matters, our analysis scrutinises the processes between the 'official' policy fields and the 'pedagogic' fields wherein different forms of 'health education' (anti-obesity campaigns, interventions, school policies, etc.) are performed. In so doing, we trace the ways in which multiple, and at times competing, ideals associated with the body, weight and health are recontextualised as they are communicated through the pedagogic device of anti-obesity policy.

The pedagogic device of anti-obesity policy: a three rules approach

Drawing on the above literature, this section advances the following argument: the pedagogic device, which shapes the formation of policy solutions, controls certain principles that come to constitute what is widely regarded as 'valid' or even 'sacred health knowledge' (Evans et al., 2008: 24). Such principles matter insofar as the pedagogic device influences how legitimated health knowledges are to be enacted or taught (public pedagogy) and evaluated across populations, providing a 'symbolic ruler for consciousness' (Bernstein, 2000: 36).

Divided into three, the following considers (i) the distributive rules in the ORF of anti-obesity policy, (ii) the recontextualising rules of anti-obesity policy and (iii) the evaluation and symbolic control of obesity through the PRF. Throughout we recognise these rules are *interrelated* and integral to the definition of obesity as a contemporary health concern, calling forth 'new policy initiatives' (OECD, 2017: 8) comprising 'the transformation of [obesity knowledges] into pedagogic communication' (Bernstein, 2000: 25). We examine how the anti-obesity offensive has been reshaped within the ORF and PRF, filtered through ubiquitous neoliberal market logics emphasising comparison, individualism and measurement (reflective of Bernstein's 'evaluative rules'), alongside more recent emphasis given to 'environmental influences' on obesity. However, in drawing from Popay et al. (2010) and others (e.g. Warin and Zivkovic, 2019), we also argue that the current recontextualisation of issues of structural inequalities fails to redress problems attendant to lifestyle drift, the reproduction of weight-related stigma and the projection of policymakers' values onto other people's bodies and lives.

The distributive rules in the ORF of anti-obesity policy

Bernstein's (1996) theory of the pedagogic device prompts us to think about how the distributive rules have shaped the ORF of anti-obesity policy. Crucially, distributive rules 'mark and distribute who may transmit what to whom and under what conditions, and they attempt to set the outer limits of legitimate discourse' (p. 31). The distributive rules comprise 'two classes of knowledge': 'the *thinkable*' and 'the *unthinkable*' (Bernstein, 2000: 28–9, emphasis in original). Official (thinkable, state-backed) obesity knowledges are distributed and specialised in specific health fields via particular agencies and actors who enact 'legitimate' claims. Increasingly, government health policies have been influenced by transnational actors, such as the OECD (2017) and WHO (2018) (similarly, with reference to the ORF of Australian school education, see Loughland and Sriprakash, 2016). Furthermore, following our discussion on the global circulation of obesity discourse and its recontextualisation (Chapters 1 and 2), policies have a history enacted in *national contexts*. In Anglophone neoliberal societies, such processes are shaped by individualistic discourses, reductionist paradigms and disciplines. Bernstein prompts us to consider how distributive rules have shaped the ORF of anti-obesity policy in places like Britain, as governments enact certain political economic priorities and agendas. As observed in England, Scotland and Wales, national public health policies have been influenced by the distribution of knowledge associated with priorities and ideologies that have antecedents in Thatcherism, comprising 'key neoliberal strategies such as financial deregulation, trade liberalization, and the privatization of goods and services' (Scott-Samuel et al., 2014: 53).

The continued emphasis, globally, on competition, individualism, standardisation and comparison, are distributed across the ORF. Anti-obesity policies are assembled through this pedagogic discourse, establishing rules and principles of control through which some knowledges are excluded (e.g. how chronic diseases are related to power) (Aphramor, 2019a), whilst others are selected for pedagogic purposes 'by agents who have previously been legitimately pedagogised' (Bernstein, 2000: 31). When reviewing the UK policy context, Holman et al. (2018) reveal how disciplines such as psychology and behavioural economics dominate health behaviour interventions, i.e. individual-level approaches, including tactics such as 'nudging' (Mulderrig, 2017; see below), favoured within public health and policy. In contrast, disciplines such as anthropology, which could unsettle previously held assumptions by offering nuanced context-specific ethnographic knowledge, tend to struggle to get a hearing or are completely ignored (Warin and Zivkovic, 2019). The limiting effects of the distributive rules are also observable in otherwise useful academic analyses of anti-obesity policy. Boswell's (2016) study in Britain and Australia, for instance, ignores healthism and lifestyle drift; furthermore, fat studies receives scant attention despite the author's professed concern with emotions and the voice of those labelled obese.

In the ORF of anti-obesity policy, broader ideas associated with 'the neoliberal imaginary' (Rizvi and Lingard, 2010) tend to frame interventions in individualistic terms despite 'strong evidence' contradicting this depiction (Ulijaszek and McLennan, 2016: 397). Reproducing the WCHP or 'fat as fatal' frame (Kwan and Graves, 2013), pedagogic emphasis is given to a weight-centric and marketised ideology that is rationalised (deemed efficient, calculable, amenable to technological control, etc.) (Monaghan, 2008). Indeed, given the ORF's colonising tendencies, as seen in education in various nations (Evans et al., 2008; Loughland and Sriprakash, 2016), anti-obesity policies often call for the development of particular types of intervention in the PRF. Common policy prescriptions to be enacted in the PRF involve using instruments to measure and monitor (groups of) individuals as proxies for population-level concerns, rendering the public qua pedagogised subjects responsible for personally acknowledging and then fixing 'their health problems' (Dukelow, 2017).

In accord with the distributive rules alongside global ideologies of healthism and the turn to the market to 'solve' health problems, public health policies prioritise measurability, commensurability, comparison and performance. Examples include setting 'targets' to reduce obesity prevalence (e.g. lowering numbers by a specified date); continuous measurement of bodies (e.g. the UK's National Child Measurement Programme) and techniques of 'comparison' such as presenting data on national levels of obesity, with nations seemingly pitted against each other on league tables of shame (e.g. World Population Review, 2021). Different 'locations' are also compared within countries, as seen in a report identifying 'England's obesity hotspots' (DOH, 2008). Embodying marketised logics, these measures and comparisons promote not only the imperative of health but also the centrality of 'healthy' (inter-)national competition, evaluation and success via modes of entrepreneurship on and by human bodies. Recently reflecting on such practices, Evans and Davies (2020: 737) write:

> Policy-makers' obsession with 'weight issues' and national obesity stan-
> dards, especially when reported as international league tables comparing
> 'their' nation's/populations' collective girth size, has been remarkable.

In sum, distributive rules within the ORF shape what is (un)thinkable as obesity knowledges are transformed into pedagogic communication. These rules define who can transmit knowledge (relations of power) and which knowledges (relations of control) are deemed legitimate. Such relations set the conditions for the selection of 'evidence' presented in anti-obesity policy documents. This point pertains to which disciplines (or who) can transmit what (knowledges) and the conditions for that transmission. To use Bernstein's language, legitimate obesity discourse is framed by the distributive rules through which particular forms of evidence continue to be transmitted to and embraced by policymakers, whilst others do not have such access or have limited influence. As noted, it is through these rules within the pedagogic device of anti-obesity policy that neoliberal values prevail plus disciplinary practices aligned with individualism, commensurability and (inter-)national competition.

Recontextualising rules of anti-obesity policy: pairing structural inequality and individualism

Bernstein's (2000) 'recontextualising rules' also form part of 'the pedagogic device' and provide instruction regarding how discourses from the ORF are interpreted, adapted, accommodated and responded to as they are moved and (re) appropriated. Recontextualising rules comprise instructional and regulative discourses, with the former geared towards creating skills in relational context whilst the latter is a 'moral discourse which creates order, relations and identity' (p. 32). In this subsection we explore how the emergence of what is now commonly recognised as 'a lifestyle drift' within health policy (Popay et al., 2010) reflects the ways in which certain health knowledges are recontextualised, selected and organised for these pedagogic purposes. As we will see, dominant discourses from the ORF are brought into new relationships with widely circulating discourses surrounding the social determinants of health. Arguably, this frame seems 'progressive' but, to adapt Moore (2013) when reviewing Bernstein's critique of British education, there is an 'invisible pedagogy' at play that needs to be explicated and challenged in the context of class reproduction and (as we explain shortly) symbolic control.

The context for our discussion can be sketched as such: much concern surrounds what Kelly and Barker (2016: 110) term the 'epidemic' of 'non-communicable diseases' (e.g. cancer, type 2 diabetes, obesity) and so-called drivers such as 'smoking, diet, alcohol consumption and physical inactivity'. Yet, such behaviours do not exist in a power vacuum; they are not free-floating choices made by equals sharing similar material conditions of existence (Graham, 1994; Scambler, 2012). Offering a radical reading, Aphramor (2019a: 38–9) frames non-communicable diseases as 'an epidemic' of 'power-related diseases' (e.g. the harms of subsisting on zero-hours contracts, racism, discrimination and structural injustice more generally). Of course, in accord with the more politically palatable framing (one that apparently makes it easier to mobilise support in policy-related circles) (Boswell, 2016), concerns about non-communicable diseases, rather than power-related diseases, shape government calls to promote healthier populations and tackle 'the social determinants of health' (Medvedyuk et al., 2018). The focus on healthy populations and social determinants is a seemingly progressive move within the ORF. However, as we will explain, it reproduces class-based assumptions about unhealthy (impoverished) bodies and lives, promoting ultimately individualised and typically marketised interventions.

We hinted at such definitional practices in Chapter 1, citing the US CDC's 'health frame' and how their reference to the complexity of obesity is belied by injunctions for individuals to make better choices in line with an 'energy balance' model of weight (Kwan and Graves, 2013). Such matters relate to the 'instructional' component of 'pedagogic discourse' as constituted through 'recontextualising rules' (Bernstein, 2000: 31–2). Social policy analyses in Britain and Australia point to similar enactments by 'public health experts' with reference to environmental *and* behavioural narratives (Boswell, 2016). Both narratives 'ultimately, claim to advocate making "healthy choices easier"' so that 'performing political narratives in practice represents less a perfect or pure manifestation of a distinct discourse, and more of an effort to "bridge" distinct discourses in order to better mobilise broader support' (p. 20). Whilst building bridges is laudable, these policy discourses tend to be premised on a 'thin' understanding of 'the social' wherein society is conceptualised as an aggregate of individuals, or groups of individuals, behaving more or less 'rationally in their own declared self-interests' (Hansen et al., 2016: 241). This thin understanding, entwined with the moral or regulative discourse of obesity within the ORF, is traceable not only to disciplines such as social epidemiology and the 'tradition of methodological individualism' commonly informing it (Medvedyuk et al., 2018: 575), but also to the growing influence of behavioural economics and cognitive psychology (Hansen et al., 2016). These approaches fail to offer a nuanced view of society as a network of structured power relations with emergent and consequential properties for health inequalities independent of individuals' so-called lifestyle 'choices'. If read with reference to Bernstein's concept of the pedagogic device, this is a recontextualising process that reproduces new middle-class interests and rhetoric, for example, concerns to tackle social injustice via policy prescriptions and other means that 'help' or 'empower people' to 'do the right thing' (eat well, be active, be well). We would refer the reader back to the OECD (2017) report as an example, where reference to 'the population' is a gloss for individuals qua 'consumers' (p. 8).

As the discourse of market rationalism, individualism and consumer choice moves from its original site to the pedagogical site of health education and policy (via recontextualising rules), it has had profound effects on shaping obesity knowledges and communicative practices. Because of the above epistemological

or methodological issues and politically expedient priorities (an ultimately atom-
istic view of society), pedagogical enactments of public health discourses and
policy approaches to structured health inequalities do not seriously address or
redress matters pertaining to social justice (O'Hara and Taylor, 2018). Such matters include, inter alia: the moral meanings of fat and the structural underpinning of stigma relations, the material conditions of existence that impact life
chances independent of body composition and personal behaviours, the indebt-
edness of lifestyles to social structures and 'the epidemic of power-related diseases' (Aphramor, 2019a: 39). Necessary political responses, which cannot be
marketed and 'sold' in the interests of accumulating profit, therefore tend to be
ignored, denied or silenced. This alternative class of knowledge would be categorised as 'unthinkable' as distinguished by the previously described distributive
rules (Bernstein, 2000: 29).

It is through recontextualising rules that neoliberal tenets of competition and
standardisation move from wider fields (e.g. the market) into anti-obesity policy
and establish new relationships with discourses ostensibly focused on addressing structural inequalities. In other words, the recontextualising rules refer here
to the way in which discourses of inequality are moved and re-appropriated by
state-backed 'legitimators' and 'administrators' (Monaghan et al., 2010), with
such idea-elements brought into relationships with discourses of neoliberalism
and healthism. This recontextualisation, reflected through a 'lifestyle drift' and
associated notions of 'citizen shift' oriented to consumer practices (Williams and
Fullagar, 2019), means that policies seemingly attuned to social determinants of
health are refracted through self-responsibilising and market-based logics (see
also Baum and Fisher, 2014). As such, many national policies now group together
structural inequality and neoliberal targets and practices intended to tackle obesity. The elaboration of the goals of many government policies to achieve such
ends include an intriguing mix to reduce 'environmental influences' (structural
determinants) and to ensure better 'individual lifestyles'. As these discourses are
coupled, the problem of individual decision-making becomes the implied or
preferred target for pedagogic strategies intended to ameliorate environmental
issues. In effect, the guiding principle for those administrators/enforcers in the
PRF (schools, teachers, clinicians) is that even structural inequalities ultimately
become an issue of 'teaching' individuals to make 'better choices'. Less is offered
in terms of addressing structural inequalities driven by economic rationalism and
market ideologies. This point is worth stressing in political contexts such as the
UK amidst significant cuts to welfare and public services, including austerity
policies that have 'inflicted "great misery" on citizens' (Booth and Butler, 2018)
and especially disadvantaged families.

In short, the recontextualising rules of the pedagogic device of anti-obesity
policy are consequential. These rules shape an understanding of how to address
health inequalities not as a structural or systemic issue but as an issue of individualised, measured and competitive obligation. The instructional and regulative discourses of anti-obesity policy are enacted as such: teachers, parents and

individuals qua entrepreneurial and totally pedagogised selves are charged with the responsibility of negotiating the environment and making healthy choices, albeit through policy 'prescriptions' (Warin and Zivkovic, 2019: 212) which might 'guide' them. None of this is politically neutral, and this is not lost on other social researchers. Warin and Zivkovic describe the attendant politics as 'unpalatable' with reference to an anti-obesity intervention that originated in France and was recontextualised in Australia.

Building on Warin and Zivkovic's (2019) recent uptake of the *lifestyle drift* concept in relation to obesity and public health, we are interested in how recontextualising rules get behavioural discourses 'inside' ostensibly progressive anti-obesity policy as pedagogy. Lifestyle drift is a problem pertaining to what we call 'type two' (T2) approaches to public health pedagogy. T2 approaches begin 'upstream' and supposedly advance knowledge of and action towards so-called non-communicable diseases with reference to an encompassing complex system, or socio-economic environment, which impacts everybody's health (we will return to this below). In contrast, 'type one' (T1) approaches do not drift 'downstream' towards lifestyle because they already explicitly locate the causes of non-communicable diseases within individuals, or groups of individuals, whilst also foregrounding the locus of prevention and change there. Stated crudely, T1 approaches posit that bad outcomes (disease and early death) are due to risky behaviours – pedagogically framed as the result of ignorance (in relation to health knowledge), complacency and/or irresponsibility – and these problems must be changed in the interests of health (promotion). Given the pervasive moralisation of health (Metzl and Kirkland, 2010), T1 approaches represent forms of symbolic control, if not communicated violence (Bourdieu, 2001), through pedagogic means. Regardless of individuals' intentions, these recontextualising rules of obesity blame victims of structural inequality whilst charging them with the task of 'pulling themselves up by their bootstraps' in line with self-responsibilising neoliberal logics (see also Mannion and Small, 2019).

In contrast, T2 approaches might be considered more compassionate or ethical, and of universal relevance. Ostensibly articulated at the population rather than individual level, T2 approaches focus on the broader environment and locate health-related problems as originating and requiring solutions there. However, regulated through a pedagogic device aligned to neoliberal globalised discourses, lifestyle drift means that it is not always possible to clearly distinguish between T1 and T2 approaches as they are enacted through policy (for empirical evidence of this in Australia and Britain, see Boswell, 2016). Through an analysis of recontextualising rules we are sensitised to tensions, contradictions and paradoxes in this pedagogic discourse. Even where policy ostensibly recognises environments as being a *problem*, or limiting in terms of health opportunities, they tend to 'call up' (Maguire et al. 2015) enactments that legitimise individual-level *solutions*. Baum and Fisher (2014: 216) consider this lifestyle drift 'a by-product of the appeal of behavioural health promotion', revealing how there are strong incentives for governments to adopt this line. They add that

ideology is a powerful driver of policy and political actors with a strong commitment to neoliberalism and individualism are very likely to be drawn to
behavioural solutions and to use power over the representation of social issues
to maintain this stance.

(p. 220)

Williams and Fullagar (2019: 21) also shed empirical light on the nuances of
this drift, referring to the 'complexities of advanced liberal governance that help
explain discrepancies between policies that address health inequalities and the
interventions designed to reduce them'.

Specific reference to anti-obesity policies and related critical literature is
instructive. O'Hara and Taylor (2018) give examples of the two main approaches
outlined above, approaches which, in practice, meld into one WCHP. They refer
to a technical report on weight and well-being by the Provisional Health Service
Authority (PHSA, 2013) in British Columbia, Canada, which, encouragingly,
asks whether it is 'time for a shift in paradigms?' The first, T1, version of the
WCHP seeks to promote a 'normal weight', as defined by BMI, 'through limiting caloric intake and increasing energy expenditure' (O'Hara and Taylor, 2018:
2). The PHSA (2013: 36) notes that this individual-level paradigm 'is particularly
well-established within the health care system'. Of course, this paradigm also
extends beyond Canada and healthcare settings. Referring to 'elite or expert-
dominated policy settings' populated by 'scientists and medical professionals' in
Britain and Australia, Boswell (2016: 20) refers to this approach as an 'Individual
Intervention' narrative. However, as stated by Medvedyuk et al. (2018: 577): 'The
emphasis on behavioural remedies set the stage for continued stigmatization and
victim blaming when weight reduction regimens fail'.

Given the ineffectiveness of this approach and feelings of personal failure that
typically accompany it, a second version of the WCHP has emerged. This T2
approach offers a systemic perspective by approaching 'the medically problematic
categories of "overweight" and "obesity" through an ecological lens addressing the "obesogenic" environment' (O'Hara and Taylor, 2018: 2). This framing,
which transforms the issue from a private trouble to a collective problem of global
proportions, has contributed to the success of the 'obesity epidemic narrative'
as evidenced in (inter-)national policy within and outside of Europe (Boswell,
2016; Schorb, 2013; Chapter 1). The PHSA's (2013) report explains that whilst
this so-called population and social level approach 'broadens' the 'options' (p. 7)
to tackle obesity, it requires co-ordinated action that is difficult to achieve and has
not, to date, proven successful in any nation. The report adds that the ecological approach 'is almost completely focused on issues of weight, obesity and poor
physical health with limited protection and promotion of mental well-being'
(p. 7). Reference to 'limited protection' might be considered an understatement
insofar as weight-centric approaches are 'pathology focused' (p. 52).

The WCHP might be pathology-focused and, when framed as a T2 approach,
is based on a thin understanding of the social, but it has traction and is widely

communicated with authority and conviction. Various actors or 'recontextualis-ers' function as 'reproducers' of this health knowledge in 'the pedagogic field' (Bernstein, 2000: 37), ranging from obesity scientists to slimmers (Monaghan et al., 2010). It is these actors who come to distribute, enact and embody sacred health knowledges about weight management and lifestyle choices, constituting what is deemed legitimate 'health education' as formulated within policy goals and weight-centric interventions. For example, the policy conflation of individu-alism with structural inequalities has come to influence the way in which obesity should be both 'measured' but also how solutions should be implemented.

Examples of the above abound in policy reports and the recontextualisation of obesity knowledges in countries allegedly in the grip of an epidemic. For instance, the Parliament of Canada (2016), in a report that addresses T2 issues (the obesogenic environment, food labelling, taxation), quickly places responsi-bility onto individual citizens: 'Canadians must renew their efforts to eat healthy (*sic*) and to get active — and government and industry must give citizens the means and motivation to make informed lifestyle choices' (p. iv). In America, calls to combat childhood obesity in Michelle Obama's *Let's Move!* campaign paid lip service to ecological T2 concerns (e.g. supporting access to affordable and nutritious food), though the pedagogy of healthy choices, parental responsibil-ity, agency, lifestyles and good citizenship (T1 concerns) prevailed (Backstrom, 2020). Moreover, Backstrom's framing analysis of *Let's Move!* reveals that the First Lady 'rarely advocated for policies' such as those designed to 'combat poverty, or better support working families' (p. 15). In Australia, Lupton (2014) analyses two high-profile government-funded national anti-obesity campaigns: *Measure Up* and *Swap It, Don't Stop It*. These campaigns, as enacted within the PRF, again suggest that behaviour change entailed making the 'right choice' and, moreover, there is no 'attempt to deal with the social determinants influencing body weight and health status' (p. 39). In Ireland, the *Stop the Spread* campaign, similar to *Measure Up* in Australia, urged the public to measure their waist size and reduce this if necessary. In so doing, an overweight majority allegedly in 'denial' about their girth was instructed by a state-sponsored agency to regulate their bodies/ lives (Dukelow, 2017).

Several UK public health policies within the ORF and interventions within the PRF have also attempted to change the 'obesogenic environment' via an approach that initially appears to challenge common 'myths' and 'presump-tions' (Casazza et al., 2013; Chapter 2). Consider the government-commissioned Foresight Report *Tackling Obesities: Future Choices* (Foresight, 2007). The report sought to refocus attention on complex environmental factors, in line with the policy and biomedical framing of obesity as a 'wicked problem' (Boswell, 2016). In short, it aimed to 'challenge the simple portrayal of obesity as an issue of per-sonal willpower – eating too much and doing too little' (Butland et al., 2007, cited in Ulijaszek and McLennan, 2016: 407). The report used systems map-ping, drawing together a range of evidence and expertise to identify biological and social influences. Kelly and Russo (2018: 87) observe that despite its whole systems perspective and identifying the complexities of obesity 'the relational and dynamic nature of the problem as spelt out by the Foresight Report is entirely absent' in the policy action 'driven by what amount to simple heuristics'. Ulijaszek and McLennan (2016: 17) note various problems here, such as a failure to engage 'the moral implications of obesity' or 'examine values and norms surrounding large body size, including blame and stigma'. There is growing evidence of this trend (Kelly and Russo, 2018; Lupton, 2014; Mulderrig, 2017; Ulijaszek and McLennan, 2016; Williams and Fullagar, 2019) through which policies identify obesity as a complex systems-level problem, with such concerns recontextualised to offer a behavioural solution that is 'firmly individualistic' (Mulderrig, 2017: 472). More recently, the UK Government released *Childhood Obesity: A Plan for Action, Chapter 2* (DHSC, 2018), an update on their 2016 strategy. Both documents emphasise the role of 'healthy choices' in reducing obesity, despite attention also being given to T2 concerns (e.g. regulating the food industry). We will turn to the most recent iteration of such pedagogy in Chapter 8 when critiquing anti-obesity policy and COVID-19 preparedness.

Despite invoking the complexities of environmental influences, there continues to be pressure from the ORF, often via governments and their health agencies, to use evaluative measures in publicly funded institutions such as schools (e.g. the National Child Measurement Programme; see also Chapter 5). This pressure persists, even though governments often acknowledge that, for many individuals, 'healthy lifestyles' are constrained or negated by structural inequalities. Moreover, reviews have found that interventions have had limited success in reducing inequalities in childhood obesity associated with socio-economic status (Hillier-Brown et al., 2014). Consequently, policy responses represent pedagogic methods comprising unproven interventions *and* contradictory tendencies for citizens' subjectivity. On the one hand, policies emphasise an increase in modes of responsibilisation and self-regulation, yet they also tout the need for dependency on governments to intervene (change the obesogenic environment).

This contradictory constitution of the imagined pedagogic subject, or entrepreneurial self, is also reflected in the increasingly common policy focus on 'nudge' techniques (see Mannion and Small, 2019). Nudging aims to subtly direct people towards approved behaviours. It includes discounting, temptation, repositioning products and so on within the 'choice architecture', i.e. the environments in which people make decisions. As Selinger and Whyte (2011: 924–5) explain, the notion of 'choice architecture' entails viewing the masses as 'irrational' and 'biased' in their decision-making. Elsewhere, Quigley (2013: 592) describes how research in the behavioural sciences suggests we are 'imperfect decision-makers. We do not always act rationally in our best interests […] we all fall foul of a number of cognitive biases which affect the way we make decisions'. By seemingly taking such 'biases' into account when formulating health policy, neoliberal governments seek to 'nudge' citizens to make 'better' decisions. Such pedagogy is ostensibly 'framed' as facilitative, unlike authoritarian/enforced enactments as reported in Japan, for example, where firms risk penalties if their workers are overweight (McCurry, 2008). Alongside so-called hugging (see Mannion and Small, 2019), where attempts are made to reward individuals, nudging encourages people to learn to make particular choices in an almost effortless way.

In short, rather than forcing the public to make 'better lifestyle choices', the recontextualising rules of anti-obesity policy comprise ostensibly softer tactics. These include steering people, perhaps in a passive way and based on a seemingly 'intuitive response' (French, 2011: 158) through, for example, environmental prompts. Such approaches have proven influential in the policy field post-2008 in nations such as the UK and the USA. However, as explained above with reference to lifestyle drift, in practice distinctions between these different pedagogies are blurred. Moreover, ethical concerns still arise in relation to supposedly subtle, supportive and gentle efforts to redress obesity. As discussed below, anti-obesity policy cannot be disentangled from a broader pedagogical context of bodily evaluation and symbolic control wherein relations of shame and blame are enacted and/or felt (Scambler, 2018).

Evaluation and symbolic control of obesity through the PRF

In his theory of a 'totally pedagogised society', Bernstein (2001) points to the reduced power but not influence of the nation-state. Rather than direct governance and sanctioning people's behaviours, Bernstein argues that nation-states more often seek to influence the production, recontextualisation and evaluation of discursive codes. This is significant in view of how nation-states, noted above with reference to distributive rules, are often ranked internationally (and in ways that exceed indicators of health) (Loughland and Sriprakash, 2016). In this regard, we argue that state (supported) attempts to address obesity increasingly occur via new symbolic orders of regulation and control through pedagogic means, albeit still reflecting the discourse of neoliberalism and notions of 'free choice' described above. Symbolic control, as Evans and Davies (2020: 738) remind us, also incorporates fields of 'economic control'.

Specifically, the third aspect of Bernstein's pedagogic device is the *evaluative rule*. This dimension refers to the process through which particular discourses are appropriated, how they come to be reproduced and transformed into 'pedagogic practice' (Bernstein, 2000: 35). In relation to obesity, the evaluative rule plays a crucial role in terms of the constitution of the norms associated with (de)valued personhood; for example, the healthy responsible citizen versus the fat individual who is deemed lazy and lacking self-control. The evaluative rule, which 'condenses the meaning of the whole device' (p. 36), produces new modes for institutions and subjectivity; expectations and expressions through which *symbolic control* over cultural definitions (of weight/obesity) and practices take place. As we explain further below, anti-obesity policies and interventions are increasingly assembled in ways that reflect this mode of control, including social marketing through which pedagogies and 'perfection codes' (Evans et al., 2008; Evans and Davies, 2020) can operate in different social sites. On the latter concept, Evans and

Davies explain that such codes 'have their social bases outside formal education in the economic interests of business, industry and the media and the medical and health fields' (p. 738). Here anti-obesity policies reflect this decreasing state control through direct regulation of individual behaviour, moving instead towards forms of 'social marketing' in order to influence embodied cultural practices.

Mulderrig (2017: 472) explains that social marketing involves 'the merging of government and market-based social practices, and as such potentially creates contradictions and tensions as the assumptions, values, and interests of these different social fields are brought together'. Enacted through the PRF and utilising approaches from commercial marketing, public health behaviours are 'advertised' through different media to encourage the uptake of those behaviours, alongside related products and services. Dukelow's (2017) governmentality analysis of Ireland's publicly funded *Stop the Spread* social marketing campaign is illustrative. She observes how the exercise of power and pedagogy included the distribution of 250,000 measuring tapes through pharmacies, 'emulating the "free gift" tactic frequently used by companies to promote their products' (p. 86). Such approaches are not only legitimised by state agencies and those receiving public funds, but also, following the reference to pharmacies, private entrepreneurs/groups/interests seeking to influence the ORF.

To the extent that direct state control is diminished in advanced liberal nations (a contingent situation, to be sure), there is a proliferation of marketised attempts to exert greater control over the public's everyday embodied social practices and consciousness. The rules of the pedagogic device of anti-obesity policy call forth 'continuous evaluation' (Bernstein, 2000: 36), albeit through what initially seem like softer forms of governance that are more-or-less visible as public health pedagogy. Practices include not only the evaluation of those agencies/organisations charged with tackling obesity but also the evaluative rule which 'refers to all processes of knowledge acquisition, and the formation of the self-governing pedagogic subject, who is open to continuous and ongoing evaluation' (Singh, 2015: 359). To return briefly to Foucauldian analyses, we are reminded of how 'gentler' public health approaches are reflective of 'modern state power as pastoral power' that 'cannot be exercised without knowing the inside of people's minds, without exploring their souls, without making them reveal their innermost secrets' (Foucault, 2000: 333, cited by Dukelow, 2017: 90). Such constant self-regulation and monitoring is a form of this symbolic control of evaluation. Critically, such control also reproduces the stigma and deviance of obesity as an abject and blameworthy condition that threatens individuals, their social networks (as seen when obesity is deemed contagious; see Brown, 2014; Dukelow, 2017) and the 'vulnerable' nation-state.

Reflecting the multiple, diffuse and fluid circulation of knowledge-claims about health, the self-governing pedagogic subject qua entrepreneurial self is increasingly expected, or at least encouraged, to learn about health through a range of new evaluative monitoring devices. Note the popularity of digital health technologies, devices designed for continuous self-evaluation and improvement as discussed in Chapter 2. Wearable digital media collect data on the users' bodies and health practices (weight, steps taken, heart rate, etc.), conceptualised elsewhere as 'McDonaldizing the body' via rationalising processes (Monaghan, 2008). Understood through a pedagogical lens, embodied subjectivities are constituted by comparative performances or displays related to data about weight and 'lifestyle choices'. Such pedagogic practices, we would suggest, reflect the sort of symbolic control achieved through evaluative rules in a 'totally pedagogised society' (Bernstein, 2001). Here medical surveillance is no longer confined to the health professional, but via diffuse measuring and monitoring practices that pedagogised subjects are encouraged to undertake on their own and perhaps with other virtual bodies within a shared (online) 'assemblage' (Rich, 2010) (see also Chapter 4, on Canadian women's use of technology). It is through such evaluation that we can determine 'the whole purpose of the device' which 'is to provide a symbolic ruler for consciousness' (Bernstein, 2000: 36).

Our key argument is that these methods are instructive, regulative and generate forms of (self-)governance in the pedagogic field – on the one hand, they instigate a turn towards the environment in health policy, and on the other hand, they reduce this concern to self-regulation and symbolic control. Rather than directly disciplining and regulating bodies, techniques such as social marketing and self-evaluation promise a seemingly progressive mode of regulation and route to 'redemption' (Raisborough, 2016). Such pedagogies are, after all, 'sold' to consumer citizens as a means to maximise health, well-being and productivity in performance-oriented societies. These evaluative rules are therefore crucial to the processes of symbolic control of bodies through 'legitimate' discourses of obesity. As described by Monaghan et al. (2010), these body-subjects include diet club members whose interests include mitigating disease risk, displaying 'moral worth', negotiating weight norms and avoiding/managing stigma (p. 46). In short, these discursive practices, codes and pedagogic methods produce affective intensities; these not only define and (dis)credit 'knowledges' but also come to impact ways of feeling, relating to the body and shaping particular affects and desires (see Bernstein, 2001; Fullagar et al., 2022).

Critically, and in following Chapter 2 on various media and stigma, we would stress that many of the irrationalities of obesity discourse are reproduced and reinforced by ostensibly well-intended health policies, prescriptions and practices. Relations of affect are lived out through people's emergent feelings of shame, guilt and anxiety about their 'impure' flesh. Such feelings are experienced within potentially oppressive social structures, or legitimised 'boundaries' that are (re)produced through power relations (Bernstein, 2000: 5), including the intersections of class, gender, ethnicity, age and national identity (we explore these empirically in Part 2). Indeed, the evaluation and symbolic control of obesity through the PRF of obesity can have particular consequences for specific groups of people and, for those without the relative social, economic and other forms of capital, these mechanisms can exacerbate their 'multiple stigmatised statuses' (Puhl and Heuer, 2010: 1021). Understandably, then, Colls and Evans (2014: 742) critique the popular ecological (T2) framing which, they argue, 'exacerbates' rather than challenges 'the marginalization of communities already stigmatized along racial and class lines through pathologizing their places as obesogenic'.

There is growing critical commentary and scholarship on such matters. In advancing a pedagogical reading of obesity as a 'regulative discourse', Evans et al. (2008) refer to Aphramor (2006), who challenges the imagery used in various campaigns in Britain. These educational materials include paraphernalia from the British Dietetic Profession urging people that 'Now is the time to deflate those spare tyres' and an advertisement from the World Cancer Fund, posted on London buses, advising: 'Don't look like the back end of a bus, obesity can cause cancer: take control, find out how' (cited by Evans et al., 2008: 56). These are not isolated examples of symbolic control or violence. Elsewhere, in her analysis of anti-obesity campaigns in Australia, Lupton (2015) suggests 'the pedagogy of disgust' is used as a motivating force, involving graphic and confronting images. She critiques, inter alia, the assumption that the public lack knowledge, the use of unpleasant images to motivate lifestyle change and the empirical inaccuracies of paternalistic health promotion pedagogies that present behaviour change as easily achievable. Similarly, in the context of health education, Leahy (2009) reveals how disgust and shame are used as teaching tools.

The above examples from the PRF are obviously 'harder' (confrontational, shocking) pedagogies. However, they are recurrent within a larger context, or 'emotion-risk assemblage' (Lupton, 2015: 6) wherein ostensibly benevolent representations, or softer strategies (pastoral forms of power, one might suggest), are less than convincing. Of course, following our discussion on misrecognition in Chapter 2, there are symbolically violent (class-related, gendered) processes at play here that have pernicious consequences independent of social actors' intentions. Accordingly, we are not claiming policymakers and public health workers necessarily seek to stigmatise people through evaluation and symbolic control of obesity through the PRF. Indeed, as demonstrated in Warin and Zivkovic's (2019) research, these recontextualising agents may be expressly committed to avoiding such harm. However, weight-related stigma is so pervasive within the obesity assemblage that even when public health workers seek to 'hide or erase' discrediting images and text this 'only serves to make visible that which has already been construed' (p. 177). We would remind readers of those 'invisible pedagogies', alluded to above, when scrutinising the pairing of structural inequality and individualism within the recontextualising field of anti-obesity policy. To adapt Bernstein, seemingly progressive public health policy enactments within the PRF and evaluative rules of the pedagogic device comprise tacit meanings. Such shared meanings do not need to be spoken in order to be understood and exert inclusionary/exclusionary effects and psychosocial affects.

We will finish this section by returning to and underscoring the question of values, which, as noted by others (Ulijaszek, 2014; Warin and Zivkovic, 2019), tend to be ignored even in 'sophisticated' public health policy documents and projects. In part, this problem reflects our earlier point about distributive rules and who transmits legitimated knowledge. In all of this, one might consider how values, more so than evidence, infuse not only obesity science (Bombak, 2014b; Gard and Wright, 2005; Chapter 2), but also supposedly gentle forms of governance, such as nudging, within the invisible pedagogy of public health messaging. Reviewing and adding to various ethical critiques (e.g. regarding nudging as shoving), Selinger and Whyte (2011) discuss what they term 'semantic variance' (p. 930). Their point relates to the dramatically differing ways in which people may interpret situations within which choices are made and nudges are introduced, incorporating gaps between how choice architects and members of the public might define and respond to context-dependent meanings. One of their examples relates to the possibility of reproducing sexism through technology (referring to efforts to promote driver safety), though they stress '[t]he point, here, is not merely that well-intentioned nudges can perpetuate harms through unintended consequences' but rather 'choice architects may project their values on others. In this case, choice architects' having different life experiences from those they nudge may prevent them from foreseeing how certain nudges may be problematic' (p. 931). A concrete example of this in the context of the Obesity Prevention and Lifestyle Program researched by Warin and Zivkovic (2019) is the ways in which public health workers could not appreciate how class structures have material effects and affects. Social class, for instance, influences taste as embodied and relished within disadvantaged lives geared to surviving in the present, rather than a projected 'healthy' future as valued within middle-class reasoning and recontextualised pedagogies. Recognising such matters, we would contend, is crucial if health equity is a serious policy concern. After all, health and risk behaviours are indebted to social structures, with such behaviours only partially explaining the disproportionate burdens experienced by people in poorer socio-economic circumstances (Bacon and Aphramor, 2014; Scambler, 2012). It is these people who mainly suffer 'the weight of the world' (Bourdieu et al., 1999) and the 'bodily injuries of class' (Warin and Zivkovic, 2019: 185). Disturbingly, such harms appear to be exacerbated, not ameliorated, within the pedagogic device of anti-obesity policy that is now entangled with COVID-19 'patrician policymaking' (Dingwall, 2020b).

Discussion: from policy analysis to social research

This chapter analysed anti-obesity policymaking and its implications for 'policy enactments' (Maguire et al., 2015). Our eclectic approach entailed synthesising studies of obesity discourse (Evans et al., 2008) and entrepreneurship (Monaghan et al., 2010) with an embodied reading of Bernstein (1996, 2000, 2001). Like others who have analysed national educational practices within marketised global dynamics (e.g. Loughland and Sriprakash, 2016), we utilised Bernstein's theory of the pedagogic device and the distributive, recontextualising and evaluative rules to examine policymaking processes. Substantively, we scrutinised the pedagogising of obesity knowledges and the recontextualisation of policy across various nation-states. In so doing, we went beyond viewing pedagogy as a mere epiphenomenon of neoliberalism, instead explicating the mechanics of policy processes as enacted, embodied and emplaced (Evans et al., 2013). Through this analysis we became sensitised to various tensions, including contradictory health messaging or the discrepancy between assumed causes and prescribed solutions to the putative obesity crisis.

These pedagogical processes are inseparable from politics and thus power and control. Our analysis has highlighted the 'distribution' of these relations through the ORF and PRF (e.g. in the form of social marketing campaigns via government-sponsored health agencies). To this end, certain disciplines, organisations and institutions exercise more influence than others to construct 'legitimate' or even 'sacred' health knowledges (Evans et al., 2008). We have highlighted how, within a complex and contested arena, particular discourses are recontextualised in ways that emphasise hegemonic logics associated with healthism and the economisation of human relations. In particular, Bernstein's concept of distributive rules reveals how wider discourses of neoliberalism, economic rationalism and the new public health are realised in the 'legitimate discourses' of (ultimately) individualising, consumer-oriented health education and promotion. Crucially, here we discerned how the pedagogic device recontextualises the social determinants of health as matters requiring embodied, easily measurable and competitive obligation among responsible consumer citizens. Through such mechanisms, and similar to 'policy moves' in the formal educational arena, the pedagogic device 'deflects attention from the real human consequences of long-term structural inequity' (Loughland and Sriprakash, 2016: 243).

The previous point is worth stressing. A key problem that we identified is the way in which neoliberal discourses acquire and recontextualise social inequality and its relationship to health inequality. Complex understandings pertaining to health, if not ignored or silenced in policy circles populated by the privileged (Dingwall, 2020b), are recontextualised and appropriated as they meet with pervasive discourses of competition, comparison and surveillance; so much so that they become part of the 'legitimate discourses' of obesity and inequality but in ways that are politically neutered. As explained above with reference to the obesogenic environment ('T2 approaches' within the recontextualising rules of obesity policymaking), an ostensibly progressive public health pedagogy melds with 'T1 approaches' where self-responsibilising subjects are obliged to combat their own and/or their kid's weight problems by exercising better lifestyle choices. Yet, as argued over a decade ago by Popay et al. (2010), 'with lifestyles in the ascendancy, action to address the upstream determinants of inequalities in health is at best neglected, at worse undermined' (p. 148). The continued centring of individuals' or consumers' choices in the ORF and PRF, in an effort to 'mobilise broader support' (Boswell, 2016: 20), is thus deeply problematic. Rather than promoting social and, by extension, health justice, these fields reflect and reproduce embodied neoliberal values, ideologies and (dis)advantages.

As Rizvi and Lingard (2011: 8) explain when analysing the education policy assemblage, neoliberal values can be re-imagined because 'public policy formations that appear stable, potentially even complete, are never so settled'. To be sure, whilst dominant pedagogies, through which various publics might come to learn about obesity via policy formations, are part of a range of 'heterogeneous elements' (p. 8) that are assembled so as to suggest 'discursive coherence' (p. 20), this front stage presentation requires considerable backstage political work. We would return here to the OECD (2017: 8) report, which claims '[c]ommunication policies to tackle obesity are advancing' – a statement denoting progress and consensus whilst eliding controversy within global/ising obesity knowledges and the 'fracturing' (Scambler, 2018) of social relations within and between member states. In short, whilst our analysis, like Evans et al. (2008) and Monaghan et al. (2010), is not premised on the idea of political mischief, conspiracy or malicious intent, it cannot be denied that public representations of policy mask the political work that is 'done in drawing heterogeneous elements together, forging connections and sustaining them in the face of tensions' (Rizvi and Lingard, 2011: 8). The problem here is that if anti-obesity policies are seen as 'coherent' and part of a 'linear' process of policy formation (see Maguire et al., 2015) then the complex, scientifically uncertain, politically fraught and ethically questionable processes pedagogising obesity knowledges will likely go unrecognised and unchallenged. A case in point is the continuous evaluation of bodies through seemingly progressive, invisible as well as digitally mediated pedagogies that are implicated in stigma and symbolic control. These processes might be felicitous to the new inequality and 'the weaponising of stigma in neoliberalism' (Scambler, 2018: 141), but they also leave us hankering for tools to disrupt such pedagogy.

It is with this disruptive spirit in mind that we would point out something that might be considered almost blasphemous by pedagogues who are structurally comparable to priests in relation to laity in 'the religious field' (Bernstein, 2000: 37). Namely, whilst the pedagogic device has 'origins' in religion (p. 36), obesity knowledges and policy prescriptions are not God-given truths. These are social products, 'fabrications' even (Evans et al., 2008). As with any human product, policies emerge from social life, replete with history, hierarchies, boundaries, constraints, contingencies, uncertainties, presumptions, myths, blind spots, emotions, structured interests, tendencies, etc. Other critics recognise such matters. Ulijaszek and McLennan (2016: 397), for instance, state that weight-centric public health ideology and policies 'reflect the landscape of policymakers, advisors, political pressures and values, as much as, if not more than, the landscape of evidence'. In a similar vein, Marmot (2004b), when commenting upon the relation between science and policy, writes: 'Scientific findings do not fall on blank minds that get made up as a result. Science engages with busy minds that have strong views about how things are and ought to be' (p. 906). Accordingly, efforts to rethink obesity necessitate grappling with the complex interplay between the ORF and PRF.

It is within this pedagogical context that Bernstein's rule-bound approach has explanatory value. Bernstein 'is good to think with', enabling us to highlight how seemingly competing ideas associated with structural inequalities and individual behaviours appear in the policy arena not only through lifestyle drift but also nudge and other 'progressive' practices. These approaches influence the pedagogic fields and modalities through which health education and promotion occur, suggesting that obesity and the inequalities that might influence it require amelioration through particular norms, technologies and communication practices, i.e. those that are predominantly directed at (groups of) individuals who should know and behave better. Our critique does not imply that we are endorsing a collective, over an individual, approach to *tackling obesity*. Questions remain as to whether higher weight is intrinsically and necessarily a massive problem (see Chapter 2), or whether it might instead be considered a crude proxy for power-related diseases and thus socially structured practices that require targeted policies (e.g. exploitative employment practices, resulting in precarity and sleep debt; food insecurity that may be especially deleterious for pregnant women and subsequent generations). Rather, our argument, following Bernstein, is that the pedagogic device exerts effects that are officially legitimated but, insofar as these are political, they are open to disruption and transformation.

We would add a critical realist argument here, which is compatible with Bernstein's approach (Moore, 2013). Insofar as the enactment of obesity discourse recurs in a regularised and patterned manner across different formations, it is reasonable to infer that this is reflective of underlying macro-social structures (notably, relations of class/command and stigma/blame) (Scambler, 2018). Social structures generate potentially oppressive tendencies that may be exercised (un) realised by actors across myriad assemblages or configurations of practice. As with racism, which may or may not emerge in specific situations but is relatively enduring across time and space (Porter, 1993), tendencies towards size-ism manifest in various ways, ranging from pedagogies of disgust at an organisational and embodied micro-level, to ways of 'knowing' an ostensibly encompassing obesogenic environment that is ultimately individualising and stigmatising. As such, the above analysis speaks to the relevance of Bernstein's thinking within a broader meta-theory. Via such work, we examined consequential rules beyond schools/curriculum or educational inequality and scrutinised 'general principles underlying the transformation of knowledge into pedagogic communication' (Bernstein, 2000: 25). Like critical realism, such theorising provides intellectual ammunition to challenge potentially oppressive structures that underpin the persistent (thinly veiled) focus on the supposed deficiencies of overweight/obese/ fat individuals (Monaghan, 2017). As per critical realism, the Bernsteinian 'rule-driven' model is not a 'deterministic' approach. Rather, it serves to highlight the nuances of anti-obesity policy as pedagogy in a broader context. It does this by facilitating close examination of the operations of the ORF and PRF as multiple agencies draw from, reproduce and legitimate marketised understandings and a lifestyle drift response to obesity.

Through such an analysis we presented various critiques, ranging from how symbolic control operates in relation to an imagined 'totally pedagogised self' to the problem of semantic variance. One response to such ethical matters, proposed by Selinger and Whyte (2011) when critiquing nudging, entails undertaking localised sociological studies to explore social meanings in context. Sociologists, alongside colleagues in disciplines such as social anthropology, are well equipped to bring to view not only discrepancies but also possible points of overlap between policymakers' values and those of their intended targets. However, from what we have discussed, we recognise that those with 'a seat at the policymaking table' do not necessarily welcome nuanced social scientific insights (Warin and Zivkovic, 2019), a point that Warin (2020: 672) subsequently underscored with reference to what she terms 'the "gentle and invisible" violence of obesity prevention'. Besides Marmot's (2004b) reference, above, to time and 'busy minds', absorbing these issues typically runs counter to structured interests, education and culture – for instance, the influence of healthism on those in the PRFs, such as dietetics and nutrition professions (Aphramor, 2019a; Overend et al., 2020). In Bernstein's (2000) sense, this is about the classification of knowledge, its relative strength, with power creating boundaries between the inside/outside (legitimate/illegitimate, good/bad, sacred/profane), within a division of labour and cosmology comprising 'psychic defences' (p. 7) (see the admonishing reactions to critical perspectives, reported in Chapter 2 and revisited in our epilogue). Nonetheless, such 'defences are rarely wholly effective and the possibility of the other, the unthinkable, the yet to be voiced, is also rarely silenced' (p. 7).

In view of such matters, which could no doubt be expanded upon with reference to other critical writings on 'strategic ignorance' and 'oracular power' (the almost mystical authority to determine boundaries between knowledge and ignorance) (McGoey, 2019; see also Dingwall et al., 2013, and Chapter 8), we remain hopeful. By explicating mechanisms of power, presenting empirical observations and making connections across diverse contexts, there is the *potential* to prompt those in the ORF and PRF to recognise, inter alia, the hidden injuries inflicted in the name of health and the need for a different approach. In so doing, researchers may promote an ethically defensible stance towards, for example, pervasive gendered body dissatisfaction, dieting cultures and childhood obesity. Insofar as society is an open system populated by reflexive agents, such research points towards the possibility of countervailing tendencies and meaningful resistances that could help to reshape the PRF (e.g. by introducing students to critical health and 'fat pedagogies' amidst problematic educational efforts to redress disordered eating).

Part 2 of our book partly takes up this challenge of exploring diverse embodied social realities, drawing from research that we have undertaken separately in various domains. These studies focus upon Canadian women (formerly) identifying as obese (Chapter 4), girls who were introduced to fat pedagogy in an English secondary school (Chapter 5), and a right-wing online US news media platform that degraded fat studies professors during the early COVID-19 lockdown (Chapter 6). Advancing theoretically informed empirical studies, which are not beholden to biomedical and public health frames, Part 2 demonstrates the necessity of critical social research when rethinking obesity in crisis times.

PART 2
Researching matters of fat

4

OBESITY, BODILY CHANGE AND HEALTH IDENTITIES

A study of Canadian women

As noted in Part 1, Canadians alongside citizens of other neoliberal nations are continually exhorted to combat obesity. Following ominous warnings from the Canadian Medical Association (Wisniewski, 2013), we observed that the Parliament of Canada (2016) further legitimated medicalised concerns about weight/fatness as a costly public health crisis. Here, as elsewhere, radical bodily change is championed via an assemblage of policy interventions, clinics, weight-loss clubs and reality television shows such as *The Biggest Loser*. In this narrative, a 'fat person', through guidance, using particular products and concerted effort, sheds a lot of weight and passes irrevocably into a socially approved slim physique. Audiences are instructed that these transformed champions will be healthier and stigma-free, thus redeeming themselves rather than being continually weighed down by the guilt, shame and blame attendant to unwanted fatness (Raisborough, 2016). However, weight-loss targets are seldom sustained; dieters usually regain, if not increase, weight in the medium- to long-term (Gaesser, 2009; Mann et al., 2007; Rothblum, 2018; Chapter 7). Defining obesity as a chronic disease (Mauro et al., 2008) is a staid way of describing the life-colonising struggles that such individuals are expected to embrace in order to produce and maintain presumably 'healthier bodies'.

Limited research on embodiment and shared experiences of fatness has incorporated a consideration of biographical time, the malleability and elasticity of the body as an unfinished 'project' and, conversely, the limitations of bodies in terms of 'frequently refusing to be moulded in accordance with our intentions' (Shilling, 2012: 10). For example, partly reflecting their own gendered biographical situations and social identities as overweight or fat, researchers have explored women's struggles in commercial weight-loss clubs on both sides of the Atlantic (O'Toole, 2019; Stinson, 2001). Such work provides insights that resonate with feminist scholarship on how 'weight' is 'unbearable' for many women in Western culture (Bordo, 2003). Similar to Stinson (2001), scholars have also discussed their

DOI: 10.4324/9781315658087-7

own ambivalent experiences of weight-loss – feelings that were compounded by their critical orientations to weight-related messaging (Heyes, 2007; Longhurst, 2012). However, that even critical scholars yearn for a thinner body should not be the last word in explorations of weight trajectories and bodily transformations, especially given the ineffectiveness of weight-loss dieting. Bodily transformations may take many forms beyond fat and thin and manifest differently across the lifecourse. Bodily changes may potentially be accompanied by feelings of triumph or disillusionment with unanticipated alterations in tone, muscle mass and skin, and these feelings may be further affected by the passage of time. In line with nascent body studies that foreground embodied agency, action and change (Shilling, 2008), this chapter argues that critical weight and fat studies scholarship would benefit from a more nuanced exploration of bodily transformations and the habitation of bodies that were somehow different but still the same. Do dieters try and recapture a thin body that no longer exists and wind up with something totally different? Does the passage of time and experiences of ageing exacerbate feelings of dissatisfaction with one's fatness or lead to resignation or acceptance? Do hopes for a thin(ner) future lead to feelings of disillusionment or triumph? How are such experiences mediated by gender, the division of labour and healthcare systems? We will aim to address such questions with reference to Canadian women identifying as (formerly) obese.

Conceptual and substantive matters

Before describing the research informing this chapter, we will first situate our work in a larger body of literature to highlight not only what is particularly useful in these studies but also their limitations and thus the academic import of our contribution. There is no need for us to reiterate key themes from literature discussed in preceding chapters, such as Evans et al. (2008) on obesity discourse and disordered eating among young women. Much has also been written in earlier chapters on aesthetic concerns and stigma, particularly as these processes affect women and girls (Kwan and Graves, 2013; Lewis et al., 2011; Monaghan and Malson, 2013). Rather, our intention here is to selectively review the sociology of the body/embodiment (e.g. Shilling, 2008; Watson, 2000) and the embodiment of health identities (James and Hockey, 2007). These writings relate to the conceptual and substantive matters that preoccupy us in this chapter, notably widely circulating expectations to *change* bodies through lifestyle interventions.

Insights from the sociology of the body/embodiment are noteworthy. These include interactionist insights on 'the looking-glass body', which comprises reflections and imaginations of the corporeal self (Waskul and Vannini, 2006), the body in consumer culture (Featherstone, 1991), health fascism (Edgley and Brissett, 1990) and qualitative analyses of modalities of the body in health and illness (Watson, 2000). The latter study offers a particularly useful body schema, based on research among men that could also be extended to women (for an application of this schema in research on young people with asthma and their

invocation of obesity discourse, see Monaghan and Gabe, 2016). This schema incorporates: the visceral (a material, medically visualised body), the experiential (emotions), the pragmatic (a body that acts in the world) and the normative (the size, shape and weight of bodies) (Watson, 2000). As with social studies of chronic illness, which attend to bodies, changing self-conceptions and their relation to biographical time (Corbin and Strauss, 1987), such literature sensitises us to processes reported in our data that may otherwise go unnoticed.

Shilling's (2008) book on changing bodies is especially apt in this chapter. Shilling does not subject weight-loss and the obesity epidemic to critical empirical exploration, but he does offer a useful means of conceptualising embodied action and selfhood. Indeed, there are broader lessons here that could be extended to more specific fields of study. Informed by a pragmatist focus on human agency, change and the construction of identities, Shilling explores different contexts that shape embodied subjects and which are themselves moulded by corporeal dimensions of social action. Attending to sport, illness and gender non-conformity, for instance, Shilling discusses the dynamic relations between external and internal environments, or the dialectical interplay of social structures and frameworks with embodied actions, emotions, cognition and selfhood. The themes of crisis, habit and creativity also run through his book; for instance, when an otherwise taken-for-granted body ails and feelings of being ill at ease (dis-ease) emerge. Unifying Shilling's interest in these disparate domains is a concern with the meanings of life, phases of embodied action and how environments affect bodily transformation and human potentiality.

Yet, more could be written about other contexts wherein changing bodies are central and potential exists for broader social transformations in bodies of health knowledge, policy and practice. What about biomedicalised consumer culture wherein actors feel obliged to fight weight and dis-ease – or the appearance of the body as dysfunctional, its 'dys-appearance' (Leder, 1990) – given the conflation of physicality with social acceptability, desirability and moral worth? Whilst Shilling (2008: 1) immediately refers to '[b]ody modification and transformation' and their significance 'in contemporary consumer culture', the obesity epidemic is ignored. This, we would argue, should be redressed in an external social environment wherein 'the health role' (Frank, 1991, cited by Shilling, 2008: 6) and expectations of performativity are breached by 'ailing' bodies (or bodies projected to ail as they age whilst obese). Given the ongoing political significance of obesity as a costly public health issue (e.g. Parliament of Canada, 2016), everyday orientations to weight (loss) represent a suitable domain for advancing a pragmatist-informed approach to body studies. Accordingly, this chapter aims to complement Shilling (2008) by researching an arena wherein bodily change, or expectations of and resistance to such change, are organising features of everyday life. To that end, we foreground themes such as restrictive dieting, appearance, health and weight-related stigma as voiced by women when discussing their past, present and projected futures. If relevant and useful for comparative purposes, we will also draw from other embodied sociological studies on the meanings and vicissitudes of intentional weight-loss among other groups (e.g. Monaghan, 2008; Stinson, 2001).

Finally, we aim to complement writings on 'embodying health identities' (James and Hockey, 2007). Similarly concerned with the social and physical aspects of human life, James and Hockey draw from various theories when conceptualising the body as an existential 'reality' that 'comes into being through the process of objectifying our embodied experiences as participants in the social world' (pp. 54–5). This literature, in turn, leads to an appreciation of how the body 'can take many forms' as part of a dynamic, socially embedded and contingent process. Part of their discussion concerns 'health experiences across the life course' (p. 148), the accumulation of 'biographical information' upon the body (e.g. old scars on aged bodies), and the co-production of age-related health identities. Their discussion also flags the hegemony of Western medical science, which 'produces the concept of the "healthy" body via objectifications' (p. 141). Older age is a period of instability and may be challenging for biomedicine, although it also reinforces elite professional status by providing a time of increasing surveillance. Geriatric medicine, for instance, medicalises old age as 'later life is collapsed into illness' and is used to 'divide normality from pathology' (p. 152). Accordingly, older adults must often negotiate their embodied health identities within the institutionalisation of chronological age and the (bio)medicalisation of older age. Such practices also dovetail with representations of health, as observed when James and Hockey mention obesity and how 'idealised images' of slim, taut bodies in consumer culture do not necessarily translate into actual embodied actions (p. 98). In that respect, both older bodies and fat bodies risk being labelled aberrant in an era in which 'sickness, illness or impairment of *any kind* [is framed] as a moral deviation from the ideal [...] of the embodied subject able to exert control over his or her own organism and over the wider social and physical environment' (Shilling, 2008: 105). Accordingly, our research is offered against the background of these broader socio-cultural and embodied concerns.

The research

This chapter draws from a qualitative study undertaken by Andrea in Canada between 2013 and 2014. The study explored self-identified obese persons' health perceptions and experiences across time and different weight trajectories (Bombak, 2014e). The following reports on the experiences of 13 women. Sample size was dictated by pragmatic concerns given the abundance of data produced by repeated interviews and fieldwork, and a theoretical sampling approach designed to obtain divergent and fluid perspectives on obesity and weight-loss. Andrea did not halt recruitment until the sample included individuals who, during screening and the first interview, identified themselves as: (i) trying to achieve or maintain *weight-loss*, or (ii) focused on diet and exercise in order to achieve *healthiness* (but remained weight neutral), or (iii) politicised size activists who rejected thin ideals and/or healthist edicts. For many participants, orientations to weight (loss) changed during the research, illustrating the processual and unfinished nature of the body (Shilling, 2012).

Participants were recruited via posters and an electronic mailing list. The mailing list was directed at a healthcare audience, whilst the posters were placed at various sites (e.g. fitness centres, community centres, campuses and clinics). When recruiting participants, Andrea stated that she was interested in the views of people classified as obese according to the BMI (≥30 kg/m²), or who had been classified as obese in the past. We remain critical of biomedical labels and the BMI (see Monaghan, 2007b); however, Andrea worked in a Faculty of Medicine and the study was approved by her institutional ethics board with the stipulation that posters should refer to standardised measures of obesity. Whilst that stipulation in itself raises ethical questions (e.g. regarding the epistemic authority of medicine to define research agenda whilst pathologising larger bodies, the pervasive problem of 'ethics creep' in health studies), there were some advantages. It facilitated discussion with participants on the medicalisation of body size and the meanings of labels such as obesity and language around fatness. Additionally, it ensured participants had embodied knowledge of societal reactions to non-normatively large (censured, discredited) bodies.

The sample was predominantly White. Many healthcare-affiliated employees were recruited from a related listserv, incorporating various occupations, including accountant, receptionist, transcriptionist and frontline healthcare provider. Interestingly, those recruited via posters were also often employed in the health field. This was not a criterion for inclusion, though their self-selection is an interesting sociological finding, reflecting the relevance of obesity discourse among such workers who, as suggested in other research (Thomas et al., 2008), tend to construct a humiliating environment for people categorised as obese. One interviewee was registered as disabled. Interviewees were in their 30s, 40s and 50s. The median age was 49, the mean age was 45 and the modal age was 54 years. Participants were diverse in terms of living and family circumstances, socioeconomic statuses and experiences with, and perspectives on, weight (loss). At the same time, there were discernible patterns; for example, only two women had lost a significant amount of weight and had kept this weight off.

Participants' perspectives on health, obesity, weight trajectories and changes over time were first explored using a semi-structured interview schedule. This enabled Andrea to elicit in-depth understandings and generate rich qualitative data. Four women were then chosen for repeated, in-depth interviews and participant observation. These women demonstrated the maximum range in the sample in terms of weight-related perspectives and experiences. Repeated interviews were conducted every three to four months over the course of a year. Interview guides for repeated interviews were constructed in an iterative process and informed by prior interviews. All interviews were audio-recorded and transcribed verbatim.

Participants were asked about sites meaningful to them as larger persons and consent was obtained to join them at some of these sites. Venues included restaurants, family homes and workplace cafeterias. Andrea also grocery-shopped, participated in menu planning and food preparation, and exercised with contacts during their fitness and group classes. Public venues such as the grocery store or gym have been identified in other research on obesity as potentially stigmatising arenas (Lewis et al., 2011). Detailed fieldnotes were written up after every fieldtrip in order to capture observations, situated accounts and other details.

All data were indexed using NVivo 10 software and analysed thematically. Themes included bodily function and mobility; compulsion, addiction and validation; social impacts of weight-related changes; size acceptance and mood. An explicit analytical lens was brought to embodied change (or lack of change) and different weight trajectories, including women's focus on the ageing body. The study's qualitative longitudinal design proved particularly valuable in this regard (Saldaña, 2003). Data were analysed across and between time points, and participants and were systematically reviewed to construct an ideal typology of changing orientations to weight (loss). Ideal types are a heuristic device, enabling researchers to reconstruct intersubjective realities (Aronovitch, 2012). Ideal types provide a tool to explore and describe empirical data and help generate hypotheses whilst acknowledging that models strive to represent, but not stereotype, necessarily fluid, messy and contingent phenomena. As observed in this study, ideal types could be overlapping, and participants could embody multiple ideal types when describing various periods of their weight history. Participants' weight and expressed attitudes towards weight also changed during the period of data collection. The descriptions of what follow therefore depict types derived inductively from the data as well as the divergence of the empirical data from these types over time.

From hope to resignation: changing orientations to weight (loss)

Whilst Amelia and Harmony had lost what they defined as a significant amount of weight and had kept this off for a year or more, they were unusual. Most participants would be medically defined as chronically obese and/or perpetual weight cyclers, much in line with what is known more generally about intentional efforts to lose weight (Mann et al., 2007; Rothblum, 2018). Three women (Melissa, Matilda and Clarissa) reported previous eating disorders, and they no longer sought to lose weight. Another, Rachel, reported a past eating disorder but vacillated between wanting to lose weight and advocating a weight-inclusive approach to health, HAES (Burgard, 2009; Chapter 7). Most participants, however, hoped ultimately to permanently lose unwanted weight in line with conventional narratives of healthy embodiment. At the same time there was ambivalence and perhaps realistic scepticism regarding the likelihood of achieving this goal. The overlapping, non-mutually exclusive patterns in which weight-related talk manifested were as follows: (i) hopeful narratives, (ii) disordered eating distress and (iii) weight-cycling or stagnation. These are summarised in Table 4.1 and elaborated upon below using data. Our analysis also includes cases that departed from the ideal type, reflecting the messiness of the empirical world.

TABLE 4.1 Typifying Common Orientations to Weight (Loss)

Common Types	Defining Elements
Hopeful narratives	Seeking to lose and/or maintain weight-loss in the hope of a sustained thin(ner) future body and consequently better life.
Disordered eating distress	Resistance to weight-loss and the expectation to restrict one's dietary intake in order to shed weight. Past experiences of extreme restriction were thought to contribute to poorer health and current larger size.
Weight-cycling or stagnation	Stalled future due to perpetual weight-cycling, weight gain or chronicity of fatness. Typically framed in terms of innate biomedical or behavioural attributes. Resignation to living 'large' but also critical of stigma.

Hopeful narratives: embodying a thin(ner) body and the good life?

> Harmony expressed commitment to maintaining her much slimmer body. Her intonation suggested considerable aversion to her formerly fat body. Adamant she would not regain weight, she said: 'The only reason that I can do it probably is because I recognise it [weight regain] and I won't give up. Most people who lose weight, they give up and they just gain it back'.
>
> *(Fieldnotes)*

Hopeful narratives express interviewees' confidence and desire to achieve and/or maintain a thin(ner) body. Such talk, in its ideal typical sense, ascribes value to a culturally normative body qua 'passport to all that is good in life' (Featherstone, 1991: 186), incorporating health, well-being and social acceptance. Hope was expressed in terms of how the narrator's current weight-loss would be maintained, unlike prior episodes that resulted in weight regain, disappointment and sense of failure. Insofar as hope was independent of continued weight-loss, we also include here accounts from women, such as Harmony quoted above, who intentionally lost weight and was currently maintaining a lower weight. At the beginning of this study, approximately a third of participants said they were losing weight or maintaining lost weight. Yet, whilst such talk tended to emerge at and consti-tuted certain stages in women's dieting careers, there was also fluidity regarding the actual stage in an individual's weight-loss trajectory in addition to variability in their personal history with weight (loss). For example, women voiced hope-ful narratives when *presently gaining weight, weight stable or experiencing an episode of weight-cycling*. Regardless, hope became a means through which women with a biography disrupted by 'weight-related troubles' sought to construct positive meaning, viability and identity for the present and foreseeable future.

Consider Rachel's experiences. She focused on currently losing weight, mostly in the hope of maintaining mobility as she aged. Invoking pragmatic, experiential and visceral modes of embodiment (Watson, 2000), Rachel stated that her health was good despite her size (in line with her endorsement of HAES) but felt weight reduction might aide her functioning body. Her current regime was conveyed as a meticulously planned 'body project' (Shilling, 2012). Andrea was invited to go grocery shopping with Rachel and into her home for meal planning and food preparation. Bread was baked in a kitchen featuring a whiteboard that outlined daily meal plans for the week. Cookbooks and health food paraphernalia were also on display. Recipes were often taken from websites with names that suggested a focus on low-calorie meals, and these recipes formed the basis for grocery lists. Rachel also demonstrated how her online fitness community worked, giving concrete expression to those various digital media and body pedagogies that we introduced in Chapter 2. Community membership entailed religiously entering a log of diet and physical activity, with the software calculating nutrient values and energy balance. Other members would then comment on these endeavours, a source of praise to which Rachel felt 'addicted' in a positive sense.

The centrality of food and the pleasure Rachel derived from it were apparent, but so too was the enshrinement of dietary self-monitoring, the energy imbalance model and their conflation with health and morality. When reflecting critically on her *past* weight-loss efforts, which also entailed calorie-counting, Rachel described these as disordered (see the next subsection). However, she claimed her *current* approach was different; it was more 'ordered' (sensible) because of the aforementioned software. Lest this be construed as a Weberian iron cage of rationality, Rachel mentioned online community members whom she considered especially successful in achieving their goals but who were not overly restrictive and therefore unlikely to re-trigger disordered eating. Rachel believed that a thinner, healthier and more mobile future was possible for her if she followed a very narrow line of rigorous self-monitoring that did not descend into her past obsessive disordered eating habits. Similar to other contacts, Rachel's reconstructed past reflexively informed her present and projected future.

The positivity of hopeful narratives must be understood in relation to not only the negativity of past weight-loss endeavours (those defined retrospectively as obsessive and dangerously restrictive) but also the negativity of what it means to be obese in societies such as Canada. Participants, in reproducing the pejorative status of fatness and implied notions of gluttony and sloth, often attributed their heavier or weight-cyclic pasts to improper 'obesogenic' behaviours. In compounding the 'deviant' or 'sorry' nature of their past 'obese selves' and thus the imperative to bring forth and maintain 'positive' physical change, these women also recounted how they had experienced a history of stigma (see also Lewis et al., 2011; Puhl and Heuer, 2009; Thomas et al., 2008). In view of these hurtful realities, hopeful narratives captured the possibility of a positive yet fragile metamorphosis: the present involved careful self-monitoring and a perpetual awareness that 'small slips' could jeopardise new or newly emerging embodied selves. Just as the beautiful butterfly emerges after spending most of her restricted life as a hungry caterpillar, these women projected themselves into a brighter future wherein lightness of body facilitated freedom to experience the external environment. At the centre of this preferred future was an imagined 'looking-glass body' (Waskul and Vannini, 2006) with an improved physical form, having conquered what many described as addictions to food. What we call hopeful narratives were thus infused with anticipation and expected triumph as part of a delicate and carefully nurtured body project that also gives concrete expression to behavioural approaches to public health (policy), as discussed in Chapter 3.

Megan's account exuded a high degree of hope for a thin future. Throughout her interview she projected positivity and energy. In her 50s, Megan had previously weight-cycled. She attributed periods of weight regain to her limited willpower but also blamed external factors, including a car accident that inhibited her ability to exercise (for comparable accounting among men when 'excusing' their unwanted weight, see Monaghan, 2008). At the time of interviewing, Megan was a member of a commercial weight-loss group. Five months into her membership, she believed she would finally succeed in maintaining lost weight, due to the group's ongoing monitoring and accountability (see also O'Toole, 2019; Stinson, 2001). Megan now felt able to 'more strictly watch my calories and control things', adding that she would 'not let it [weight-regain] get to the point where it's … you know, it's just so insidious that you turn around and you think "how did I get here?"' In short, Megan's imagined future self had become successfully habituated to her weight-loss group's edicts, which would keep her 'suitably thin' rather than subject to chronic relapse. Like several other participants, Megan also faithfully assumed weight-loss could forestall bodily decline associated with ageing. Echoing anticipatory medicine (Evans and Colls, 2011), Megan sought to lose weight in the hope of combating possible future health problems. In that respect, she was comparable to some of the men interviewed in Monaghan's study regarding their reasons for going on a diet (e.g. the biomedical health rationale) and (often unsuccessful) efforts to sustain a (modified) diet (see Chapter 2 of Monaghan, 2008). According to Megan, her health was presently good, but she felt she would be gambling with her future health if she did not act now:

> I think it [weight] is just a smoking gun [laughs]. I'm on no medications; my blood pressure was like 100 on 50 before I gained a lot of weight. So now it's up to like 120 on 60-something [laughs; this would be within the medically defined healthy range], so I had a lot of room to move. My sister and my brother are both on blood pressure medication. So I haven't had any problems with sugar so far but I guess that it's probably just the Russian roulette, dodging the bullet 'til you develop diabetes.

Such talk makes sense in a broader cultural context wherein type 2 diabetes mellitus is a cultural signifier of obesity (McNaughton, 2013). Even though Megan appealed to her good health, she felt a sense of dis-ease given the medically defined risk of becoming chronically ill as an obese woman. Yet, hopeful narratives were not only voiced in response to possible or actual physical illness and related concerns (e.g. in order to remain physically mobile). Weight-loss also promised a future that was void of many of the social ills that plagued their lives; for example, limited sociability, poor familial relations and/or the absence of romance.

Even so, some women, who had experienced (some) past success in becoming thin(ner), said this did not result in the positive outcomes they had anticipated. Amelia lost weight through lifestyle changes but voiced disillusionment: 'I've got this very healthy body for [my age], [laughs] but I still feel unhappy and lost and lonely and all those things are still there'. This 'experiential mode of embodiment' (Watson, 2000) incorporated a critique of medicalised measures, with biographical time and bodily change serving as crucial reference points. At the start of data collection, Amelia felt that her current weight-loss was insufficient amidst angry references to the BMI chart at her local fitness venue and her memories of a thinner past. Whilst this reflects the disciplinary power of 'normal' and 'pathological' categorisation according to the BMI (medicine's hegemony in defining 'healthy' bodies through objectification, see James and Hockey, 2007), it also suggests the evocative nature of some participants' pasts as thinner, socially acceptable, women. By the end of the study, Amelia was more self-accepting, which she attributed to changes in her fitness, health, appearance and maintaining her present lower (if still obese) size for an entire year for the first time. Time spent at her present size, less stigma and gradual habituation to ageing helped alleviate her socially constructed/embodied sense of dis-ease or corporeal 'dys-appearance' (Leder, 1990).

Other participants who had lost weight described their ongoing fear of fatness and recourse to other body modification technologies in order to remedy their appearance-based concerns. Harmony, in her 50s, underwent cosmetic surgery to remove loose skin, her so-called mother's apron, after losing weight. Reproducing the 'aesthetic frame' (Kwan and Graves, 2013), Harmony was delighted that having the skin removed meant she could wear youth-signifying clothing again, such as a bikini, which made her feel 'giddy'. Women attempting weight-loss were often trying to recapture a distant thinner past and overcome a heavier, more immediate, past. Associating weight gain with ageing, Harmony described her own negative reaction to obese women as being predicated on a universal desire to embody a much younger self: 'We all wanna be that sleek youthful beauty we were when were about like ten'. Of course, such a sentiment is by no means universal. For example, many women experience discontent from girlhood onwards amidst normative expectations to be petite and pretty (Bordo, 2003; Monaghan and Malson, 2013), whilst others resist the abjection of obesity altogether, notably activists who define 'fat as foxy' (Kwan and Graves, 2013: 34).

In summary, hopeful narratives project a preferred thin(ner) future. This future is imagined to be free of past, present and/or anticipated problems, which are reductively attributed to 'excess' flesh. Within this narrative, which implicates efforts to rationalise and streamline gendered bodies, slenderness is equated with self-improvement and a better life. However, irrespective of the narrator's current health status and possible good health (outcomes), intentional weight-loss did not necessarily produce the futures for which these women longed and prophesised. Despite their hopes and apparent success in achieving – or coming closer to – a projected target weight, many recognised that sustained, substantial weight-loss was virtually impossible. Some women described thinner childhoods, which could haunt the present, whilst others recounted being obese throughout their lives despite efforts to change this. Such embodied histories made the production of hope especially challenging in the absence of institutional scaffolding, notably the 'support' elicited among fellow members of weight-loss groups or online. Of course, this is not the end of the matter: other accounts also emerged, notably among women reporting histories of disordered eating.

Disordered eating distress: shadows of the past

> When I was not stable and not in a positive place with my body image and myself, and not feeling that HAES was a viable option for me, it really kept me up at night. Because it becomes a demon, right? Trying to lose weight at all costs becomes all-encompassing and obsessive, for me. It's something that no longer keeps me up at night, which is a real freedom and contributes massively to a quality-of-life.
>
> *(Clarissa)*

Approximately a third of participants described how their past weight-loss efforts triggered disordered eating and how this consequently shaped their present selves and their projections into the future as ageing bodies. These women were *most likely* to abandon weight-loss as a primary goal and explicitly align themselves with HAES, or implicitly adopt many of its edicts. Yet, insofar as we are offering a typology or heuristic device, it should be stressed that individuals could vacillate and shift their orientation to weight-loss over time: size acceptance did not preclude ambivalence, contradiction and ambiguity (see also LeBesco, 2010; Murray, 2005a; Chapter 7). Importantly, practices that some size-accepting participants described as 'disordered eating' were currently endorsed by women trying to 'manage' their weight.

In its ideal typical sense, 'disordered eating distress' underpinned efforts to accommodate, and even value, one's size. Such talk invoked the narrator's realisation that whilst they might have been (considerably) thinner in the past, achieving and/or maintaining slenderness was not a panacea for myriad ills and tended to be transitory. Furthermore, achieved slenderness could have serious costs and these outweighed promised benefits. It is for these reasons that narrators asserted that they were healthier at their present higher weights, or less likely to further damage their health by pursuing ill-fated weight-loss. Such talk was informed by biographical time, comprising an embodied history wherein personal weight-loss had become an organising feature of everyday life. Unlike hopeful narratives, what characterises disordered eating distress is that past weight-loss efforts effectively cast a shadow over the promissory culture of slenderness, rendering this a 'fat fabrication' (Evans et al., 2008).

The negative consequences of calorie restriction and dietary prohibitions had particular valence in that regard. Participants' histories of illness when attempting to lose weight, and the recounting of these experiences, shaped their present relationships with food and sensitised them to the potential dangers of re-engaging in dieting. Health problems associated with their previous pursuit of slenderness included: low blood pressure, lethargy, hair loss, amenorrhea and damaged metabolisms that resulted in further weight gain. Matilda painted a picture of a woman pressured by misguided people who, even if well intended, failed to appreciate that she could be 'suddenly' tipped into a state of starvation. Matilda had earlier described how her past disordered eating had resulted in dangerously low blood pressure – in effect, her 'visceral' body was jeopardised by practices that elevated appearance, or 'social fitness' (Watson, 2000), over metabolic fitness. Matilda was understandably aggrieved by medical advice to lose weight, interpreted as a manifestation of 'direct stigma' (see also Lewis et al., 2011), which could reinforce her prior conviction of not eating:

> I'm just really annoyed that the whole issue of weight keeps coming up, and it's like, you know what, I don't want to do that again so please stop talking to me about needing to lose weight. I don't want to be that person who suddenly feels like I need to not eat.

In re-ordering their visions and priorities, women voicing such words also projected a future in which they, and other people, accepted their size unreservedly. At the same time, a cautious understanding of the future was acknowledged should stigma be unremitting or if they resumed disordered eating. Melissa captured such sentiments when stating that she tried to ignore exhortations to lose weight because she felt that these would lead to inevitable weight preoccupation and cycling. As seen below, she struggled with a harsh social environment where people, much in line with 'health fascism' (Edgley and Brissett, 1990) or 'micro-fascism' (Rail et al., 2010), feel entitled to police other peoples' diets/bodies:

> But to lose that weight, I just gained back more. And that going back and forth, I believe, has been harder on my body than just staying a little overweight … Some people seem to think that it's OK that if I order the whipped cream on my hot chocolate, they should point out that's unhealthy or … I'm not stupid. My body's a different shape than yours. It doesn't make my feelings any different.

Women expressing disordered eating distress remained health conscious. Challenging size discrimination was one component of this, as per HAES (Burgard, 2009). Indeed, HAES-aligned participants often described engaging in health practices as a counterpoint to the damage inflicted by an unforgiving external environment that precipitated a crisis situation for them. These women's favoured pursuits – valued independent of weight-loss – included eating home-prepared organic food, physical activity, prioritising sleep and mindfulness.

Yet, we would be remiss if we presented all women with disordered eating pasts as advocates of healthism (Crawford, 1980), wherein health is elevated to a super-value (see also Brady et al., 2013). A minority of HAES-aligned partici-pants resisted the focus on preventive actions to ensure healthful aging. Consider Clarissa, who was probably the most unambiguous fat acceptance advocate but who was also frustrated with having to be a champion of fatness and fitness. The following talk, in foregrounding the inevitability of death, emerged as part of a broader discussion on the need to relax societal standards of 'what makes a healthy person':

> It's like in the end we're all gonna meet our same end, one way or another. And I know that our goal and everybody's goal is to sort of prolong that end from happening, but in the end we're all just gonna die.

In sum, while Clarissa was extreme in her rejection of healthism, most women voicing 'disordered eating distress' endorsed health whilst resisting injunctions to lose weight for health's sake. As with Matilda, such women feared that capitulat-ing to anti-obesity messaging could reignite pathological eating habits and resul-tant health problems that shadowed their pasts. Of course, the weight changes produced by these actions, regardless of the dangerous means required to achieve them, are often culturally valorised and could fuel the validation that many par-ticipants craved. Such approval likely contributed to the obsessive weight man-agement techniques described by women still hoping for thinner futures, actions deemed pathological by HAES-affiliated participants.

Stagnation and weight-cycling: stalled futures

Repeated weight-cycling, gain and stagnation were habitual for many partici-pants. Weight fluctuations were sufficiently common to render any *weight-loss* mundane rather than a triumphant precursor to a better future. Some of these participants, in internalising fat oppression rather than the resilience promoted by HAES, blamed themselves for their chronic or elevating weight. This is much in line with an emergent culture of blame, as noted in research on being 'fat' in Australia (Thomas et al., 2008) and writings on how relations of deviance and blame are being heaped onto relations of stigma and shame in globalised capitalism (Scambler, 2006, 2018). Women often referenced thinner pasts, casti-gating themselves for their present size and imagined fat futures with reference to 'obesogenic' habits. Hannah, a healthcare provider in her 30s, said she had always been overweight but was presently at her highest weight. Her occupation influenced her view that her good health, despite some mobility issues, would inevitably fail if she remained obese:

I find my weight has impacted my day-to-day movements, my mobility kinda thing, and so … if I continue on this path… And I see it in my patients a lot. I mean, they can't, you know, travel, they can't just walk outside, they're in wheelchairs or they can't do proper self-care. Like I'm not at that point now, but, I can see if I keep doing this, or if I keep letting it be this way, I can see what's to come.

Hannah, a former athlete, reproached herself as such: 'I don't do any sports. I don't walk to work. I avoid stairs. Every once in a while I'll eat better, like I'll change my eating habits a bit, but it tends to be more short-lived now'. Hannah described herself as an 'emotional eater' whose brief forays into healthier behaviours were hampered by periods of stress-induced eating. Paralleling observations on the effects of obesity discourse and 'constant pressures to be successful' among girls in English schools, Hannah appeared to 'give up' on pedagogies intended to promote healthful, active lifestyles (Evans et al., 2008: 125). Whilst worried about the future, Hannah said she lacked motivation to be active in the present:

> I guess barriers to doing things that promote my health concerns motivation, or lack of motivation. And also maybe the lack of consistent support to keep me motivated. And like I remember when I used to work out at the gym or go to the gym, I actually like it. I do like weight-lifting and things like that, but for whatever reason I'm just not motivated to go there. And I'm not motivated to go on a regular basis.

Even so, Hannah recognised how the external and internal environments interacted, much in line with Shilling's (2008) exegesis on changing bodies. Hannah felt that fitness venues and advertisements needed to respectfully feature larger women as a way of incentivising them to exercise and promote inclusion, a sentiment that would likely resonate with predominantly female interviewees in Lewis et al.'s. (2011) study who felt they did not belong in certain places and who even put their life on hold by not pursuing dreams and ambitions.

Yet, even participants who blamed themselves for their size remained indignant about forms of stigma, ranging from environmental (as above) to direct stigma. In her 50s, Daisy was thinner in the past but, like Hannah, felt her present was mired in stagnation and her future quality-of-life was endangered by her size. After gaining weight, she underwent weight-loss surgery and became an avid runner. Following an injury, she regained weight. She described her inactivity and feelings of uncontrollable food consumption as 'disappointing', adding that whilst she intended to 'start soon' on a weight-loss programme 'there's always something that stops you' such as work demands. Still, she was very angry about her treatment by others:

> You lose all the weight and you're proud and excited and then you gain it back. And you get really disappointed and you feel ashamed and embarrassed

because you know everybody is watching and keeping … I have a favourite [relative], and she will say to me, 'your face is getting round again'. Do you think I don't have a mirror or a scale? Like, why do people have to tell you? They do it, and it's hard, it's really tough. And there's nothing out there. People think you can go to Weight Watchers. Do you think we don't know? Fat people know what to eat and what not to eat. That's not why they're fat. It's not lack of knowledge. You know? They don't get it. People don't get it. And it sucks. I don't want to be told all my life that I'm fat.

For these women, any weight-loss occurring during the study was mentioned only briefly. Within 'stalled future' narratives, women instead focused on stigma, their food addictions or their bleak visions of ageing at a larger size. Whilst personal health concerns emerged in these discussions, much was also said about their families' health or the effect of weight stigma on future generations. Daisy, quoted above, captured this with reference to her overweight children and grandchildren. In some respects she sounded like Thomas (2016), a fat studies scholar who critiques US anti-obesity policies for failing children such as her 7-year-old grandniece. Daisy also shared similar views to Katrina, who reflected on her own experiences of feeling unwanted. In her 40s and 'chronically obese', Katrina had recently lost weight due to regular physical activity. However, she believed sustained weight-loss was impossible for her in the absence of accessible bariatric surgery. She had, over the years, lost and regained hundreds of pounds. Katrina worried about obesity as a health problem, but was most concerned about preventing stigma for future generations:

> There's always somebody who is going to have in the back of their head, 'oh God what's this fatty want?' … and just think about the perception of what is the size, and size is not right, it doesn't fit in with society today, and it's wrong, it's very wrong. Somebody has to figure out how to make this work and fix it so that little kids don't have to grow up thinking 'nobody is ever going to want me'.

In summary, 'stalled future' narratives were commonly expressed by women deemed obese and who were presently weight stable or recurrently weight-cycling. Some described thinner or more active pasts that they wished to recapture. However, they found these efforts stymied by insufficient motivation, exacerbated by stigma and structural issues. Whilst these women worried about their futures, their anxiety often focused on future generations and broader issues than weight, notably discrimination (as will be seen in the next two chapters, these are empirically warranted transnational fears). These participants had apparently habituated or resigned themselves to their sizes. The discredited meanings of fatness, in an intolerant social environment, continued to impact their lives, but these women's concerns often seemed to transcend what benefits they thought may accrue from their own (often transient) weight-loss.

Discussion: towards changing bodies of knowledge, policy and practice

Canadians have been told that obesity is an 'expanding threat' (Wisniewski, 2013: 358), with the Parliament of Canada (2016) also reproducing this frame and the WCHP. Mindful of such concerns, this chapter reported and analysed qualitative data on shifting orientations to weight (loss) among Canadian women identifying as obese, or formerly obese. In particular, we explored social meanings and practices among women whose biographies comprised a troubled relationship with dieting, food, exercise, fat and stigma. Themes included the pursuit of slenderness and experiences of typically ill-fated weight-loss attempts. This chapter thus provides grounded insights about an arena that is all-too-easily colonised by stigmatising assumptions about 'fat people' and their putatively deficient lives, 'signature elements' of 'the health and aesthetic frames' (Kwan and Graves, 2013) that resonate in North America and elsewhere (Evans et al., 2008; Lewis et al., 2011; O'Toole, 2019; Thomas et al., 2008).

Inductively generating a three-part typology of orientations to weight (loss), we offered a heuristic in order to grapple with multiple meanings of fat embodiment in a largely judgemental external milieu – what O'Hara and Taylor (2018: 4) term an 'adipophobicogenic environment' that could reduce health, well-being and quality of life. We termed the three non-exclusive and sometimes overlapping ideal types: (i) hopeful narratives, (ii) disordered eating distress and (iii) weight-cycling or stagnation. In actuality, women's orientations shifted and departures from ideal types were common. Such change is understandable given, among other things: The failure of diets in the medium- to long-term, the messiness of the empirical world and embodiment, emergent experiences of ambivalence and contradiction, the socially situated character of talk and our extended methodological focus on dynamic social processes – notably weight trajectories and dieting careers which are, by definition, contingent and mutable. A recurrent observation, however, is that body dissatisfaction was common. In going beyond Tiggemann's (2004) review, this emotion exceeded appearance-based concerns to include other (imagined) modalities of embodiment, such as a projected 'pragmatic and visceral body' (one that enacts social roles as well as being a biological reality) (Watson, 2000). Consequently, the multi-dimensional body was defined not only as an object of censure, interpersonal surveillance and (dis)satisfaction but also as at risk of biomedical health problems in the pre-emptive war on obesity (O'Hara and Taylor, 2018).

Attendant to the reflexive nature of the looking-glass self/body (Waskul and Vannini, 2006) and biographical time (Corbin and Strauss, 1987), the above has furthered a temporal focus on bodily change and health identities. In so doing we referred to and sought to advance a field that is relatively neglected in studies of the body-health-society nexus (James and Hockey, 2007; Shilling, 2008). Accordingly, we drew from critical weight and fat studies, incorporating discussion on framing, stigma, fat acceptance, HAES and the consequences of anticipatory medicine that collapses time. Studies of women and dieting culture were also noted, which ask whether feminism and intentional weight-loss are compatible (Stinson, 2001). However, amidst a raft of unanswered questions (e.g. regarding women's possible disillusionment after repeatedly dieting, resignation and ongoing dis-ease), our chapter offered an explicitly sociological discussion on bodily change and (abandoned) efforts to bring forth such change. In so doing, we contributed empirically to interactionist writings on embodiment, health (fascism) (Edgley and Brissett, 1990; Waskul and Vannini, 2006) and managing potentially spoiled identity (Goffman, 1968 [1963]).

Informed by a pragmatist perspective on human agency, identity construction and potentially transformative action, the present study has thus added further 'flesh' to various theorists' conceptual concerns. Researching women's reflexive looking-glass bodies, incorporating their imaginations of themselves and other people, is important from a pragmatist perspective insofar as these are defined as the 'solid facts of society' (Cooley, 1902: 87, cited by Waskul and Vannini, 2006: 5). Internal time-consciousness is also crucial here. As with hopeful narratives, for example, women's embodied self-conceptions were informed by their *past* as obese, marginalised women, their *present* as conscientious weight-loss strugglers and their projected *future* as victors who had achieved the good life. These obser-vations buttress the pragmatist argument that 'it is precisely this tendency towards reflexivity that characterizes embodiment as a *temporal process*' (p. 5, emphasis added). Such observations also resonate with Monaghan's (2008) ethnographic research on men's 'dieting careers', incorporating triggers for dieting, efforts to sustain weight-loss and 'the defeasibility of dietary approaches to weight-loss (and sometimes the intention to diet)' (p. 105). Of course, there is also the *longue durée* that underlies such micro-social processes. This temporal dimension includes 'the civilizing of appetite' (Mennell, 1991), itself attributable to a history of food security in the Global North, an antecedent fear of fatness among the privileged and embodied concerns about social ranking/distinction. In that regard, efforts to change bodies are *deeply* embedded and historically unfolding social practices, forming sometimes painful lived realities and memories within much larger 'fig-urations' or chains of interdependency (Elias, 2000 [1939]). We have only hinted at such processes here and there is much more that could be written on the larger social body wherein weight struggles unfold for women, men and children (on the use of an Eliasian perspective when researching the civilising of boys' bodies during the anti-obesity offensive in Northeast England, see Monaghan, 2014a).

Whilst there are other limitations to this study, such as the tendency for spe-cific types of worker to self-select for interviewing, it has nonetheless provided rich insights on changing orientations to weight (loss). Building on the theme of change and the materials introduced in Part 1 of our book, we think it is apt to finish this chapter by furthering calls to reflexively change bodies of health knowledge, policy and practice. Whilst we will elaborate upon this call later in our book, we will stress here the importance of recognising gendered power as a political impediment to rethinking obesity. Such power pertains not only to the operations of masculine domination and misrecognition (Bourdieu, 2001) but also to a failure to appreciate that women and girls may be especially vulnerable in the war on obesity (Evans et al., 2008; Herndon, 2014; Monaghan and Malson, 2013; Murray, 2008; Chapter 5). Unfortunately, though, this point is likely to be eclipsed by a combative (ruggedly masculine) biomedical health frame that has broad cultural resonance alongside aesthetic concerns in a consumer culture wherein existing feelings of vulnerability and powerlessness are reproduced, amplified and exploited. Such preoccupations impact myriad people, including workers in the health field who participated in the present study and, despite repeatedly failed diets and attendant harms, often hoped to slim down and experience a better life.

The next chapter reports on a study undertaken by Emma among schoolgirls in England who were introduced to fat pedagogy and critical health education. In so doing, the chapter continues with a gendered lens on power and inequality, furthering an empirically grounded and theoretically informed approach to matters of fat and critical weight studies.

5

EXPLORING FAT PEDAGOGY AND CRITICAL HEALTH EDUCATION WITH SCHOOLGIRLS

Rethinking 'Britain's child obesity disgrace'

Concerns about 'fat kids' (Boero and Thomas, 2016) and 'governing children's bodies' (Lupton, 2018: 37) saturate obesity epidemic discourse. For example, the WOF (2016) dedicated its second World Obesity Day to ending obesity among children and adolescents. Shortly thereafter, the Chair of NHS England claimed 'childhood obesity is an "absolute scandal"' when discussing the importance of behavioural health interventions and providing 'intelligent guidance' to parents (Campaign for Social Science, 2017). Schools constitute a key domain for recontextualising such concerns, furthering the anti-obesity offensive via 'body pedagogies' or educational practices and policies 'oriented towards defining and shaping particular bodies' (Rich, 2010: 147). School-based strategies have included 'lunch box surveillance' and making larger children run 'fat laps' (Gard and Wright, 2005: 185), whilst more recent and 'inclusive' disciplinary techniques include the use of 'fingerprinting technology' in canteens (Evans et al., 2013: 325) and other 'digital devices' and software (Lupton, 2018: 38). Schools have also sent 'warning letters' to parents of children deemed overweight or obese. This practice was endorsed by England's Chief Medical Officer, despite the letters annoying some parents who expressed their grievances on social media (Boseley, 2016b). More recently, when reporting on the National Child Measurement Programme, which calculates pupils' BMI by measuring their height and weight in reception (aged 4 to 5) and year 6 (aged 10 to 11), the *Daily Mail* proclaimed: 'Britain's child obesity disgrace: first official figures reveal 170,000 leave primary school overweight – and 22,000 are dangerously fat' (Borland, 2018). Such headlines compound the harms associated with the WCHP, including growing levels of body disaffection, particularly though by no means exclusively among girls and women (Evans et al., 2008; Monaghan and Malson, 2013; Rich et al., 2011; Chapters 1 and 2).

In this context, various school-based programmes are being developed in an attempt to prevent eating disturbances and what are referred to as 'body image'

DOI: 10.4324/9781315658087-8

problems (Wright and Leahy, 2016). However, besides a general failure to connect the intensification of gendered body dissatisfaction among today's youth to the war on obesity (Greenhalgh, 2015), there is little research on the effectiveness of programmes, policies and practices intended to prevent eating disturbances. This paucity needs to be redressed, particularly at a time when obesity prevention dominates public health, policy and media discourses and is likely to intensify in the (post) COVID society (see Chapters 6 and 8). Given these gaps, this chapter reports on a study with girls aged 12 to 13 years attending an English secondary school. The study involved workshops designed to introduce girls to critical health education and fat pedagogy approaches that challenge dominant obesity discourse. In so doing, the study sought to heed Kirk's (2006: 123) call for a critical pedagogy in physical education 'that might provide a morally and educationally defensible form of engagement with obesity discourse'.

This chapter is structured into four main sections. First, we briefly summarise insights from relevant literature, including the limitations of school 'body image' programmes as a way of addressing disaffection in 'postfeminist times' (Gill, 2016). Second, we outline the study methodology, including focus groups in the school setting and a description of how these data were subjected to a feminist poststructuralist discourse analysis. Third, we examine themes ranging from the girls' initial representations of health to how being introduced to critical fat pedagogy influenced their talk regarding various biopedagogical practices in an educational setting comprising contradictory expectations. Finally, we reflect on the opportunities and challenges of enacting fat pedagogies in schools, prioritising relational considerations.

Body pedagogies in schools: from obesity discourse to critical health education

Concerns about childhood obesity, as articulated in the school context, 'are driving what might be described as "new health imperatives" which prescribe the choices young people should make around lifestyle: physical activity, body regulation, dietary habits and sedentary behaviour' (Harwood and Wright, 2012: 611–2; see also Rich, 2012). Whilst approaches might differ, tackling obesity has become a prominent feature of health education in schools worldwide, particularly in the Global North. The previously described tenets of the WCHP 'inform' many of these school-based anti-obesity programmes. Such understandings are also entwined with public pedagogies that cultivate a certain 'bodily sensibility' (Monaghan and Hardey, 2011), or 'fat sensibility' (Raisborough, 2016), that is antecedent to but is furthered in schools. As Shilling (2010: 163) claims 'school body pedagogies often reinforce rather than challenge teachers' and pupils' pre-existing thoughts and feelings about culturally stereotypical body ideals'. Indeed, evidence has emerged demonstrating how very young children exposed to obesity discourse have begun to judge their health according to weight and body size (Burrows and Wright, 2004; Burrows et al., 2009; Evans et al., 2008). Furthermore, research has highlighted the harms of obesity discourse on various groups, including detrimental effects on children's subjectivities and sense of their body (Evans et al.,

2008; Larkin and Rice, 2005). In particular, concerns have been raised about the extent to which young people's bodies are being monitored, surveilled, governed and stigmatised in relation to weight and through particular (contestable, ethically suspect) health norms (Evans and Colls, 2011; Rich and Evans, 2005; Wright and Harwood, 2009). Chapter 2 reviewed some of this literature, with the general conclusion emerging that schools are potentially unsafe environments.

At the same time, schools are implementing 'body image' and 'eating disorders' programmes. Approaches include critical media literacy, self-esteem enhancement skills and body acceptance. Wright and Leahy (2016) offer a compelling critique of school-based 'body image' programmes, revealing the extent to which such curricula are rooted in individual psychology. This individualism is deemed highly problematic, insofar as it includes a 'psychological view of individual change' and assumed 'validity associated with measurable outcomes based on psychological scales' (p. 147). They argue that whilst many of these programs are well meaning, they 'do not engage with the complexity of the discourses shaping body ideas' (p. 148). Interventions are typically premised on the abstracted idea of a rational child who, through self-determination, can learn to resist potentially harmful socio-cultural messages. In short, such perspectives are deemed to be insufficiently relational and assume too much: 'body image interventions, assume individuals who can separate themselves from the social pressures and constraints of life, individuals who can abstract themselves from their lived body experience' (p. 143). Elsewhere, given the pervasiveness of digital media in young people's lives, Ni Shuilleabhain et al. (2021) question the adequacy of current media literacy–based programmes in schools to address body image concerns.

Similar problems have been noted before, with such critique resonating with our discussion in Chapter 3 on the lifestyle drift that pervades public health policy and anti-obesity campaigns. Although written over a decade ago, Harrison and Leahy's (2006) assessment seems as pertinent today: 'the health field is still dominated by psychological models that focus on individual behaviour change while playing lip service to the social determinants of health' (p. 152). Despite the large volume of critical pedagogical perspectives, health education seems focused on helping children to make 'the right decisions' either in terms of resisting body norms or conversely ensuring they meet the expectations of health imperatives. As Cliff and Wright (2010: 230) observe in their study in Australian schools, 'the intersection of long-standing concerns around eating disorders with the newer, more urgent and more prevalent "obesity discourse" has left at least some HPE [Health and Physical Education] teachers in a position they cannot easily reconcile'.

In view of the above, burgeoning 'fat pedagogy' literature challenges weight-based oppression. Recognising the harmful effects of the WCHP, as promulgated through 'body pedagogies' (Evans et al., 2008; Chapter 2) within educational settings, fat pedagogy 'draws attention to the ways in which weight-based oppression, often expressed as fat phobia, fat hatred, and fat bullying can be addressed within spaces and places of teaching and learning' (Cameron and Russell, 2016: 9). This scholarship has prompted the development of various courses within post-secondary education, with a focus on exploring alternative perspectives that challenge weight-related discrimination. Cameron and Russell's edited book, *The Fat Pedagogy Reader*, provides multiple examples of storying, practicing, researching and expanding fat pedagogy. Although challenging weight-related discrimination, many of the examples within that book, and fat pedagogy research more widely, remain focused on post-secondary education. Hence, there is a need for research that examines how different groups respond to these alternative discourses. Other scholars share this view. For example, Cain and Donaghue (2018) examine responses to the fat acceptance movement via a critical discourse analysis of focus group discussions with 21 women, between 18 and 69 years of age, who were undergraduate psychology students in an Australian university. The authors conclude by suggesting that future studies are needed to explore how fat acceptance messages are received among more diverse audiences.

Such a conclusion is worth noting whilst also recognising myriad constraints on alternative body pedagogies in a health field striated by gendered power and inequality. Constraints include not only weight-centric ideologies and pervasive public health messaging that are invariably recycled in schools but also, and as we will elaborate with reference to girls' understandings, the nature of relationships between teachers, subjects and students (Lusted, 1986). What we will also explore is how the individualism noted above is entangled with a 'postfeminist sensibility' (Gill, 2007, 2016; Ringrose, 2013) and 'postfeminist healthism' (Riley et al., 2019). Such concepts refer to a 'set of dominant discourses that infuse and shape the zeitgeist of contemporary culture' (Ringrose, 2013: 5), including 'forms of surveillance, monitoring and disciplining of women's [and girls'] bodies' (Gill, 2016: 613). Postfeminism denotes ways of being and not just understanding fatness (Raisborough, 2016) and is 'deeply enmeshed with neoliberalism' (Gill, 2016: 613) with its focus on individualised subjectivity, freedom, choice, flexibility and optimal living (Harris, 2004). We recognise that postfeminism, like neoliberalism, is a contested concept. However, just as we agree with Bell and Green (2016) who consider neoliberalism to be an indispensable concept despite certain problems (e.g. contradictory invocations in health studies; see also Monaghan et al., 2018), we concur with Gill (2016) who defends 'postfeminism' as a useful analytical category.

Methodology and analysis

This study involved delivering two collaborative workshops (see also Francombe-Webb, 2016), designed to introduce participants to fat pedagogy and critical health education perspectives. The research, undertaken by Emma in 2016 in an all-girls school with a mixed sixth form, was funded by the Public Engagement Unit at the University of Bath. The sample consisted of 24 girls. Most identified as White British, though the group also included participants who identified as Mauritian, Turkish, half French, German and Indian. In their 'systematic review of classroom-based body image programs', Yager et al. (2013) suggest that most success was achieved with youths aged 12–13, hence focusing on participants of this age seemed especially apt. Ethical approval for the study was received from the Department for Health at the University of Bath.

In each of the two workshops, the girls participated in several activities including dance, social media and a focus group. Here, we report only on the focus group data. Focus groups provided a shared space for young people to exchange views, and Emma moderated these using 'activity-oriented questions' (Colucci, 2007) and a flexible interview schedule, which can be helpful for exploring potentially sensitive topics and engaging children and young people. This method also enabled Emma to compare and contrast students' engagement with the different health discourses across the groups (Krueger and Casey, 2000).

A total of four focus groups took place over two days of engagement and research activities, with each participant taking part in two focus groups, each comprising 12 students. In the first focus group, students discussed health issues they deemed important, including their understandings of health, and views on current school health education, body practices and frameworks. Discussion was facilitated via a drawing-based activity where they were each asked to sketch a 'healthy person' and then reflect on how their ideas about health were formed. One of the key ethical concerns was ensuring the use of research techniques that engage young people (Christensen and James, 2008). Drawing methods are being increasingly used within PE and Health Education Research (MacPhail and Kinchin, 2004; McEvilly, 2015). MacPhail and Kinchin (2004: 91) suggest these methods have various benefits, such as potentially making activities fun, providing a comfortable way for young people to express their views and an opportunity for them to offer more of their own retrieval cues. Furthermore, drawing activities can act as resources through which to 'help address the adult-child power imbalance in the interview situation' (McEvilly, 2015: 343).

In the second focus group, Emma adopted a fat pedagogy approach, introducing the group to material (e.g. slides and interactive tasks) developed from HAES, fat/size acceptance and critical health education perspectives. The fat pedagogy approach adopted in the workshops therefore aligned with the socio-critical approach suggested by Wright and Leahy (2016: 149) which 'addresses the issues of body weight and size more broadly, indirectly and educatively'. A number of tenets proposed by Fitzpatrick (2014: 184) were also adopted:

1. Being focused on health issues (local and global) deemed important by students.
2. Viewing health education as a discipline of study NOT as a means to make students healthy.
3. Rejecting health-based, rather than education-based, outcomes (fitness, BMI, eating habits, etc.).
4. Focusing on how health issues in the local community came to be diachronically (i.e. through poverty/wealth, resources/lack of resources/cultural patterns/hierarchies) rather than the all too often synchronic 'snapshot'.
5. Questioning how health issues intersect with gender, racism, social class, sexuality and culture.
6. Question the inter/national status and social construction of health issues.
7. Viewing health issues as inherently political.

The material introduced in the second focus group addressed the following themes: healthism; contesting the science and the relationship between weight and health; developing HAES; social and material determinants of health; enhancing health and well-being; engaging in critical thinking; (re)imagining school policies and practices to enhance body confidence. Through this workshop style approach, several activities (watching videos, group discussion and drawing) provided prompts to explore these themes.

All participants were provided with child-friendly information sheets and assent forms. Parents/carers were also provided with information sheets explaining that focus groups would be recorded and all participants would be rendered anonymous. Discussions from each focus group were transcribed, and participants were asked to complete an evaluation questionnaire at the end of the study.

A feminist poststructural discourse analysis (Petherick, 2013, 2015; Rail, 2009; Weedon, 1997; Wright, 2004, 2009) was undertaken on the focus group data, informed by the approach developed by Carabine (2001). The qualitative analysis software NVivo was used to manage the data and develop initial codes. This began with a careful reading of each of the four focus group transcripts and developing key codes through a poststructural reading. This involved careful identification and classification of health discourses. The interrelationships between key discourses were then explored (e.g. postfeminism and biopedagogies of health). The next stage involved identification of discursive strategies through which knowledge about 'fat' was developed and the subject constituted through particular discourses. More specifically, this involved examination of the ways in which discourses of health and of fat pedagogy were resisted, negotiated and/or subverted (Rail, 2009; Wright, 2009). Finally, the transcripts were analysed in terms of notable absences or silences (e.g. what was not spoken), based on the literature informing the research. This analysis involved multiple readings of the transcripts, and looking across the data set for similarities, silences and anomalies. Following Carabine (2001: 281) this approach can be considered an overlapping and iterative process, taking us back and forth between data, analysis, theory and literature. At the centre of this process was the concept of discourse, which 'provides a means to understand what resources are available to individuals as they make sense of the world and themselves in the world' (Wright, 2004: 20). Specifically, in using discourses analysis, this chapter interrogates how students responded to and negotiated more critical knowledge about bodies/embodiment grounded in fat pedagogy. Similar to Cain and Donaghue (2018), the aim here is to understand why girls accepted or rejected particular aspects of fat pedagogy. To do so, we needed to understand how reception of fat messages was mediated by their engagement with other health discourses, biopedagogical practices about fat and participants' own subjectivities.

Girls' understandings of health and critical perspectives

Through the adoption of the above theoretical framework and analytical approach, we were able to identify discourses through which these particular girls made sense of health and their bodies, and which were reproduced – but *in tension* – with more critical fat pedagogies. As Weedon (1997: 35) suggests, '[discourses] consist of competing ways of giving meaning to the world and organizing social institutions and processes'. This discursive approach enabled us to identify why some aspects of fat pedagogy were rejected and others adopted. Grounded in data, this empirical section of our chapter is subdivided into four parts: (i) negotiating postfeminist imperatives, (ii) critical engagement with obesity discourse and its harmful affects, (iii) exploring the complexities of the obesity debate and (iv) reflecting on opportunities for critical health pedagogy.

Negotiating postfeminist imperatives

Emma began the workshops by asking students about their own understandings of health, seeking to identify from the outset what socio-cultural factors influenced their response to the critical material introduced in the subsequent workshops. Participants were initially asked to draw a 'healthy person' and then to explore what influenced their ideas in a broader context:

> So I've drawn someone who isn't ridiculously skinny or isn't like fat, she's just a normal nice average size.

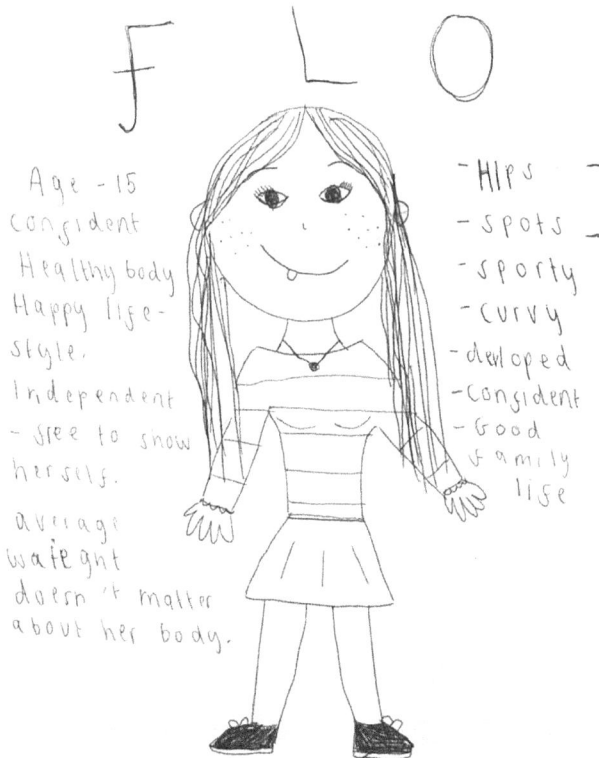

F L O

Age -15
Confident
Healthy body
Happy life-
style.
Independent
- free to show
herself.

average
weight
doesn't matter
about her body.

- Hips
- spots
- sporty
- curvy
- developed
- Confident
- Good
family
life

Mine is called Flo. She's 15. I just thought that, I looked at ideas of what somebody at the age of 15 would I think be like. She's quite confident; she's got a healthy body and a happy life. She's independent and she's free to show herself, average weight and doesn't matter about her body. [...] And also I think you have to be like a healthy person if you have a good family life as well, or you can't be like happy around you if stuff's going on as well.

(Respondent 3)

These comments, while pointing towards the significance of relationships and institutions (family life) that impact well-being, also reflect an individualising neoliberal logic. This is an ideology of empowerment and 'free-choice' but also of the need for monitoring and working on one's body in order to achieve a 'normal' weight that is neither 'fat' nor 'skinny'. This logic was even applied to girls as young as 8, as expressed by another participant:

Mine's called Hannah and she's 8 at the moment. And she likes a balanced diet, happy, quite sporty, has got some muscle but she's like not an over exerciser. She's just healthy.

(Respondent 6)

Another respondent (10) offered the following with reference to a 9-year-old girl:

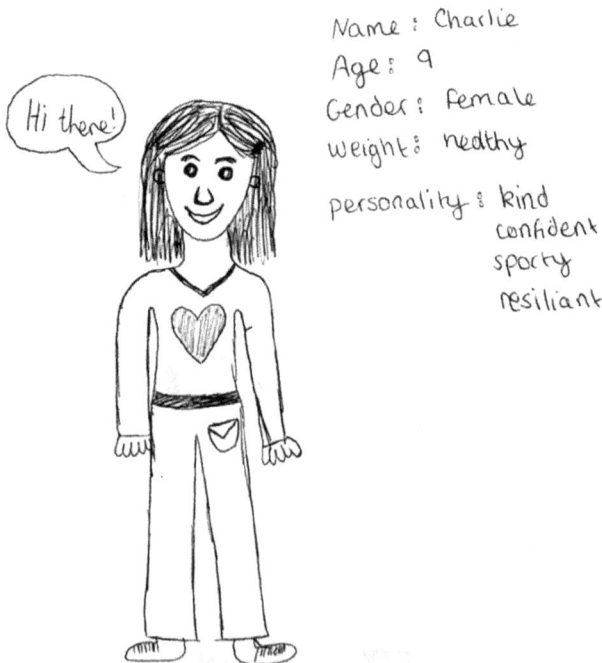

She's her proper weight and she's confident in her life, quite resilient.

Such expectations were not just about achieving 'the correct' or 'proper' weight but spoke to elements of health as optimal living, reflecting the postfeminist sensibility described above (see also Fullagar et al., 2018; Toffoletti et al., 2018). Through these discourses, the girls were constituted as consuming subjects who should demonstrate a range of sometimes contradictory imperatives (be happy but have a perfect, or at least normative, body) even before reaching adulthood. For instance, another girl said about her idea of a healthy person: 'So mine is Jeanette. She's 14 and normal weight and she's happy and stuff' (Respondent 2).

Such positioning reflects Harris' (2004: 8) claim that young women are often 'doubly constructed as ideal flexible subjects; they are imagined as benefiting from feminist achievements and ideology, as well as from new conditions that favor their success'. When discussing their drawings, many described 'the healthy girl' as someone who was able to flexibly perform this sort of continual self-improvement (see also Azzarito, 2009, 2010). Furthermore, whilst the participants did not talk about race and ethnicity, they all drew White people, reflecting normative health as constituted through racialised discourses. Azzarito (2009) found similar results in her study on young people's social construction of the ideal body in PE, where White students resisted talking about race in relation to the ideal body, but their ideal body choices tended to be representative of White bodies:

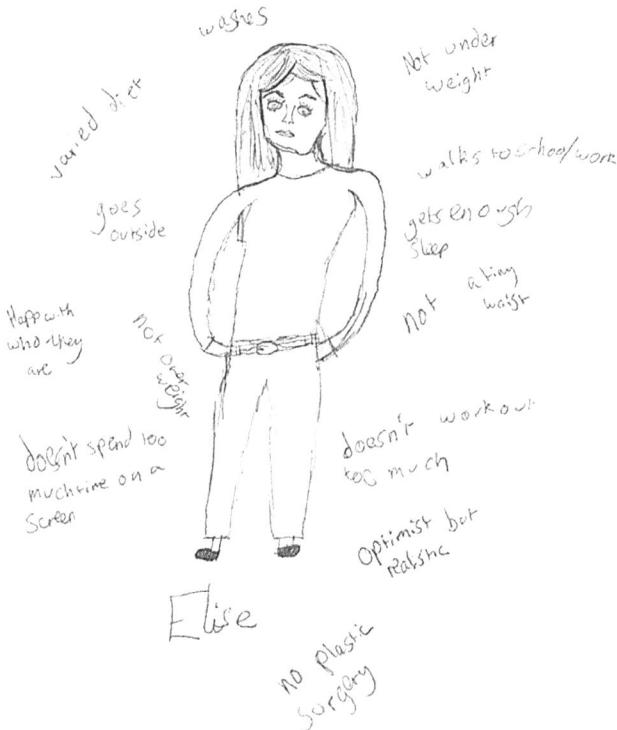

> I've got a person called Elise, like 13 plus. She's not majorly underweight or overweight, she's got a varied diet, she goes outdoors, she treats all illnesses properly, like she takes medicines carefully. She's mentally healthy, realistic, optimistic […] she's positive, has healthy relationships, is hygienic, street-smart and a good competitor.
>
> *(Respondent 11)*

In the above comments, Elise is not only the 'correct weight' but also meeting a broad range of features of a postfeminist subjectivity which reifies the need to work on oneself, find solutions and negotiate problems – to be 'street-smart' and 'competitive'. The references to activity, diet, particular sizes (not to be fat or thin), and a variety of personal, physical, and psychosocial characteristics, are similar to those described by Canadian youths, who tended to conflate appearance, health and morality (Rail, 2009). Importantly, when asked to draw a fit or healthy youth, in a subset of the Canadian study no participants drew what might be characterised as a teenager in a larger body (MacNeill and Rail, 2010). All participants in the present study apart from two drew a girl, all of which were of a normative appearance which tended to be 'pretty active and ideally white' (Azzarito, 2009: 19). Such normative depictions reflect Azzarito's observation that at 'the intersections of gender, dominant discourses of race in society link to girls' construction of the ideal female body' (p. 22). Such discourses perhaps compound a depoliticised view of health, influencing what the girls in the present study imagined or hoped their own health to be like. We would also remind readers here of observations made in Chapter 4 on 'the looking-glass body' (Waskul and Vannini, 2006), comprising a reflected and imagined view of embodied, gendered selfhood.

The girls' careful rejection of extremes in bodies and behaviours is also noteworthy, resonating with observations among other samples. Elsewhere, the ideal body size was described in focus groups by European American college women as a flexible, elusive ideal (Webb et al., 2013), which, like the girls' figures and drawings in our study, is 'curvy-thin but fit'. Whilst the ethnically circumscribed ideal captured in Webb et al.'s study suggests a rejection of thin extremes, it remains a modestly proportionate figure that is still thought to be representative of one's health status and was on average smaller than the women's actual bodies. The college women also acknowledged that one's ideal was a shifting, unachievable target (Webb et al., 2013). In Emma's study, the girls' emphasis on, for instance, variation in diet and not spending 'too much time on a screen' is suggestive of the disciplinary nature of 'the war against obesity' and is concordant with Welsh's (2011) reference to women's pleasures. In this schema, personal behaviours are coded as healthy/good and unhealthy/bad, ranging from the 'self-indulgence' of dieting for aesthetic (not health purposes), to satiating one's 'unhealthy' appetites excessively (p. 42).

In this regard, even pleasure, and as described by the girls in the present study, happiness, can become health imperatives when constituted through 'postfeminist healthism' (Riley et al., 2019). Accordingly, they were not just expected to monitor their weight and be thin, in line with what Raisborough (2016) terms a 'fat sensibility', but also to 'experience themselves as fun, valued and empowered' (Riley et al., 2019: 7), happy, carefree, positive and resilient (see also Rich, 2018) so as to negotiate problems and transform themselves. Such perspectives and ways of being overwhelmingly locate problems related to health within the individual, rather than social structures. To this end, notable silences in both the drawings and focus groups were any comments about socio-economic status or ethnic inequalities.

Critical engagement with obesity discourse and its harmful affects

In the second focus group, Emma attempted to 'disrupt' obesity discourse by introducing and discussing weight-based oppression. Despite the prevalence of post-feminist health imperatives, the girls welcomed these more critical perspectives and indicated it was important to develop ways of learning in school that helped them challenge weight stigma. For the girls in this study, concern was expressed around the increased surveillance and inequalities that might be experienced by people with non-normative bodies and which, as O'Hara and Gregg (2012) explain, are inconsistent with a human rights approach to health. The girls spoke of examples of weight-related discrimination they or others had experienced. In short, they engaged with a socio-critical approach by identifying how educational practices in their own schools contributed to the marginalisation of particular bodies:

> Like also some of the [PE] teachers have a specific [idea] what they have to have as somebody running, for example, they will never pick someone who's a bit bigger because they will think that that will let the team down.
>
> *(Respondent 13)*

Several participants raised specific concerns about the negative experiences of being measured and weighed in school, and some spoke critically about the National Child Measurement Programme. Evans and Colls (2011) also critique this policy, questioning the value afforded to the BMI. In view of such literature, participants' talk can be easily appreciated as meaningful and reasonable rather than irrational youthful intransigence requiring correction by adults:

RESPONDENT 1: I refused to do it [being weighed].

RESEARCHER: You refused to do it. Yeah, why is that?

RESPONDENT 1: Because I know that they'd tell me I was overweight and I just didn't want to hear that … Because that would just make my self-confidence go down even more. Like I don't think it matters, like I don't care how much I weigh, it's what I look like. So I do know they're going to tell me I was obese so there's no point in doing it because …

RESPONDENT 2: Their standards of weight are like these really tiny little girls and then that's what they call normal.

By the second focus group, the girls seemed more comfortable critiquing messages about managing one's weight and examining the detrimental effects of new health imperatives. This orientation is noteworthy when considering what it is in relation to; namely, emotionally abrasive processes, personally embodied and publicly enacted, wherein some bodies come to matter more than others. As Hickey-Moody et al. (2016: 213) argue: 'bodies involved in such generative processes of mattering can become controlled by fear such that what is made to matter can become (self-)policing'. In these examples, participants discussed the extent to which fears circulating about weight could propel some towards harmful body practices:

RESPONDENT 6: In year 6 [students aged 10 to 11] there was a girl and she wasn't medium, which is only a tiny bit, she was like ... And they labelled her in capital letters in red, 'obese', and she went anorexic or something in less than two weeks, and that was year 6.

RESPONDENT 4: It's quite hard to like just give someone labels, like be put into a category because it means you lose your confidence in yourself. And just suddenly being told that you're overweight or underweight, that can make you think, 'Oh I need to change that'.

Others pointed to the ways in which thin girls' bodies continued to be normalised across a range of social contexts and pedagogical sites. One participant had observed the way in which thin bodies were used in some of the educational material focused on enhancing body confidence, material which was promoted in their school: 'On the like "I love my body" page, it's always a thin person saying "oh, I love my body". And it's like you love your body because you're thin!' (Respondent 1). In that respect, thinness became a passport to body confidence – a covert form of moral censure or oppression for girls who do not happen to conform to this ideal. Yet, and to continue with Respondent 1, there was a critical understanding of how fat is often associated with lack of moral responsibility (Rice, 2007) in ways which circulated across family, school life and other social contexts:

RESPONDENT 1: Well I think that personally, because for example my mum and dad are doctors, but I don't think they're very good counsellors because they're so rude [...] sometimes when I see people who are slightly larger or curvy at the beach they're like, my dad says, 'hippos,' to them. [...] How mean is that? And I think, no offence to my mum and dad, but I think a lot of doctors, because they've got this idea of being healthy and stuff, they judge people too quickly and stuff.

RESEARCHER: Yes. So that's going back to those –

RESPONDENT 1: I have to eat this stuff in secret because my parents are like, 'No you can't have that'. And I'm like, 'But I've been good all day so I'm going to have this cookie'.

Through these discussions, participants made connections between school-based health imperatives and intersections with class, culture and families. These 'connections' reflect assemblages through which body pedagogies are formed, often constituting emerging independent relations between schools and families (see Rich, 2012).

Exploring the complexities of the obesity debate

During the second focus group, students were introduced to critiques of obesity discourse and alternative perspectives on weight/fat. This exercise entailed exploring some of the 'truths' about the relationship between weight and health, claims which often fail to acknowledge how weight-centric approaches are especially uninformative for racialised individuals (Gujral et al., 2017). Participants were asked to discuss some of the so-called paradoxes to the 'obesity canon' (Moss and Petherick, 2016; Chapter 2). They were introduced to such paradoxes with reference to studies revealing the large component of overweight and obese populations who are metabolically healthy (Bacon and Aphramor, 2011; Flegal et al., 2013; Lavie et al., 2015; McAuley and Blair, 2011; Tomiyama et al., 2016). On a reflexive note, we recognise that discussions limited to critiquing the WCHP may reproduce the 'good fatty' archetype without problematising the structural contexts in which participants are embedded. Enacting 'contrition' (Monaghan, 2008), the 'good fatty' seeks or promises to take control of their health whilst also being physically presentable and active (Pausé, 2015). For participants new to critical approaches to weight, however, these critiques can serve as a valuable starting point for challenging the WCHP (Gard, 2016). For many of the participants in Emma's study, the idea that someone does not necessarily need to be thin to be healthy was a new and positive way of thinking, possibly to be shared. For example: 'I like learning about the thing about you can be healthy if you're bigger because I'm going to tell my sister that' (Respondent 4).

Participants also explored health outcomes, raising questions about somebody's assumed health status because of their weight. The dominant rendition is that 'fat bodies' not only look and feel bad, but they also die sooner and suffer more illnesses than their 'normal weight' counterparts. Some participants countered this frame with reference to an antithetical image of a 'much thinner' body that was at greater risk of illness than a bigger built, robust body that adhered to daily routines:

> I swear, though, if you're much thinner than you should actually be it will put you in like more harm, that you'll actual live less because your body's more fragile as it doesn't have like stuff on it, while instead of someone who's like got a bigger build and like healthy in the way they actually are, well maybe some people think they're actually overweight but they're healthy. They could live longer because they've got stuff on them and they're like sticking to a routine.
>
> *(Respondent 7)*

Girls reported that after engaging with material introduced in the workshop, they were more aware of the complexities of health which were often absent in circulating obesity discourse. By the second focus group, they also began to explore characteristics related to biological factors, health practices, genetics and social determinants:

RESPONDENT 1: Sometimes skinnier people, they might have a very fast metabolism so their heart may be rather unhealthy but it doesn't show, which is actually a bit more dangerous than if you're overweight.

RESPONDENT 2: In the media we're being told that if you're overweight or if you're underweight it's a bad thing. But everybody's body is different so it doesn't necessarily mean that if somebody, if two people are the same weight it doesn't mean that one of them is healthy and one of them is also healthy. One of them could be unhealthy at the same time.

These girls began to talk about health in terms of socio-cultural influences, in particular how class, place and space intersect to produce different health practices and opportunities:

RESPONDENT 1: Like if there's facilities nearby then you're obviously more 'I'll just go to the gym' because it's five minutes [away], but if it's like half an hour [away] then you think 'actually, I can't be bothered'.

RESPONDENT 2: I mean now you can go into town, you can get some drugs [medicines] just as easily, just like for a pound you can whatever. If you're in another place, say the countryside, then you won't have that just on hand.

As the discussions progressed, these and other participants began to consider what prevented some groups from accessing particular physical activity sites:

> Yeah because like all those sports … All sports clubs and things like outside of school like you have to pay for. But like people might not be able to afford that stuff.
>
> *(Respondent 3)*

Similar observations were made about the opportunities for 'eating healthily' at school:

RESPONDENT 1: Well this isn't really being fat, but at school they're like, 'oh eat healthy', but they sell unhealthier stuff.

RESPONDENT 2: Yeah.

RESPONDENT 1: Yeah, they're like five a day.

RESPONDENT 3: They had five a day and then like …

RESPONDENT 1: And there's no fruit, there's actually no fruit.

RESPONDENT 2: There is but I bought it once and it was totally off.

RESPONDENT 1: Yeah. It's always like off.

RESPONDENT 2: And their sandwiches are like stale.

RESPONDENT 1: Yeah. I think the main meal is slightly okay.
RESPONDENT 2: Depending on what they are.
RESPONDENT 1: I mean most of them are ready meals.

In short, in the context of a focus group wherein students had been introduced to materials that challenged obesity discourse and an attendant fat sensibility, participants felt enabled to critique the WCHP. In so doing, they flagged the contradictions of various imperatives associated with body size, diet, physical activity and care of the self.

Reflecting on opportunities for critical health pedagogy

RESPONDENT 11: I think PSHE [Personal, Social and Health Education] needs to be more relevant to teenage girls.
RESPONDENT 12: Yeah […] Like the subject at our school doesn't really matter.
RESPONDENT 9: They don't really cover it, to be honest.
RESPONDENT 8: They try and avoid it.
RESPONDENT 7: Yeah.
RESPONDENT 1: And when they do it they just like brush it off and then that's it.
RESPONDENT 9: PSHE teachers, yeah, they're telling you what to think and what to say and how to manage everything.

Tinning (2014: 209) refers to how critical pedagogy raises opportunities for teachers working in the areas of health and physical education 'to tackle issues related to the cult of the body and to educate students as critical consumers of physical culture'. Whilst the data above suggest some girls in our study welcomed the idea of introducing critical pedagogy and even sharing this outside of the group, many were also sceptical about its implementation within the current school context. This was for two reasons, pertaining to the contradictory content of the students' health-related education and, furthermore, the impersonal nature of staff-student relations. We will elaborate upon these in turn.

First, students were aware of the 'new health imperatives' that were promoted across the school, shaping their own understandings of health. Some participants were critical of how these imperatives were constituted as the morally 'right' choices to make (Harwood and Wright, 2012), based on biomedical categorisations such as overweight:

> I think they should, instead of telling us … because what they always say, they always say, 'We're not deciding for you, we're just giving you the information that you need to make a decision'. But in that they are kind of telling you, 'This is wrong, this is right, you should probably follow this path'. And I think instead they should be telling you to learn to love yourself as you are, so not saying that, 'Oh you're overweight. You're underweight', you need to find a medium. They're, 'Oh you're OK as you are. You're OK as you are as long as you're healthy inside'.
>
> *(Respondent 3)*

In the above extract, respondent 3 is referring to the didactic pedagogies focused on weight-centric health imperatives. At the same time, they were being encouraged through the PSHE focus of the school to 'just be themselves', conversely suggesting therefore that their bodies did not require intervention. This, in turn, shaped their expectations about Emma's project. Respondent 2 remarked: 'I thought it [the focus group] was going to be like love your body, love your body, nothing else'. These comments reveal the extent to which students were also trying to reconcile health agendas in a similar way to that which has been reported by teachers (O'Dea, 2004). Cliff and Wright (2010: 230) reveal the 'inherent complications and contradictions' between these discourses of obesity and eating disorders as they are 'mobilised to teach young women about health and eating'. These are not just tensions that have to be reconciled by teachers but so too by students (see also Burrows, 2011).

Second, girls highlighted the 'disjuncture' between themselves and the school staff, symbolised and compounded by large and impersonal interactions. They pointed towards teachers' emphasis on the transmission of health knowledge, premised on a 'foundational understanding of educational activity' (Burdick and Sandlin, 2013: 145) – an approach that values the transmission of 'cognitive' knowledge to bring about health behaviour change. This approach created a barrier to developing the sort of interactive pedagogical relationality between teacher, subject and student (Lusted, 1986), which could provide a safe(r) space to explore sensitive health matters pertaining to bodyweight:

RESPONDENT 7: I think people like school nurses and stuff should, like even if we're not going to be anorexic or something, they should still I think build a bond and really get to know us. Because I don't get how, if you're anorexic … sort of thing, why would I, if I was anorexic, why would I go to someone I don't even know to ask for help? You know.

RESEARCHER: Are you talking relationships?

RESPONDENT 2: I've never met her, I don't even know where her office is.

RESPONDENT 11: Because my friend needed to talk to her. And we went, a whole lunch time, we couldn't find her room, we don't even know where she is. A bit depressing.

RESPONDENT 5: But they don't like … I don't want to say they don't do a proper job, but they don't understand the young person.

RESPONDENT 7: Yeah. They don't really like ….

RESPONDENT 8: I think professionals should be, I think involved.

Accordingly, the idea that critical pedagogy can simply be 'transmitted' to schoolgirls, such as those participating in the present study, needs to be counterbalanced with an appreciation of relational contexts of power and inequality. As indicated, these considerations also exceed the boundaries of the school as a site of learning and practice, ranging from the pervasiveness of neoliberal and gendered tenets of healthism to family life.

Discussion: tensions and opportunities when teaching in postfeminist times

Schoolgirls participating in this study negotiated contradictory health discourses, reproducing the dominant WCHP but also demonstrating a willingness to engage productively with critical pedagogies on the body, health (practices) and weight (Leahy et al., 2013). Whilst the goal of critical obesity scholars might be to 'offer resources for understanding rather than recruiting students to particular points of view' (Gard, 2016: 249), evidence suggests teachers may struggle to translate critical theory into pedagogical practice (Croston and Hills, 2017). Indeed, the present study reveals that even where girls might be receptive to fat pedagogy the complexity of their lives belies any simple notion of transmission of knowledge that adopts a humanistic approach, i.e. wherein students are positioned as rational autonomous learners (Burdick and Sandlin, 2013). The present study also revealed how gender, ethnicity and social class intersect and feature in the 'reproduction and resistance to dominant health discourses' (Van Amsterdam and Knoppers, 2018: 130). As discussed with reference to Whiteness, for instance, constructions of health were just as much a product of what was not said, or silenced, within taken-for-granted ideologies and representations of virtuous, morally credited citizenship, reflecting how 'monocultural' ideals about health 'erase difference' (Azzarito, 2010: 262).

The potential success for teaching fat pedagogy remained constrained by girls continually negotiating the expectations of 'postfeminist healthism' (Riley et al., 2019), comprising individualising, self-responsibilising expectations to work on the self and be 'just the right weight' and at the same time be 'happy' with themselves. These postfeminist imperatives clashed with messages reportedly promoted through PSHE, namely that students should 'just be themselves' and 'love their bodies' regardless of external dictates. This tension reflects the observation that much of what happens within health education might be well intended but it is shaped by broader assemblages, including a contradictory and ethically suspect policy terrain (Evans and Colls, 2011; Chapter 3). This is a terrain in which teachers are expected to ameliorate body dissatisfaction and obesity (see Pringle and Pringle, 2012) within the 'disturbing systemic pressures, born of neoliberalism' (Evans and Davies, 2017: 687). Furthermore, a 'disjuncture' between students, subject and teachers (Lusted, 1986) was repeatedly identified as a barrier to girls being able to safely engage with critical perspectives. This problem was not isolated to the subject of PSHE but a feature of the way in which 'health' pedagogies were enacted across the whole school and by multiple staff, including school-based health professionals, notably nurses. As such, even where, as is the case in this study, students might be receptive to fundamental shifts in thinking about health, success also hinges on the social relations and configurations of schooling through which fat pedagogy can be enacted.

In view of the above, those enacting a critical pedagogy should seek to avoid reproducing the same modernist narratives of learning which, as noted by Sandlin et al. (2011: 5), assume 'more unitary notions of the self and posits that critical transformational learning is the result of rational dialogue facilitated by an educator-as-interlocutor'. They suggest that an 'alternative vision focuses more on embodied, holistic, and aesthetic aspects of learning and development and sees transformation, learning, and development as more tentative and ambiguous' (pp. 5–6). In these moments, there may be opportunities for 'learning about the in-between and otherwise' (Rice, 2015: 392), which seem so central to helping girls better deal with the embodied complexities and uncertainties of health in postfeminist times. In that respect, complex and contradictory social relations should be recognised and debated via socio-critically informed perspectives, in favour of individualising, psychologising tendencies characterising much work in the health field.

Whilst the research informing this and the previous chapter were completed before the COVID-19 pandemic, the next chapter shifts to an online study of fat degradation enacted during the early stages of the mass lockdown in the USA. This research, we would suggest, underscores the need for those critical perspectives and pedagogies discussed above. Indeed, as the obesity and COVID-19 crises become increasingly entangled and provide the conditions of possibility for ever more disturbing expressions of cruelty towards gendered bodies, there is a dire need for critical perspectives and, as we will explore thereafter in Part 3, alternative approaches to health that are not premised on the tenets of the WCHP.

6
DEGRADING BODIES IN PANDEMIC TIMES

Politicising cruelty during the COVID-19 and obesity crises

Mass communications frame fatness and COVID-19 as a dual threat. This discourse furthers well-established tendencies to degrade bodies labelled overweight or obese, positioning them as deficient and requiring correction. Following the declaration of the coronavirus pandemic, fear-based public health messaging and mass media quickly posited a putative relationship between overweight/obesity and COVID-19 (increased risk of severe illness, of being hospitalised and death) (e.g. Brooks, 2020; Donnelly and Newey, 2020; Chapter 8). As Pausé et al. (2021) explain, such claims further 'problematised fatness' in line with the tenets of the WCHP. In short, in the absence of certain science and much prejudice, obesity epidemic entrepreneurs reproduced the 'fat as fatal' and 'frightful' frames (Kwan and Graves, 2013), which, as explained in previous chapters, are gendered and especially corrosive for women and girls.

Add to this mix pervasive concern about *unwanted weight gain* during government-imposed quarantines, or mass lockdowns, intended to limit the spread of SARS-CoV-2. Fat activists responded to such concern and derisive humour by reframing the problem as one relating to socio-cultural fears about fatness, or fatphobia (Pausé et al., 2021; Thoune, 2020). According to such reasoning, if such fears are socially constructed then they can also be deconstructed and reconstructed in positive ways via education, self-acceptance work and declaring fat pride rather than shame (Cooper, 1998; Chapter 1). The Fatosphere is one domain wherein such identity work and associated body pedagogies are enacted. As explained in Chapter 2, burgeoning literature on media and bodyweight explores such matters (e.g. Lupton, 2017). However, little is known about the intersection of the declared COVID-19 and obesity crises as enacted online, and how this dual crisis frame might be weaponised for political ends.

Empirically, this chapter aims to advance knowledge on such matters via a case study of communications that were primarily published by an online right-wing

DOI: 10.4324/9781315658087-9

US news media platform, Campus Reform. Backed by 'big money', Campus Reform caters to conservative students and is known to manufacture ideologically motivated attacks against faculty (Hamera, 2019; Kamola, 2019). This chapter scrutinises a particular Campus Reform story (Dallmeyer, 2020) and readers' comments (n = 135) denouncing a blog post from a professor working in fat studies during the early COVID-19 lockdown (Thoune, 2020). The denunciation might be conceived ethnomethodologically as an attempted 'status degradation ceremony', defined as 'communicative work between persons, whereby the public identity of an actor is transformed into something looked on as lower in the local scheme of social types' (Garfinkel, 1956: 420). However, rather than a purely localised matter, the vitriol expressed on Campus Reform radiated towards other professors, various academic disciplines, universities and social justice agenda amidst perceived threats to the body politic. Analytically, this chapter not only draws from ethnomethodology but also scholarship on meddling and health fascism (Edgley and Brissett, 1999), the weaponising of stigma (Scambler, 2018), and the politics of cruelty, defined as infliction of pain, including emotional pain, with the purpose of achieving 'some end, tangible or intangible' (Shklar, 1989: 29, cited by Kivisto, 2019: 191). When looking beyond the flesh and a particular case study, this chapter challenges the ways in which cruelty enacted towards those deemed fat (especially women) can spiral into corrosive nationalist discourse.

Research context, data generation and analysis

After reports of an initial outbreak of pneumonia of unknown cause in Wuhan, China, in December 2019, the WHO declared COVID-19 a global pandemic in March 2020. Research for this chapter commenced one month later, a period when responses to this novel coronavirus had profoundly affected everyday life. Many governments claimed healthcare systems could collapse if otherwise uninfected people's movements were not curtailed. Lockdowns or 'shelter-in-place orders' became the primary public health intervention. As noted above, concern also emerged about weight-gain, a topic subsequently attracting the attention of psychologists interested in 'health behaviours and wellbeing during COVID-19' (Ruiz et al., 2021).

It was in this context that Lee's curiosity was piqued. How was fatness and COVID-19 being discussed online during the early stages of the lockdown? Was such discussion implicated in intense forms of stigmatisation, a feature not only of the enduring 'war on obesity' (O'Hara and Taylor, 2018) but also of what Strong (1990) calls 'epidemic psychology' that comprises fear-based psychosocial response to a large scale, novel infectious disease (see also Chapter 8)? If fatness was being further denigrated during the COVID-19 lockdown, which actors were involved and what did this mean in a broader political economy? Might sociology offer a lens on such matters, just as health offers a lens on society (Scambler, 2018)?

Such questions prompted Lee to undertake an exploratory online search on 15 April 2020. He typed 'fat shaming AND COVID-19' into Google's search engine. The top ten results included an attention-grabbing article from Campus Reform. Dated 5 April 2020, the article was titled: '"Two Fat Professors" are afraid of COVID-19 causing "fatphobia"' (Dallmeyer, 2020). Rather than expressing empathy, the article, as with other Campus Reform publications, sought to fuel suspicion and derision (see Hamera, 2019). Indeed, the article, in keeping with the general tenor of that platform, gave expression to the 'US campus culture wars' wherein those with right-wing political allegiances attack public intellectuals and institutions with progressive or left-leaning sensibilities. Followed by 135 reader comments, Dallmeyer (2020) centred Thoune's (2020) blog post on diet culture during the COVID-19 lockdown (discussed further below). No further comments were posted during the next two months when Lee undertook a thematic analysis of these materials. Interestingly, when Lee revisited Dallmeyer's (2020) article 12 months later, there were 127 responses (suggesting moderators had removed some). Some paratext had also been deleted, including editorial statements claiming 'the radical left' were intent on intimidating conservative students and Campus Reform relied on readers' donations. The proceeding analysis focuses on the originally published text.

Given the foci of the Campus Reform article and readers' comments, Lee also visited Thoune's (2020) blog post and co-hosted website: Two Fat Professors (www.twofatprofessors.com/). The blog post was published on 1 April 2020. Still publicly accessible when Lee finalised his study 12 months later, Thoune's post had reportedly been viewed over 3,000 times (the second most viewed on that website), though there were no reader comments. The website homepage declared that its two hosts were dedicated to 'fighting fatphobia with education, community-building, and A LOT of sass'. The menu linked to an 'about us' section (containing the hosts' scholarly profiles), another on 'publications' (academic writings, news reports, external blogs), 'resources' (their favourite readings, videos, links to other websites, etc.) and blog posts dated from 1 March 2019. Rather than geared towards direct income generation and monetisation via advertising or donation requests, the website was focused on the unremunerated work of public intellectuals.

After reading materials on www.twofatprofessors.com several times, Lee sent Darci Thoune an introductory email on 5 May 2020. Lee explained his interest in and support for her work, and he subsequently obtained permission to refer to her blog post in his own academic writing. These exchanges furnished Lee with additional insights on the hostile conditions under which fat studies professors do the work of public intellectuals, including receiving hate mail. Lee also corresponded with Thoune's co-host, Laurie Cooper Stoll, who, interestingly, has published on fat as a social justice issue and fatphobia within health research (Cooper Stoll, 2019; Cooper Stoll and Egner, 2021). In view of Campus Reform's modus operandi and after reading literature from academics who have first-hand experience and knowledge of their inflammatory journalistic practices (Hamera, 2019; Kamola, 2019), nobody was contacted on that platform. To be sure, the ethics of digital research cannot be ignored. Lee would, however, defend his decision with reference to not only the aforementioned literature and personal communications with fat studies scholars but also what was observed in respect to Dallmeyer's (2020) article and her readers' comments (see the analysis below). These communications are treated in this study in the same way as any other views would be if they were published in traditional print media (on the 'situational ethics' of digital research, see the British Sociological Association, 2017). Materials from Campus Reform are quoted below verbatim without correcting the originators' grammar, spelling and other errors.

Data were analysed using an abductive approach. For Scambler (2001), abduction entails identifying underlying generative mechanisms that may, at least in part, explain observed events in the empirical world as analysts seek to construct 'second-order' accounts of what people say and do (p. 35). As also explained by Timmermans and Tavory (2012), abduction requires an awareness of existing theoretical frameworks or models when interpreting data. Certainly, Lee remained open to being surprised by what he observed, seeking to discern emergent patterns and themes when reading and re-reading data. However, he did not wear theoretical blinkers, as might be the case with a purely inductive approach. Accordingly, Lee drew from and sought to further critical scholarship on the already existing problems encountered by those writing about and seeking to rethink what biomedicine calls obesity (e.g. in terms of pathologising assumptions, moralising actions and stigma) (see Chapter 2). Such literature is also part of the social world and is invaluable when making sense of and ultimately challenging ways of knowing fatness in contexts of culture, power and difference. The outcomes of this research and analysis inform the remainder of this chapter.

'Diet culture at the end of the world': insights from the Fatosphere

> The most obvious problem with jokes about the 'quarantine 15' or 'the COVID 19' is that gaining weight is framed as an inherently bad thing – an idea that's steeped in fatphobia.
>
> *(De Elizabeth, 2020, cited by Thoune, 2020)*

Thoune (2020) offered an early intervention during the COVID-19 lockdown, derived from her own experiences as a self-identified fat woman in America. She spoke to concerns about unwanted weight-gain and derisive humour, often expressed online, that mock fat people for their putative deviance. In her blog post, 'Diet Culture at the End of the World', Thoune stated the title 'is a bit of an overstatement, but in many ways everything in my life has changed as a result of this global pandemic'. She acknowledged that her 'privilege' enabled her to manage various changes, some of which were 'pleasurable' (e.g. wearing comfortable pyjamas and watching Netflix). However, the pandemic also surfaced 'deep-rooted American cultural values', including those relating to 'diet culture'. Immediately after joking about her compatriots' fear of running out of toilet paper (an item that quickly disappeared from supermarkets during this time), Thoune stressed the serious side to her message: 'Before I go any further, I want to emphasize how important it is in this moment to lead with kindness and compassion – not just for others, but for ourselves as well'. She continued:

> Based on what I'm witnessing in the news and on social media, many of us are legitimately and justifiably freaked out. And, I don't mind confessing that over the course of my life, in my most desperate, anxious, and freaked out moments, my default mode has been to find ways to hate or to be cruel to myself. The scenario generally goes like this: Life is fucked up? This means I'm worthless. The math has always been easy. Although, the older I get the longer it takes to get to this point. And, I'm guessing the math must be easy for others too – the number of posts that have popped up on my social media sites addressing fears about weight gain has been astounding. In the midst of a global pandemic, for many their greatest fear is gaining weight. Or, having too much food around. Or, not being able to exercise enough. Or, not having easy access to 'healthy' food. Or, doing too much stress baking. Or, of being worthless. And on, and on, and on.

> In addition to comments from people I know online, I've also noticed a sizable (no pun intended) uptick in the number of 'funny' memes about weight gain during the Covid-19 crisis. These memes seemingly poke fun at diet culture and shame viewers for: not going to the gym, eating 'too much,' for getting fat, and for not starving ourselves at the end of the world.

It is in this context that Thoune reflected candidly on disordered eating and its connection to trauma. Taking a non-judgemental stance towards people's coping mechanisms, Thoune stated that comfort eating was 'OKAY', but, perhaps more importantly, 'Now is the time to connect with others and to support each other however we can (from a distance)'. In advancing such concerns, Thoune challenged not only online '"funny" memes about weight gain' in the time of COVID-19 but also the more general and already existing system of cultural values and norms that degrade 'fat people'. Suggested antidotes to such degradation and negative emotions included expressing 'love, empathy, and understanding', albeit whilst acknowledging likely difficulties during a time of mass panic and anxiety.

Furthermore, Thoune's blog post urged readers to reflect upon how their own 'health talk' during the crisis could make others feel 'terrible' about their perceived or assumed failures, possibly contributing to disordered eating and social isolation rather than connection and hope. Obvious linkages could be established here with fat studies scholarship on the problem of fatphobia before and during COVID-19 (e.g. Cameron and Russell, 2016; Pausé et al., 2021). A sociological reading of Thoune's (2020) position would also suggest that she was asking her compatriots to avoid 'meddling' or 'thrusting of oneself, often boldly, into the affairs of others' (Edgley and Brissett, 1999: 4). Meddling, which incorporates 'health fascism' and 'the cult of the perfect body' (see also Edgley and Brissett,

1990), has historical roots in Puritanism and efforts to purify the moral fibre, spirit or soul of America. Meddling gained momentum in the last decades of the twentieth century with the rise of health and fitness movements, including injunctions and interventions that could be experienced as 'unwelcome, if not downright improper, and certainly unnecessary, annoying or offensive' (Edgley and Brissett, 1999: 5). Indeed, health fascism and meddling invite, demand even, extreme opprobrium from the broader community towards those believed, or assumed, to have reneged on their duties as responsible biocitizens. Fat people are obvious targets here. In response, Thoune (2020) finished her blog post on a compassionate and optimistic note:

> When we creep out of our shells to look at the Internet with one eye open, it would be wonderful to see signs of help, encouragement, nurturing, kindness, and generosity. As much as trauma and anxiety are contagious, I also believe that hope can be equally contagious. Let's be hopeful. Let's be kind. Let's be the very best versions of ourselves that we can be as we face down what feels like the end of the world.

An unconvincing status degradation ceremony: critically analysing Campus Reform

Thoune's calls carried no weight on Campus Reform. Rather, communicated violence emerged comprising misrepresentation, silences and cruel denouncement. In grounding analysis of what might also be termed a 'status degradation ceremony' (Garfinkel, 1956), the success of which is never guaranteed, this section is divided into three parts. First, it will critically outline Dallmeyer's (2020) piece; moving, second, to the publishing context; and finally to an analysis of core themes derived from readers' comments. As will be shown, this ceremony was irreducible to any particular individual or even fatness. Rather, there emerged a spiralling of vitriol that spoke more to the denouncers' organisational context and a broader political economy comprising vested interests, shared anxieties, tensions and (potential) conflict. Furthermore, contradictions emerged that rendered this assault unconvincing for those not sharing Campus Reform's conservative standards of preference.

The Campus Reform article

Published under Campus Reform's logo, resembling a circular target from a shooting gallery, Dallmeyer's (2020) headline proclaimed 'Two Fat Professors' were 'afraid of COVID-19 causing "fatphobia"'. Whilst the headline might be considered successful, if judged as 'click bait' intended to grab potential readers' attention and attract traffic to Campus Reform, it was misleading. Thoune's (2020) blog post was single-authored, and she was not claiming COVID-19 (a biomedical disease) caused fatphobia (an already existing, socially constructed problem). Rather, the post foregrounded embodied social relations, practices and (dis)connection, not crude biological pathways construed within a reductionist, temporally and thus causally flawed model of emotional life. Two bullet points then followed the headline:

- A blog post on a website owned by a pair of professors who proudly call themselves 'fat,' laments that too many people are advising others on how to stay healthy during social distancing.
- The post argues that speaking about health is 'traumatizing' for some who are impacted negatively by 'diet culture.' (Dallmeyer, 2020)

These bullet points, whilst introducing scepticism and implied derision by inserting scare quotes around certain words (similarly, see Hamera, 2019), incorporate certain truths. As already noted, fat activists substitute pride for shame, and Thoune (2020) was concerned about trauma in the context of diet culture and COVID-19. The remainder of Dallmeyer's (2020) article also had superficial plausibility insofar as it referred to the two fat professors' publications and presented direct quotations. However, Dallmeyer did not acknowledge Thoune's *central message about the need for compassion and kindness.* Indeed, there was complete silence on this. Instead, various framing devices established a preferred reading.

The Campus Reform article featured a photograph, directly taken from two-fatprofessors.com, immediately after the bullet points. It showed the smiling scholars in graduation gowns with the word 'professors' in bright pink plus two pastel-coloured iced doughnuts replacing the letters 'o'. Readers were invited to interpret the image as such: witness two professors who cannot be taken seriously, especially in the midst of declared public health crises. Similar to other articles on this platform, the story was interspersed with numerous 'related' hyperlinked reports that were again littered with scare quotes: '[RELATED: Colleges dropping "Fat Studies" courses in 2018]', '[RELATED: "Fat" is the new "f-word" at this Ivy League University]', '[RELATED: Princeton to host "fat positive" dinner for "fat identified" students]'. An italicised text box also warned: '*The radical left will stop at nothing to intimidate conservative students on college campuses. You can help expose them.* Find out more »'. Such paratext and hyperlinked materials positioned Campus Reform's intended student audience as victims of various wrongs (for instance, exposure to and expectation to support ridiculous ideas and activities). Here Campus Reform created the impression that such wrongs were commonplace, even in elite institutions, and they should be investigated, reported by the media and widely condemned.

Furthermore, Dallmeyer's (2020) piece, which read like a prosecution in the court of public opinion, included testimony from two ostensibly credible witnesses: a Campus Reform correspondent who was a sophomore at Thoune's university, and a 'Fitness coach and former college cross country athlete'. The sophomore's testimony included his repeated complaint that Thoune 'is portraying something that isn't an issue' and 'is expressing an issue that isn't relevant' (cited by Dallmeyer, 2020). Such words were suggestive of his social distance from Thoune's situation, his own embodied privileges and unfamiliarity with critical literature on weight-related issues (e.g. O'Hara and Taylor, 2018; Chapter 2). Implicitly referring to Thoune's (2020) use of the word 'fat', he also went from the singular to the plural when complaining: 'I also think it's unprofessional where [the author] uses derogatory terms' (cited by Dallmeyer, 2020). Yet, rather than using terms such as 'overweight' and 'obesity', implying pathology and disease (risk), 'fat' is the preferred word among fat activists, fat studies scholars and others (e.g. 'plus-size' fashion bloggers; see Limatius, 2019) who reclaim it as a political act. Any apparent concern here about Thoune's alleged 'derogatory' and 'unprofessional' language was thus based on strategic ignorance and was also betrayed by the fact that the sophomore was participating in a potentially harmful status degradation ceremony.

The fitness coach, another man, predictably issued lifestyle advice. In so doing, he could be compared to those 'field experts', discussed by Setälä and Väliverronen (2014), who are mediators of science and biological citizenship. The coach's 'expert' advice, as reported by Dallmeyer (2020), conflated health with weight (loss) and presumed fat people were inactive and ignorant. He warned: 'Obesity leads to a majority of our health problems here in the States. We shouldn't be praising or shaming obesity but we must educate'. The hardly flattering corollary of such pedagogy, of course, is that if fat professors are intervening in public health debates then they should learn some basics about healthy lifestyles and put this acquired knowledge into practice. Yet, Thoune's (2020) blog post did not ignore health, nor was it 'against health' broadly defined (including mental and physical health). Thoune repeatedly mentioned 'health', though she avoided conflating it with weight-loss unlike the fitness coach and other advocates of the WCHP. Instead, Thoune raised concerns about unsolicited and unhelpful advice, especially 'health talk' on avoiding *weight gain* amidst widespread fear, anxiety and stigma. She supported a weight-inclusive and relational view of health, which entails being surrounded by 'people with love, empathy, and understanding so we are all able to get through these next couple of months without losing our minds' (Clarishka, undated; cited by Thoune, 2020). The erasure of such concerns on Campus Reform contradicted its assurances of accuracy and objectivity through 'rigorous journalism', as outlined below.

The publishing context: Campus Reform as a political economic project

Campus Reform identifies as 'a project of the Leadership Institute'. Founded in 1979 and backed by wealthy US donors, the Leadership Institute's website states that it 'trains conservatives'. Its expressed goal is to teach 'conservatives of all ages how to succeed in politics, government, and the media', focusing on 'campaigns, fundraising, grassroots organizing, youth politics, and communications'. The website's 'about' section, accessed when researching the background to Campus Reform, boasted that the organisation offered almost 50 'types of training schools, workshops, and seminars', alongside other services and that, over the past 40 years, it had 'trained more than 200,000 conservative activists, leaders, and students. The Institute's unique college campus network has grown to more than 1,700 conservative campus groups and newspapers' (Leadership Institute, 2020). Kamola (2019: 10) offers further context:

> The Leadership Institute is part of the State Policy Network, a group of think tanks and political groups funded by the Koch donor network. The LI's primary source of funding comes from the Donors Capital Fund, Donors Trust, and the Charles Koch Foundation. Donor Trust and its affiliated Donors Capital Fund have been called the 'the Dark-Money ATM of the Conservative Movement,' taking hundreds of millions of dollars from donors and channeling these anonymized funds into groups advocating free-market and ultralibertarian political objectives. In 2016 the Leadership Institute spent $15.8 million on its political campus activities, much of it coming from dark-money sources.

Despite Kamola's ominous reference to 'Dark-Money', some details on the Leadership Institute's finances are publicly available. The most recent audited financial statement, for the years ending 2017 and 2018, lists 'total assets' exceeding 23.5 million US dollars (this was just shy of $28.4 million in 2017) and in 2018 the Leadership Institute contributed almost $1.5 million to CampusReform.org (Independent Auditor's Report, 2019: 3). Thus, Campus Reform's online media platform, as a project of the Leadership Institute, has received significant financial support.

Like other well-funded conservative and libertarian media in the USA, Campus Reform has manufactured stories with an eye on Fox News as a 'final destination' (Kamola, 2019: 14). Campus Reform has been a 'go to' source for other conservative US populist media, such as Breitbart News, as explained by Hamera (2019) with reference to anti-feminist and anti-fat coverage. It is in such a context that Campus Reform proudly claimed to be 'America's leading site for college news'. Offering a narrative of grievance and putative abuses against conservative students, the website mission statement, accessed in 2020, proclaimed:

> As a conservative watchdog to the nation's higher education system, Campus Reform exposes liberal bias and abuse on the nation's college campuses. Our team of professional journalists works alongside student activists and student journalists to report on the conduct and misconduct of campus administrators, faculty, and students. Campus Reform holds itself to rigorous journalism standards and strives to present each story with accuracy, objectivity, and public accountability.

The above statement contains certain facts about the organisation's operational structure; specifically, Campus Reform relied upon student labour, as per Dallmeyer's (2020) article. Yet, the above excerpt and the impression it creates regarding an unsavoury university system are problematic. This is because this 'watchdog' has acted, in concert with others, as a politically motivated antagonist rather than an objective reporter. Kamola (2019) provides ten examples of 'right wing attacks' against academics from organisations, including but not limited to Campus Reform. As part of a more detailed discussion, which seeks to defend academic freedom, Kamola also offers an 'autopsy' of an episode initiated by Campus Reform that resulted in the victimisation of Johnny Williams, a Black Trinity College Professor. Campus Reform initially targeted Williams in 2017 for allegedly advocating for violence against White people. This high-profile story, which was subsequently discredited, followed a 'common script' (p. 3) used by right-wing media. The script not only aims to stoke outrage against professors deemed 'recklessly irresponsible and dangerous' but also 'generally discredit universities and colleges, painting them as places that shelter and enable deviant and socially unacceptable ideas' (p. 9). Such reporting has proven consequential. Just as Williams received threats of physical violence (death even) after right-wing media attention, academics like Thoune and her colleague, as noted above, have also been targeted with hate mail 'from the alt-right crowd' (Thoune, personal communication, 2020).

In sum, the above has provided context to Campus Reform's communicative practices, and why the Two Fat Professors were denounced therein. The remainder of this empirical section critically explores how readers of Dallmeyer's (2020) article were active participants in this theatre of cruelty. As will be observed, members' responses 'instructed' readers that fatness was shameful and deviant alongside other intersecting identities and practices such as: being a woman who looks and feels a certain way, being a feminist and having credentials in 'useless' or 'risible' academic disciplines (notably sociology and women's studies). Here, fatness became a peg to hang myriad grievances, ranging from suspicion that US universities host 'unreasonable' ideas to the charge that these allegedly inferior – rather than world-leading – institutions are responsible for the nation's declining hegemony.

Scrutinising readers' comments

Consider three comments, posted under Dallmeyer (2020). These words advanced a symbolic assault that was irreducible to any specific individual and fatness. Indeed, one may discern here a spiralling strategy, comprising foreboding meanings that gave cruel expression to shared anxieties about the US body politic. Stated differently, fat bodies were denigrated and then discarded by readers when constructing a particular vision of how the world should be. Infused with racist, sexist, ableist and nationalist ideology, the comments below also incorporate neoliberal tenets that extol personal responsibility for status, fitness and health:

> We live in a liberal dominated fictional world where no one is responsible for their status. Fat people, Africans, etc. are all relieved of their responsibility for their poor performance.
>
> *(gsh)*

Very fit guy here. Proud of it. And I LOATHE fat people. I wish they'd all just die. They use more resources, hospital stays are more expensive and they're just ugly and useless.

(j James)

Here we have a Dean of — wait for it — Diversity & Inclusion in the Med School ….and she's a virtual Laff Riot! https://campusreform.org/?i…

I'm guessing if we combine 'em…and let the cute D&I Dean do an interchange with the Fat 'Profs' (and I use that word loosely)…we could generate an entire 15 minute skit for Ye Olde Monty Python: Fat Shaming the Wuhan Virus is Racist & Dangerous Fat Phobia at the End of Time!

(bdavi52)

Based on several readings of the 135 comments, it was possible to discern three generic themes that captured the vast majority of the data: (i) size-ism/fatphobia, (ii) health fascism or meddling, and (iii) pedagogical gripes. Each theme consists of several subthemes or defining elements. These insights are summarised in Table 6.1, which is a heuristic device or second-order analytical construct for orienting to messy discursive terrain. Before discussing each of these themes in more detail, we will offer four general observations.

First, comments varied in length, ranging from one derogatory word, intended to dehumanise fat people, 'Oink!' (FreeManinAmerica), to a protracted response (227 words) that conceded 'Eating healthy can be somewhat challenging' but then dispensed highly moralising advice on diet and physical activity plus a religious injunction: 'don't forget' that '[g]luttony is a sin' (Higgs Boson). Other comments typically consisted of one or two sentences, usually comprising insults or grievances. Second, none of the comments directly engaged with Thoune (2020) and her core message. Rather, they were one stage removed, drawing from and filtered by Dallmeyer's (2020) story. Accordingly, comments such as the following emerged, which appear to be personalised but lack credence insofar as the author failed to establish certain publicly verifiable facts, notably Thoune's status as an English professor: 'Sociology is garbage. They are fat because they are physically lazy and have no will power. They are sociologists because they are intellectually lazy and could (*sic*) hack it in a real science' (sunny). Third, commentators often mixed elements for rhetorical effect. For example, size-ism was combined with health fascism, though the latter was not dependent on the former as seen in a comment that incredulously positioned those calling for compassion and kindness as such: 'Anyone who's traumatized by speech needs to take it up with a mental health practitioner and not act like a Nazi' (SGT). Fourth, a small minority of comments diverged from or contradicted the in-group's primary concern to pillory fat women academics and what they might symbolise. For example, after somebody expressed internalised weight-stigma, another replied: 'If your (*sic*) not setting fires or killing kids you're OK with me'

TABLE 6.1 Readers' Comments under Dallmeyer (2020)

Generic Themes	Defining Elements or Subthemes
Size-ism/fatphobia, intersecting with other forms of oppression	• Expressing internalised weight stigma or fatphobia • Ridiculing their targets' physical appearance (fatness), assumed character and ignorance • Discrediting fat people (mainly women) and 'body positivity' more generally via anti-fat jokes, sarcasm and expressed incredulity • Blanket vitriol directed at fat feminists and others who might challenge conservative agenda (liberals, socialists)
Health fascism or meddling	• Extolling one's own virtues as a fit person (man) and expressing disdain for those who allegedly deviate from healthist dictates and/or 'slim ideals' • Expressing apparent health concerns regarding the alleged medical dangers of obesity and connections to COVID-19 (also framed in Sinophobic terms) • Appeals to personal responsibility and appending individual blame onto shame for the putative problem of obesity/fatness (weaponising stigma) • Dispensing unsolicited lifestyle advice on diet and physical activity – weight-loss as a desirable and achievable goal for improving health • Rejecting victimhood and instructing the traumatised to consult a mental health professional rather than act like Nazis • Viewing fat people as costly on the healthcare system, American society and even the eco-system – a crime against humanity, requiring a punitive response • Wishing harm and even death on those deemed medically and intellectually 'unfit' • Explicitly nationalist concerns – anxieties about the fitness of the USA relative to other rising powers (China)
Pedagogical gripes	• Rejecting their targets' capacity to teach – their alleged indoctrination rather than education of young people, and at tax payers' expense • Attacking academic disciplines, notably literary studies, sociology and women's studies • Lamenting the state of US higher education and the 'scary' future it portends, especially in a competitive world-system

(Michael Sullivan). Another worried more about the US opioid crisis than obesity: 'Chemically enhanced lifestyles carry the real risk. Like overdosing or fatal dependency' (catapult). Although limited, 'deviant cases' should be noted in any credible thematic analysis.

Table 6.1 refers to size-ism/fatphobia, intersecting with other forms of oppression. Elements or subthemes range from internalised fatphobia to blanket vitriol towards feminists and others considered 'left of centre' on the political spectrum. Personal weight concerns are worth underscoring because they indicate that Thoune's (2020) troubles, if directly engaged with and recognised as public issues, could potentially resonate with Campus Reform's readers. Indeed, consider the possibility that few readers embody normative ideals of health: most of the US population is, after all, medically classed as overweight or obese. Consequently, securing 'distance' between the denouncer and the denounced, a necessary condition for a successful degradation ceremony (Garfinkel, 1956), might be viewed as an unsustainable fiction. In such a context, some commentators offered concessions albeit whilst reproducing the idea that fatness, framed as obesity, is undesirable. For instance: 'It's ok to be imperfect because that is all of us [and] obesity is a very hard way to live' (YrMum).

For Hamera (2019), anti-fat vitriol could prompt right-wing media supporters to reconsider their allegiances: the intense degradation of fatness therein could spoil their own identities and/or others whom they know and love. However, there is no evidence from this analysis that such concerns were to the fore. What did emerge, in line with other research on media audiences, was internalised weight stigma or 'anti-fat bias' (Holland et al., 2015: 439). Another commentator wrote: 'I have "fat phobia" whenever I look in the mirror and see a roll of it [fat] developing' (RealityCheck04). However, whilst some commentators admonished themselves for their own fatness and unhealthy lifestyles, they also turned their self-disdain towards fat studies professors and activists *whose standards of preference elevate pride over shame*. This observation does not undermine Hamera's (2019) point that attacking fatness, notably women's fatness, serves right-wing groups' affective investments. However, greater emphasis should perhaps be given to displayed attitudes to fatness rather than fatness per se – the 'sin' is to unapologetically accept adiposity rather than 'do contrition' by waging a quasi-religious 'war on obesity' (Monaghan, 2008). Accordingly, other commentators scoffed:

> LOL, you cannot make this stuff up. I almost feel bad for all the young people that fell for the whole body positivity movement and ar enow fat and in bad health. Oh well, good luck fatty.
>
> *(Esaelp_Aggin)*

Size-ism/fatphobia also intersected with other forms of oppression. Reference was made above to racism, ableism and sexism, though the latter was most apparent and leveraged for political ends. Whilst several commentators attacked feminists for being, in their estimation, 'ugly' another focused on the two fat professors and attributed their fatness to 'all the socialism and feminism they've ingested' (Sns_of_Lbrty). Arguably, the reference to various 'isms' here reveals more about this group's need to construct an imagined enemy against which to define itself rather than targeted professors' actual political views and affiliations.

Moving to health fascism and meddling, Table 6.1 lists various subthemes. Some have already been illustrated above with reference to data; for instance, the commentator who extolled their own healthist virtues in contradistinction to fat people who were wished dead (j James). Furthermore, whilst some dispensed unsolicited lifestyle advice in a somewhat patronising manner, others used COVID-19 as ammunition. In so doing, they also evidenced anxieties about the health and future of America: 'A very bad thing (one of dozens) about this virus is that one wishes it would wipe out these idiots, so that America itself can have a fighting chance to stop committing suicide' (Don Reed). Others cited coronavirus whilst expressing Sinophobia, implying that even if one is not prejudiced against fat people there is an 'objective risk' emanating from China that needs to be reckoned: 'Fatophobe or not. If you're obese you're at greater risk of a terminal Wuhan virus outcome' (koz). After scoffing that 'proud fatties' inevitably suffer serious health problems, another mentioned hospitals under strain: 'it's gonna be tougher for them to find an ICU [Intensive Care Unit] bed these days' (Lamontyoubigdummy). Another ignored fatness but they conflated health with healthism, whilst also alleging ingratitude and assumed political allegiances: 'When a virus targets you, blame those trying to help, they must be liberals' (jgilman1). Consider some additional fascistic comments, infused with a 'couldn't-care-less' attitude, contempt and feigned superiority:

> Wu-Flu doesn't care about your boo-hoo, Professor screws-loose.
>
> *(Faiillia)*

> Sociology professors and Gender Studies professors really do not understand science and nature. COVID-19 will solve the problem. Do they think that COVID-19 cares about their feelings? Anyway, their unhealthy bodies will find out that obesity is not a social construct.
>
> *(failureofreality)*

The last extract, above, overlaps with the third generic theme, pedagogic gripes. This theme includes, inter alia, deriding academic disciplines that 'give' away – rather than award – doctorates. Again, readers' comments were not necessarily about two fat professors or fat people. Rather, they consisted of more generalised complaints about the social sciences, humanities, their practitioners and, as discussed further below, the very future of America:

> A PHD in gender studies? That is about as helpful as curb feelers on a baseball.
>
> *(attackslack)*

> Give someone a PhD in the Social 'Sciences'….double down if that degree
> is in Gender Women Black Latinx Studies….and you have pure, undiluted
> hilarity.
>
> *(bdavi52)*

Much in line with the broader tenor of Campus Reform, pedagogical gripes
extended to the perceived state of US higher education. Outrage was further
stoked if universities were funded by 'taxpayers who are picking up the bill for
them [educators] to spew their garbage' (chock). Such invective was directed at
many other unnamed professors, US universities and an unknown yet 'scary'
future: 'And these "professors" and hundreds of others are shaping young minds
that are to be the future of these United States. Scarier than any virus!' (L.
Hanselman). In short, Campus Reform's readers expressed fears for the national
body, a sacred entity that must be protected now and going forward. Such complaints might be read alongside recent scholarship on the enduring significance of
the nation-state and the rise of populism (Flew, 2020), or what Scambler (2020b:
147), in the UK, terms 'proto-fascistic populism' that is rooted in 'cultural nation-
alism/isolationism', 'identity politics' and 'white supremacism'.

Complaints about academic credibility, respectability and danger were recurrent in the readers' comments section. Consider a contradictory comment from
somebody self-presenting as a 'steadfast' parent who objected to 'PC indoctrination'. On the one hand, they boasted that two of their children successfully gradu-
ated, with two more about to enter higher education. On the other hand, they
complained that many professors (who, incidentally, set and grade exams) were
more interested in indoctrination rather than education. What is also striking here
is that despite enlightening their 'kids' to such 'crap', they did not publicly object
to them entering higher education and successfully completing their studies:

> Every parent with kids in college has a duty to ensure their kids are not
> sucked in by the crap that many professors spew. Talk to your kids. Don't let
> them be indoctrinated. I have 4 – two of whom have graduated and two of
> whom are about to start. I have been steadfast in my efforts to open their eyes
> and reject the PC indoctrination and it is working. Don't let your kids fall
> for this stuff.
>
> *(KSA63)*

As noted with reference to 'the future of these Unites States' (L.Hanselman), such
invective could be taken as an expression of, or proxy for, pervasive concerns
about declining US hegemony. Accordingly, commentators jumbled pedagogical
gripes with nationalist discourse that included tendencies towards health fascism
(illustrating the degree to which Table 6.1 is a heuristic device). In drawing the
analysis of these data to a close, consider a final thread on US imperial decline.
There is a discernible leap from a pedagogical complaint about 'professors like
this' to geopolitical concerns. In short, fatness was submerged under weightier

matters; it underlay a more 'alarming' problem, an imagined 'we' who were losing control and wasting time on trivia whilst a key geopolitical rival, China, conquered the world:

> With professors like this, it is easy to see why China will surpass/has surpassed America militarily and economically.
>
> *(Jewish Voice)*

> No, China has not surpassed the US in either regard. That is just fake news from the MSM [Mainstream Media].
>
> *(Reddog replying to Jewish Voice)*

> Better educate yourself on China's hegemony in Africa and South America. Not cool, and alarming. Quietly they gain control while we dither over finding toilet paper.
>
> *(Winter Tomato replying to Reddog)*

Discussion: from 'health crises' to the politics of cruelty

Campus Reform, an online right-wing student news platform that routinely attacks faculty (Hamera, 2019; Kamola, 2019), provides a case study of how fat studies professors risk vitriol amidst heightened concerns about public health. This study shows how the COVID-19/obesity dual crisis frame was cruelly marshalled for politicised ends, within a publishing context that is backed by 'big money' and antagonistic to social justice agenda. Consonant with Pausé et al.'s (2021) observations, this chapter is suggestive of the ways in which the COVID-19 pandemic response has provided fertile conditions for the *ongoing* degradation of fatness. The main focus was a media article, written by Dallmeyer (2020), and 135 readers' comments that spiralled from the denigration fat professors to US imperial decline. Accordingly, these communications were related to organisational premises and macro-social or political economic concerns. Analytically, the use of Garfinkel (1956) on degradation ceremonies is compatible with other literature comparing the COVID-19 outbreak to an ethnomethodological 'breaching experiment' that has thrown a spanner into the workings of a 'fractured society' (Scambler, 2020b). Indeed, early societal responses to and outcomes from COVID-19 – including but also going beyond providing a 'bonanza' for the billionaire-class (Collins et al., 2020) – have thrown into relief pre-existing tensions, fissures and extant health inequalities (Arber and Meadows, 2020). Amidst those changes Lupton (2020) alludes to in pandemic times, there is continuity. The latter includes the intense stigmatisation of and moralisation surrounding fatness as obesity, a symbol and crude proxy for bigger problems.

Such degradation evidently found quick expression following the COVID-19 outbreak, with digital media serving as an efficient channel for hate and abuse. Arguably, the acceleration of 'digital sociality' during the COVID-19 emergency

(Keleman Saxena and Johnson, 2020), a vector for 'epidemic' or 'pandemic psychology' (Strong, 1990; Chapter 8) amidst other declared crises (e.g. economic, interracial, geopolitical), could provide the conditions of possibility for intensified cruelty. Although unconvincing for those who do not share right-wing groups' standards of preference, such invective 'makes sense' within the cruel logics of a crudely dichotomising gendered, heterosexist imaginary that fabricates enemies to be neutralised. Within this foreboding digitally mediated landscape an ideally hard, strong and thrusting US superpower must avoid being 'weighed down' and rendered impotent by fat feminist professors, or, rather, what they represent when calling on the world to be a kinder or 'softer' place. Elsewhere, Hamera (2019), writing before COVID-19, conceptualises such vitriol as an 'accumulation strategy' (Harvey, 1998) or mechanism that has political and cultural, not just fiscal, significance. This view emerges from her analysis of populist media that 'agglomerate, then attack a wide range of other targets – most frequently feminist women and social justice activists – on the putatively obviously rational basis of "health" rather than consistent, aggressive misogyny' (Hamera, 2019: 154). Yet, as indicated above, this strategy is tied not only to misogyny or sexism, wrapped in 'health talk', but also to felt stigma, racism, ableism and other cruelties that proliferate in crisis times (Sponholz and Christofoletti, 2019).

Irreducible to any specific individual, the discrediting of fatness on Campus Reform became a vehicle for multiple grievances against a backdrop of declining US hegemony and already existing antagonisms. Here, putative health concerns, refracted through a reductionist biomedical lens and obesity discourse, enabled participants to express, in barely disguised form, cultural anxieties about national fitness and preparedness. This, we would add, is in a capitalist world-system wherein US dominance has long been in decline and, according to Wallerstein (2011), could end in the not-so-distant future. Yet, by using anti-fat invective as an accumulation strategy, *numerous contradictions emerged on Campus Reform*, exposing the Achilles heel of this political economic project and populist arena for the aggrieved.

Contradictions on Campus Reform not only included misleading and selective reporting that belied the platform's declared mission to accurately and objectively report on US higher education and (mis)conduct. More disturbingly, perhaps, Campus Reform did exactly what it condemns its targets for putatively doing, namely, *silencing* the concerns of those who typically have less power and influence within university hierarchies. Other problems noted above included: the use of symbolically violent imagery, Campus Reform's professed dependency on donations from its intended student audience despite backing from wealthy sponsors, ill-informed/hateful comments from readers and other contributors, and possible alienation of overweight/obese/fat readers who might feel especially vulnerable in the time of COVID-19. On the latter point, denouncers and denounced may have been more similar than different not only given the scale of the putative obesity crisis but also early reports in North America of widespread anxiety about coronavirus (Asmundson and Taylor, 2020; see also Chapter 8). The possibility (statistical probability) of an elective affinity emerging from shared embodied concerns was not directly investigated during this study. It is nonetheless worth acknowledging in an inequitable world where there is also likely to be a massive and widening gap in wealth and status between Campus Reform's biggest financial sponsors and the platform's intended student audience.

The degrading of bodies (women's fat bodies, bodies of knowledge, educational bodies) on Campus Reform is thus bigger than, whilst nonetheless grounded in, the flesh and its digital (de)construction. The above hopefully prompts questions that are also bigger than the competencies or otherwise of individual online media commentators, university faculty and (student) journalists. Amidst massive disruptions wrought in the wake of the COVID-19 pandemic, a big question concerns 'what sort of society are we heading towards?' This question is pertinent amidst claims from the United Nations chief that the COVID-19 pandemic has led to a 'tsunami of hate and xenophobia, scapegoating and scaremongering' (cited by Davidson, 2020), and already existing studies of how social media can be unsafe for academics researching oppressed and minority groups (Barlow and Awan, 2016). Arguably, attempts to discredit university faculty and what they symbolise (what they can be treated as crude proxies for in traumatic times) might be taken as a canary in the coalmine – a warning of worsening socio-cultural conditions and technologically mediated responses wherein embittered tribes ignore or attack other people's suffering and enact cruelties that are irreducible to a novel coronavirus. In furthering critique and supporting research on such matters, we will finish by briefly (re) connecting with scholarship on media and bodyweight, stigma, health fascism and the politics of cruelty. Whilst these reflections are theoretically informed it should also be stated that there are substantive issues, the surface of which has barely been scratched here, which also demand further empirical investigation. For example, to draw from Kivisto (2019) on political theology and cruelty, to what extent does White Christian nationalism influence Campus Reform and its supporters? Furthermore, if that line of investigation is deemed pertinent, how might a comparative historical sociology of religion and violence further critique (Collins, 1974)?

As explained in Chapter 2, there is mounting international literature on media and bodyweight (e.g. Holland et al., 2015; Hynnä and Kyrölä, 2019; Lupton, 2017). We have already reviewed core themes from literature on media and 'fat panic' (LeBesco, 2010), or what Raisborough (2016) terms a 'fat sensibility' that is reproduced through public pedagogy that 'teaches' audiences about the perils of 'excess' flesh. When undertaking research during and in the aftermath of COVID-19, insights from earlier media studies could provide a useful handle in this 'changed' context. For instance, reference was made above to research on media audiences who internalise and enact weight stigma or bias (Holland et al., 2015), an observation that extends to Campus Reform. Other noteworthy themes in existing literature range from how news media amplify anxieties, moral panic even, amidst pre-existing societal tensions (Campos et al., 2006), to the ways in which other media, including state-sponsored public health campaigns, enact 'pedagogies of disgust' (Lupton, 2015; Chapter 3). Indeed, Campus Reform could be viewed as one further medium for ethically suspect public pedagogy that compounds fatness as morally, viscerally and thus emotionally intolerable. Here Campus Reform is the antithesis, and even nemesis, of those 'body positivity blogs' explored by Hynnä and Kyrölä (2019: 1) that seek to 'open up spaces of comfort which can be radical for bodies accustomed to discomfort' (similarly, see Limatius, 2019). Yet, what is missing from existing media studies, apart from a focus on COVID-19 and its intersections with obesity discourse (understandable at the present juncture), are the ways in which declared public health crises can be layered and how corrosive psychosocial responses may be mutually reinforcing. When undertaking further research on media and fatness, the overlapping COVID-19 and obesity crises might offer a useful lens on public pedagogies, conceptualised as status degradation ceremonies enacted in broader political economic context. Interesting lines of investigation may also be pursued here in view of Flew's (2020) advice to media studies scholars not to underestimate the nation-state and 'the challenge of populism'.

As part of that endeavour, lessons might also be gleaned from Edgley and Brissett (1999) on 'meddling'. Unfortunately, meddling has proliferated in twenty-first-century, digitally mediated, society, and it could accelerate in pandemic times following government invitations to everybody to become public health advisors and informants (for example, on 'snitching' in the Canadian context, see Urquhart, 2020). Somewhat disturbingly, meddling is framed as being not only of personal but also of broader societal benefit in a manner that echoes the Nazi regime's prioritisation of the commonweal. As Edgley and Brissett (1999) remind us, meddling should not simply be equated with the honest and benevolent actions of altruistic people who are concerned for their fellow citizens. Going forward, and in taking lessons from the present study, it would be useful to return to Edgley and Brissett's work and mine it for further insights. No doubt, many parallels could be drawn with earlier crusades waged in the name of 'health' and which have 'legitimated' all manner of unwelcome and harmful intrusions (e.g. intensive surveillance, curtailment of everyday freedoms, ridiculing and censoring dissenting views, destroying livelihoods and lives, disciplining and punishing the recalcitrant). As per Campus Reform, responses to 'health matters' in the time of COVID-19 are not necessarily grounded in concerns for the well-being of people traumatised in/by society.

The above fits well, perhaps somewhat disturbingly too well, with recent literature on the politics of cruelty. Amidst the resurgence of fascism, right-wing populism and attacks on liberal democracy in the USA, Kivisto (2019) reflects critically on the Trump presidency. Reference is made to authoritarianism, nationalism, 'deliberate state-sponsored cruelty' (e.g. the removal of over 2,000 children from their parents at the US-Mexico border) (p. 192) but also voter appeal. Although only a minority of the US population voted for Trump in 2017, his success has to be placed in the context of globalisation and attendant White, nationalist anxiety. This is a world wherein relatively privileged citizens fear losing status to minorities whom they believe have been making gains in recent years. It is understandable why, in this politically divided and affective context, the vitriol expressed on Campus Reform was not confined to 'fat women' and 'the obese' but also extended to racialised others and those advocating for social justice more generally. By reflecting on how such cruelty emerges from the body politic and embodied crises, researchers will be better able to interrogate how stigma is not simply a micro-social process. Rather, it is weaponised, notably via the heaping of blame onto shame, in order to serve powerful and well-funded interests within capitalist society (Scambler, 2018; for recent discussion that connects 'the stigma system' to scapegoating, as a divide-and-rule strategy that serves elites whilst negatively impacting public health, see Friedman et al., 2022).

Finally, it should be stressed that this analysis does not presume universities are beyond reproach and there is no axe to grind with respect to higher education, within and beyond the USA. Much about university life is unpalatable. Whilst Gill (2009) poignantly broke the silence on 'the hidden injuries of neoliberal academia' over a decade ago, others have since discussed, for example, the stigmatisation of marginalised bodies within contexts of teaching, learning, research and career progression (Reidinger, 2020). Moreover, already existing 'rationalising' practices in neoliberal universities are likely to be intensified following the economic fallout from the COVID-19 pandemic (for emerging insights, see Gilbert, 2021), compounded by contractual arrangements with finance capital (Connelly, 2020) and the spectre of a 'shock doctrine' response from right-wing governments (Klein, 2020). Indeed, it is reasonable to infer that pre-existing market-oriented tendencies will prevail and in ways that threaten academic disciplines and freedoms, especially if scholars challenge extant power relations. Amidst established trends such as the use of commercial banks (e.g. leveraged financial covenants that transfer macro-economic risk to universities; see Connelly, 2020), escalating student debt, precarious academic contracts, institutionalised distrust of faculty, autocratic management and the opening of university campuses to myriad private profit-making interests, the agenda favoured by Campus Reform's billionaire sponsors could proceed unabated. A possible clarion call from 'big money' – and those university administrators who have staged a coup at the expense of faculty (Ginsberg, 2011; Graeber, 2019) – goes like this: 'universities cannot afford to support dangerous or unreasonable ideas given that public health, and, indeed, the health of the body politic, is under threat. Health must be protected as a matter of national and global biosecurity'. However, if anything has been learnt from this analysis and from public intellectuals such as Thoune (2020), who are willing to express their own vulnerabilities, it is this: there is an urgent need for alternative approaches to pedagogy, politics and public health that are *for*, rather than *against*, people. In so doing, we need to pay heed to canaries in the coalmine and amplify, rather than ignore, their calls for compassion, kindness *and* shared hope in pandemic times. Such calls provide a basis for our discussion in Part 3 of this book.

PART 3

Critically exploring alternatives, fostering collective hope

7

TIRED OF DIETS?

From HAES® to a more radical approach

Tired of diet pitches on TV? In magazines? In your spam filter and now your inbox? If anyone would prefer to pursue an endeavour that *doesn't* fail 95% of the time, I would be delighted to facilitate a 'Health At Every Size' group at MMC [Manhattan Marymount College]. It costs nothing. Weekly topics would cover healthy living in the context of social stigma, pursuing an agenda of true body diversity, understanding that thinness and health are not the same thing, and resisting specious arguments about the efficacy of dieting. Let me know if you're interested!

(LeBesco, 2010: 79)

The above message was sent via email by 'a longtime theorist of fat politics' (p. 78) to her campus community after Weight Watchers tried to sell its programme to employees at $168 per head. Efforts to promote and profit from dieting on college campuses are unsurprising. They accord with the premises of the WCHP and broader entrepreneurial moves and policy initiatives to 'tackle obesity' in the workplace (OECD, 2017: 8), with or without supporting evidence and workers' informed consent. Despite the shaky foundations of the anti-obesity offensive, previous chapters explained that weight science, popular media, educators, policy and public health give overriding emphasis to a 'problem frame' (Saguy, 2013) wherein 'fat is fatal' (Kwan and Graves, 2013). However, according to this dominant obesity discourse, redemption is possible via behavioural change, comprising modified lifestyles and exercising 'better choices' (Chapter 3). Whether this project is enacted through pedagogies of disgust, shame and blame in various media (Lupton, 2015; Raisborough, 2016), seemingly benign 'communication policies that promote healthy diets by improving health literacy' (OECD, 2017: 8), or 'nudging' people in that direction via environmental reform (Bombak, 2014c), the central message is clear: 'excess' weight/fatness must be combatted.

DOI: 10.4324/9781315658087-11

And, as explored earlier in this book, the declaration of the COVID-19 pandemic in 2020 hardly detracted from such concerns, especially in the context of mass lockdowns (Chapter 6).

Insofar as mounting research places a serious question mark over weight-loss interventions and the WCHP more generally (e.g. Aphramor, 2005; Bacon and Aphramor, 2011, 2014; Bombak et al., 2020; Calogero et al., 2019; Gaesser, 2009; Mann et al., 2007; O'Hara and Taylor, 2014, 2018; Rothblum, 2018), it is important to critically explore alternatives. Indeed, this is imperative insofar as previous chapters have referred to 'the social justice frame' (Kwan and Graves, 2013) and critical interventions, including the appeal of and ambivalences towards HAES among women self-identifying as obese and for whom dietary approaches to weight-loss (hereafter dieting) were often 'ill-fated' (Kassirer and Angell, 1998; Chapter 4).

After first questioning common weight-loss prescriptions, we will explicate HAES in social context. This weight-inclusive paradigm is currently the most well-known alternative to the war on obesity that is filtering into mainstream discourse whilst also becoming increasingly factious. This chapter focuses on principles, tensions, resonance and controversies within HAES. When discussing HAES and pointing towards more radical proposals we will also return to a key theme from Part 1 of our book: the politics of health and the need to rethink obesity in a broader social context. This discussion, by necessity, takes us to the wider implications of obesity discourse and critical weight studies in a world wherein health behaviours are indebted to and secondary to social structures and power relations. Finally, when discussing behavioural approaches to weight-loss and/or promoting health we limit our discussion to non-surgical interventions. Whilst social research on weight-loss surgery is growing (see Chapter 2) our focus here is on mundane (everyday) behavioural prescriptions, especially dietary approaches to weight-loss.

Questioning weight-loss prescriptions: from inappropriateness to possible dangers

> Promoting weight loss through exercise, dietary restriction, and behavior modification rarely succeeds. It often results in cycles of weight loss and gain, with the potential for serious physical and psychological health risks, and contributes to body hatred, dangerous eating disorders, and exercise addiction. Yet we believe that if we continue to use the same approaches, we will somehow obtain different results. Indeed, this is the definition of insanity put forth by Alcoholics Anonymous.
>
> *(Robison, 2005: 13)*

Robison's (2005) evaluation is hardly new. Writing over a half a century ago, Stunkard (1958) observed that efforts to promote weight-loss among people defined as obese were largely ineffective, if not counterproductive. Since then, mounting critical evidence has continued to challenge the soundness and ethics of instructing people to improve their health by losing weight (e.g. Aphramor, 2005, 2010; Campos et al., 2006; Cyr and Riediger, 2021; Mann et al., 2007; Rothblum, 2018; see also Table 7.1). For instance, following our review of 'obesity paradox' research (Chapter 2), it seems highly inappropriate – if not dangerous – to advise patients with cardiovascular disease to lose weight (Doehner et al., 2015). One might also question the need to advise the overweight and moderately obese, who generally enjoy relatively good life expectancy, to try and improve their longevity by getting to a 'normal weight' (Flegal et al., 2013). These clinical and epidemiological objections could also be expanded upon with reference to a history of colonialism, enforced starvation and collective trauma, as explained by Cyr and Riediger (2021) when using a feminist Indigenous lens to critique weight-centric public health interventions in Canada.

Whilst there are grounds to rethink and, indeed, reject weight-loss prescriptions, these are invariably presented as the 'solution' to the presumed dangers of having a BMI ≥25 kg/m². Tenets of the WCHP that pertain specifically to weight-loss and gain, as outlined in our book's introduction, include: changes in body weight can simply be attributed to energy in/out, there is a volitional component to weight, everybody should be weight-conscious and losing body weight is beneficial for the overweight and obese (O'Hara and Taylor, 2018). This weight-centric view dominates scientific, popular media, policy and lay discourse regardless of the fact that even medics do not necessarily agree with it. For instance, shortly after the Christmas festivities, when many Americans would likely feel guilty for 'overindulging', an editorial in the *New England Journal of Medicine* describes weight-loss as 'an ill-fated New Year's resolution' (Kassirer and Angell, 1998). The authors note the general ineffectiveness of calorie restriction, wasted money, negative emotions and other harms (including the potentially fatal consequences of taking prescribed diet drugs, which, we would add, have been

TABLE 7.1 Reasons to Question or Reject Weight-Loss Injunctions

- Accumulating critical evidence on mortality risk and survival outcomes associated with 'excess' (*sic*) weight (e.g. so-called obesity paradox research)
- Methodological issues with clinical weight-loss trials (e.g. attrition, measurement of weight and follow-up) and the epidemiology of weight (loss) at the population level
- Sixty years of evidence on the general ineffectiveness of weight-loss programmes
- Minimal evidence on the presumed benefits
- Substantial evidence of physical and mental health risks
- Risky 'therapies' intended to treat problems associated with dieting
- Wasted time and money
- Recognising 'bigger' problems: macro-social injustices against those who have historically been traumatised through starvation (e.g. young women, Indigenous people)

recurrent and have cast a dark shadow over the pharmaceutical industry; note, for example, the scandal in France over Mediator; Chrisafis, 2013; BBC News, 2021). Yet, rather than the public health establishment, governments and mass media taking heed, the war on obesity intensified post-2000 (Campos, 2004; Gard and Wright, 2005; Greenhalgh, 2015; Monaghan, 2008).

Following Robison (2005) it is tempting to psychologise the intensification of this war. Other critics appear to take a similar tack. Rothblum (2018), for instance, even challenges psychologists when stating how over half a century of critical evidence seldom registers with these professionals, despite their training on 'confirmation bias' (p. 66). This concept refers to how people filter out evidence that contradicts their pre-existing beliefs. We would, however, favour a sociological reading with reference to underlying social structures and processes that could include, for example, class-related tendencies, evaluative rules and symbolic control generated by 'the pedagogic device' (Bernstein, 2000; Chapter 3). Other useful literature points to 'strategic ignorance', which is integral to power relations in myriad domains but which does not bode well for science and democracy (McGoey, 2019). Whilst fat studies scholars, activists and others object to the oppressive consequences of such 'bias' for 'fat people' (Cooper, 2016a) and Indigenous populations (Cyr and Riediger, 2021), this problem is more expansive. Even if we bracket macro-social issues for the time being, the strategic neglect of physiological, psychological and behavioural evidence among obesity epidemic entrepreneurs seems hard to justify. Consider evidence on the dangers of weight-cycling or fluctuation. Drawing from Montani et al. (2006) and population-based studies, the PHSA (2013: 18) note myriad risks that are, among other things, highly gendered:

> [I]ncreased cardiovascular risks due to physiological changes associated with weight cycling, including insulin resistance and dyslipidemia. Fluctuations in blood pressure, heart rate, sympathetic activity, glomerular filtration rate, blood glucose and lipids that may occur during weight cycling place additional load on the cardiovascular system, particularly when repeated over time. Researchers also observed that weight cycling doesn't only affect people with obesity; rather, it also affects those of normal weight, particularly young women who diet. There is concern that the increasing incidence of weight cycling among girls and young women, at ever-younger ages, is likely to become a serious public health problem.

In a related vein, Aphramor (2010: 6–7) cites the British Nutrition Foundation (1999), further indicating that concerns about adverse effects of weight fluctuation span several decades:

> [A] positive association has consistently been observed between body weight fluctuation and all cause mortality and usually ... with coronary mortality in particular. This finding is very robust, further confirmation is found in the

British Regional Heart Study (Wannamethee & Shaper, 1990), in the Seven Nations Study (Peters et al., 1995) and in the Iowa Women's Health Study (French et al., 1997) (p. 137).

In light of such evidence, it is easy to appreciate why Calogero et al. (2019: 25) state that 'the prescription to "lose weight" is not realistic, meaningful, or justified'.

The need for a 'balanced' or 'wide-eyed' appraisal of the evidence

Whilst we will highlight various problems with common weight-loss prescriptions, as noted in Chapter 2 we remain conscious of possible misrecognition. Lest we are accused of simply underscoring negatives, as part of a fraught 'framing contest' (Saguy and Riley, 2005), it is worth stressing that we are not 'half-closing' (Gard, 2013: 108) our eyes when reviewing evidence (similarly, on the use of an ocular metaphor and synthesising ways of seeing, refer to Cyr and Riediger, 2021; Monaghan et al., 2018). Even though weight-loss is commonly prescribed and embraced (especially by individuals affected by stigma and successfully losing weight *in the short-term*: Chapter 4), evidence of medium- to long-term benefits is lacking.

One immediate issue is the actual state of knowledge. Whilst public health discourses claim '[s]ignificant long-term weight-loss is a practical goal, and will improve health', Campos et al. (2006: 57) state this is 'an untested hypothesis'. More recently, Calogero et al. (2019: 26–7) write: 'Publication bias as well as outcome reporting bias cloud our ability to judge available data. However, what the available data do show is that long-term weight loss is not possible or sustainable for the vast majority of people'. Citing clinical weight-loss trials, Rothblum (2018: 64) discusses three main methodological issues: 'very high attrition' rates, minimal weight-loss among participants and 'weight regain at follow up'. Hence, the feasibility and biomedical benefits of weight-loss are not conclusively supported by the same positivist forms of knowledge used to assign health risks to obesity, and other positivist research suggests that presumed health benefits are minimal (Mann et al., 2007; Tomiyama et al., 2013). Assumed population-level benefits are also contested – significant numbers of people have simply not been made thin given homeostatic pressures to regain weight (Campos et al., 2006; MacLean et al., 2011; Mann et al., 2007; Schwartz et al., 2017) – and any benefits experienced by individuals in clinical studies are not 'dose'-dependent. Furthermore, benefits such as lower medication use and reduced diabetes or hypertension incidence in intervention studies are difficult to disentangle from the physical activity and dietary changes that might produce (some) weight-loss (Mann et al., 2007; Tomiyama et al., 2013).

A counter-response is that 'surely some weight-loss is beneficial, especially for problems like type 2 diabetes or diabesity?' Notwithstanding what we have already written in Chapter 2 when reviewing obesity science, it is worth returning to diabetes as a justification for recommending weight-loss or management (also Aphramor, 2010; O'Hara and Taylor, 2018). The Diabetes Prevention

Program (DPP) is long touted as the study indicating that moderate weight-loss (5–10 per cent) can prevent diabetes and reduce cardiovascular disease risk (DPP Research Group, 2002, 2009; Hamman et al., 2006; Orchard et al., 2013). However, important nuances of the study's results are often missing in blanket statements about the trial's effectiveness. All participants were already considered pre-diabetic (i.e. defined as at high risk of developing type 2 diabetes), apart from American Indian participants who were deemed 'high risk' due to heritage. Again, these inclusion criteria mean that results may not be generalisable at the population level. Certainly, weight-loss was the dominant factor in reducing diabetes risk during the DPP trial; however, meeting physical activity goals also led to reductions in diabetes incidence, independent of weight-loss (Hamman et al., 2006). Critically, on average participants regained most of their lost weight (DPP Research Group, 2009). Increased weight-loss was associated with heightened diabetes risk during the Diabetes Prevention Program Observational Study – the long-term study of DPP participants (Perreault et al., 2012). As reported therein, this risk may have been the result of weight regain. Ultimately, these findings suggest the most beneficial and risk-free approach to diabetes prevention may be through physical activity whilst maintaining a stable weight (including a stable higher weight that medicine deems 'excessive') (see also Gaesser, 2002). Despite the above, findings from the DPP now serve as irrefutable 'truths'. Diabetes intervention trials that produce contrary, mixed or more nuanced results are interpreted to ensure weight remains linked (albeit through unclear mechanisms) to diabetes. Accordingly, and in line with the WCHP, weight-loss persists as the key focus for interventions by attributing trials' 'poor results' to methodological issues, or patient non-adherence and equivocating results (Bombak et al., 2020; Riediger et al., 2018).

Other studies, which attempt to discern the benefits of weight-loss, also deserve critical review. Interestingly, epidemiological studies often rely on surrogate end-point measures, not health-relevant endpoints. Altering these far more critical endpoints through weight-loss remains elusive. The problematic reliance on the use of surrogate measures is illustrated in the Action for Health for Diabetes (Look AHEAD) study (Gregg et al., 2012). This very large and long-running trial was funded by the US National Institutes of Health to ascertain whether intentional weight-loss in persons with diabetes would produce a decrease in cardiovascular events, actual endpoints that matter for people's health, such as stroke, myocardial infarction and mortality. Despite reductions in risk factors for cardiovascular disease, cardiovascular events were not reduced and few individuals experienced sustained diabetes remission (Gregg et al., 2012). That is, weight-loss did not save lives nor spare individuals from heart attacks and strokes. These disappointing results led to the trial being halted early and debate among researchers over whether the trial constituted a success or failure (Bombak, 2014b).

The findings from Look AHEAD align well with other studies on mortality and weight-loss. For metabolically healthy persons classified as obese, it seems that the most beneficial course of action is to maintain a stable weight, not to lose weight, which might increase mortality risk (Bosomworth, 2012). This has important implications for the health of larger persons given the pervasiveness of dieting and the high likelihood of weight-cycling, which, as noted above, might have independent and significant adverse effects on health (Aphramor, 2005; Rothblum, 2018). In the USA, 45 per cent of obese respondents in the nationally representative 2005–2012 National Health and Nutrition Examination Survey were found to be metabolically healthy, and 31 per cent of normal weight adults did not meet these criteria (Tomiyama et al., 2016). Therefore, advocating weight-loss for all persons labelled obese may not lead to health gains and may be harmful in some instances.

Additional problems with weight-loss prescriptions

Instructing individuals and populations to slim down has been accompanied by a long list of possible or actual problems. Aside from reproducing stigma, such prescriptions could 'nudge' people towards weight-cycling. Whilst results remain mixed (Mehta et al., 2014), weight-cycling has been found in some studies to be associated with hypertension, diabetes, depressive symptomology, endometrial cancer, cardiovascular disease, cardiovascular disease mortality and all-cause mortality (Delahanty et al., 2014; Madigan et al., 2018; Schulz et al., 2005; X. Zhang et al., 2019b; Zou et al., 2019, 2021), although not all findings held true for all weight classes (e.g. Zou et al., 2019, 2021). Other reported problems with attempted weight-loss include: low mood, loss of bone density and lean mass, compromised immunity and skeletal integrity, poor body image and the release of persistent organic pollutants into the body (Aphramor, 2005; Bacon and Aphramor, 2011; Beavers et al., 2011; Delahanty et al., 2014; Schulz et al., 2005; Villalon et al., 2011). Recent clinical evidence associating low muscle mass with 'several negative outcomes across the healthcare continuum' (Prado et al., 2018: 675) is also worth highlighting given the emphasis upon rapid *weight*-loss within rationalised, or McDonaldized (Ritzer, 2010), diet cultures (Monaghan, 2007a, 2008). Green and Buckroyd (2008) and Burns and Gavey (2004) also recount the congruence between weight-loss groups' and health promotion strategies and disordered eating. This is disturbing in view of the symbolic and economic capital enjoyed by organisations such as Weight Watchers when reproducing a 'problem frame' (Saguy, 2013; Chapter 1).

As with the reference to commercial weight-loss clubs, it is salutary to ground observations in organisational context and to do so across the lifecourse. Following what we reported in Chapter 5, evidence suggests school obesity prevention policies, programmes and pedagogies are implicated in disordered eating among students (Beausoleil, 2009; C.S. Mott Children's Hospital, 2012; Evans et al., 2004, 2008; Isono et al., 2009; Rich and Evans, 2009; Rich et al., 2004). Furthermore, the effectiveness of these childhood campaigns in achieving their stated aims has been questioned (Gard and Vander Schee, 2011; Rothblum, 2018). For example, well-publicised 'BMI report cards', a school-based strategy to 'combat obesity' in the USA, have not produced thinner children (Almond et al., 2016). Ethnographic research undertaken in an English college among teenage boys (Monaghan, 2014a) also indicates that anti-obesity interventions proceed even when most participants do not need to lose weight and negative unintended consequences, or collateral damage, include peer group bullying.

Whilst advocates of public health, without any sense of contradiction, sometimes cite the problem of bullying and associated poor self-esteem as a rationale for tackling obesity, it is worth underscoring the point that the purported benefits of weight-loss do not necessarily extend to well-being (Warkentin et al., 2014). Indeed, relatively high levels of depressive symptomology and stress characterise some clusters of sustained weight losers (Ogden et al., 2012). Individuals who do lose weight for a sustained period of time and are members of the US-based National Weight Control Registry (see Gaesser, 2009) report major lifestyle alterations, including: regular exercise, the consumption of low-fat diets with an average caloric consumption of 1381 kcal/day, and hyper-vigilance regarding food and weight (Wing and Hill, 2001). Some reported strategies to fight fat are decidedly less 'healthy', such as skipping meals (Ogden et al., 2012). Such tactics are nonetheless evidenced among people whose identities are colonised by the mantra of 'eat less' and 'exercise more' in a not-always-successful attempt to become a virtuous weight-loss champion (Bombak, 2015). Notably, many individuals from studies of the US National Weight Control Registry have not necessarily 'cracked' the coveted 'normal' BMI category but remain categorised as overweight or obese (Ogden et al., 2012; Wing and Hill, 2001). Rothblum (2018), citing methodological issues, offers an interesting critique here. She states that weight-loss programmes reporting 'success' employ criteria that would not be accepted in other interventions, such as those focused on anxiety disorders, depression, substance use and cigarette smoking. Smoking cessation programmes, for instance, measure success in terms of whether people quit the habit, rather than reducing the number of cigarettes smoked. In contrast, weight-loss programmes measure success in incremental terms (pounds lost) rather than whether participants' BMI went to 'normal'.

Alarmingly, and in reflecting tendencies towards 'health and body fascism' (Edgley and Brissett, 1990; Chapter 6), a shift may be occurring where everyone in supposedly 'fat nations' is simply encouraged to lose weight (similarly, see Chapter 8 with reference to recent UK anti-obesity policy and preparedness for further 'waves' of COVID-19). Greenhalgh (2015), for example, quotes a former US Health and Human Services secretary who asserted, 'All Americans should lose ten pounds as a patriotic gesture' (p. 19). This is a potent example of 'anorexic ideation' as described by Campos (2004: 147–9). Anorexic ideation valorises behaviours that would otherwise be deemed pathological. In the war on obesity, methods that might be considered counterproductive, unhealthy or dangerous – in short, 'ill-fated' (Kassirer and Angell, 1998) – have become commonplace or normalised. Even for people in 'normal weight' categories, questionable practices such as intermittent energy restriction (Harvie and Howell, 2017) and daily weighing (Wing et al., 2016) are becoming acceptable. Here, disturbing connections, contradictions and paradoxes emerge vis-à-vis putative medical 'conditions' such as *orthorexia* (obsession with eating healthy foods), *anorexia athletica* (compulsive over-exercising) and other restrictions on food intake. Yet, the visibly fat appear to be especially burdened in a culture that stereotypes them as morally bankrupt and failing to try hard enough to lose weight. In such a context, some researchers have analysed the discrepancy that exists within eating disorder literature when discussing body weight attitudes and weight control measures. As Gotovac et al. (2020: 126) state, 'why is an eating disorder in a thin person now a health behavior in a fat person?' Drawing from Burgard (2009), Calogero et al. (2019: 27) use the words 'hypocrisy and morally abhorrent' when stating 'the Weight Normative approach prescribes eating and weight-control practices for fat people that would warrant a diagnosis of an eating disorder in thin people'. Furthermore, risky medical 'therapies' intended to counteract problems associated with dieting are emerging, notably sex-specific drug regimens that have been discredited by other branches of medicine. For example, endocrinologists, supported by Australia's National Health and Medical Research Council and pharmaceutical industry, have administered synthetic testosterone to men in order to counteract muscle depletion caused by restrictive dieting (Ng Tang Fui et al., 2016). Yet, administering testosterone is widely condemned as steroid abuse and regarded by clinicians as symptomatic of a psychiatric disorder, muscle dysmorphia, when undertaken by bodybuilders and other gym enthusiasts for the same purpose (Keane, 2005; Monaghan, 2001, 2009).

Explicating HAES in social context

Given the above controversies, contradictions and concerns, there are justifiable grounds for proposing alternatives to the WCHP. Offering a critical appreciation of what is perhaps the most well-known 'size acceptance' health paradigm, HAES, the remainder of this chapter discusses: (i) HAES as a 'healthy lifestyle' intervention, (ii) studies of HAES interventions and reported (moderated) efficacy, (iii) the resonance and challenges of societal fat acceptance, and (iv) controversies, fractures and inconsistencies within and beyond HAES. This discussion, in addition to presenting readers with a map of HAES and a means of critically orienting to the paradigm, provides a point of departure for Chapter 8 and the book's epilogue on possible ways forward in these crisis times.

HAES as a 'healthy lifestyle' intervention

This chapter offered an immediate taste of HAES as communicated by LeBesco (2010) to her campus community. Responding to a 'Weight Watchers @ Work' group email sent by the college's Human Resources department, LeBesco describes HAES as 'my axe' to 'chop away at the links between fatness and ill health that exist in so many minds' – a fitting response because 'People want to be healthy, and who can blame them?' (p. 79). For HAES advocates, health indicators, predictors and practices are irreducible to weight or the BMI. Bacon (2006), for instance, states: 'health habits are more important than the scale'. And, as explained by Calogero et al. (2019: 33), who positively appraise HAES for therapists:

> The HAES model rejects weight and BMI as indicators of health and emphasizes access to holistic non-stigmatizing healthcare and self-care as sustainable predictors of health, wellness, and empowerment.

The HAES movement has antecedents in fat activists' accounts of 'dismal' health-care in the early 1970s (Cooper, 2016a: 176). In a related vein, LeBesco (2010: 78) describes HAES as an 'on-the-ground movement born out of frustration with traditional biomedical perspectives on health that pathologize fatness'. The move-ment basically argues for a weight-inclusive or weight-neutral, self-care-centric model of health promotion that is 'salutogenic' (O'Hara and Taylor, 2014: 272); i.e. it is geared towards factors that support health and well-being (see also Bombak, 2014a; Aphramor, 2005). Although HAES advocates recognise the importance of decent formal healthcare (a problem for many people in privatised systems, exemplified in the USA), their focus is typically directed at so-called intuitive and healthy eating, size acceptance and enjoyable physical activity (Bacon, 2006, 2010; Burgard, 2009; Robison, 2005). When reviewing HAES, Aphramor (2016: 2, our emphasis) states that it is 'primarily concerned with a (1) critical appraisal of weight science within the parameters of its usefulness *as a lifestyle change model*, (2) offering a non-diet alternative, and (3) challenging fat stigma'. For Gingras and Cooper (2013), what is or is not HAES is debatable; there is disagreement and contestation over who has the authority to define it and the attendant positioning of insiders/outsiders. However, for the ASDAH (2013) – which trademarked HAES in 2010 and which presents itself as 'a leading voice in the international HAES commu-nity' – there are five main principles (see Table 7.2).

In short, HAES promotes size acceptance over dieting as a route to health and well-being. When endorsing this, practitioners invoke the concept of 'intui-tive eating' (Bacon et al., 2005), with individuals urged to follow *internal* cues of hunger and satiety, rather than relying on *external* cues to either restrict caloric consumption or eat to excess. Here advocates cite, inter alia, research conducted on toddlers which found that, when allowed to eat from an assortment of nutri-tious foods, children would self-compensate and eat roughly the same amount of calories and macronutrients over a 24-hour period for six days, despite exhibiting considerable variation in consumption over the short term (Birch et al., 1991; Scheindlin, 2005; for a systematic review of research on 'intuitive eating' among women, including favourable psychosocial correlates and certain limitations with existing cross-sectional studies, see Bruce and Ricciardelli, 2016). HAES prac-titioners, as explained by Saguy and Riley (2005) with reference to 'framing contests', also invoke 'set-point theory' in an effort to neutralise the assumption

TABLE 7.2 HAES® Principles, as Defined by the ASDAH

1. **Weight Inclusivity**: Accept and respect the inherent diversity of body shapes and sizes and reject the idealizing or pathologizing of specific weights.
2. **Health Enhancement**: Support health policies that improve and equalize access to information and services, and personal practices that improve human well-being, including attention to individual physical, economic, social, spiritual, emotional, and other needs.
3. **Respectful Care**: Acknowledge our biases, and work to end weight discrimination, weight stigma, and weight bias. Provide information and services from an understanding that socio-economic status, race, gender, sexual orientation, age, and other identities impact weight stigma, and support environments that address these inequities.
4. **Eating for Well-being**: Promote flexible, individualized eating based on hunger, satiety, nutritional needs, and pleasure, rather than any externally regulated eating plan focused on weight control.
5. **Life-Enhancing Movement**: Support physical activities that allow people of all sizes, abilities, and interests to engage in enjoyable movement, to the degree that they choose.

that weight is entirely under personal control. Set-point theory posits that individuals will return to within a particular weight range, regardless of attempts to modify size (Bacon, 2010; Bacon and Aphramor, 2014), though there are counter-responses (Lupton, 2012, 2018; Saguy and Riley, 2005). For example, one argument is that regular exercise may reduce set-points. None of this necessarily means everybody is at a weight that is appropriate for them, though there is a rejection of rationalised, reductionist measures and proxies for health. Robison (2005: 13), advocating HAES for a medical audience, explains this as such:

> The HAES philosophy promotes the concept that an appropriate, healthy weight for an individual cannot be determined by the numbers on a scale, by a height/weight chart, or by calculating body mass index or body fat percentages. Rather, HAES defines a 'healthy weight' as the weight at which a person settles as they move toward a more fulfilling and meaningful lifestyle. This includes, but is not limited to, eating according to internally directed signals of hunger, appetite, and satiety and participating in reasonable and sustainable levels of physical activity.

Taken together, the above indicates that HAES proponents endorse a lifestyle model of health that aims to be more holistic than the WCHP and is respectful of 'natural' bodily diversity, needs and pleasures. Whilst the division between nature and culture and other dichotomies (e.g. mind/body, internal/external, biology/society) is justifiably challenged within the sociologies of embodiment (Williams and Bendelow, 1998), food and eating (Lupton, 1996), it is worth noting that the HAES emphasis on health and personal behaviours has also been critiqued (Brady et al., 2013; LeBesco, 2010). This point is worth underscoring not least given the problem of 'lifestyle drift' (Popay et al., 2010), discussed in

Chapter 3. One crucial concern is that HAES arguably continues to support pedagogies championing individualist behaviour change to the relative neglect of broader social factors; or, at least, it fosters tendencies that reproduce health as a super-value and index of moral worth, as part of an ultimately politically conservative and self-responsibilising project (Aphramor, 2016). For instance, Calogero et al. (2019: 36) endorse size activism and social justice, but they also favour the development of 'intuitive eating skills' by 'clients' so that they 'enable themselves to care for themselves as lovingly as they can'. We will return to a more politicised critique after outlining HAES interventions and reported efficacy as moderated by stigma.

HAES interventions and reported (moderated) efficacy

Two caveats are immediately in order. First, because HAES emerged outside of formal research contexts and is underfunded (relative to research undertaken within the WCHP), evidence on its efficacy is underdeveloped; for example, the studies cited below are adult-centric (though, for a recent contribution within adolescent healthcare, see Raffoul and Williams, 2021). Second, objections have recently been made not only about the ethics of weight-loss interventions but also about the problems of relying on ethically approved academic research trials wherein participants are divided into a 'conventional slimming intervention' (which is harmful) and an alternative, such as HAES (Aphramor, 2020b). Pointing to the hypocrisy and harms associated with these randomised control trials, Aphramor, to whom we will return, urges readers to reflect on the ethics of their citation practices.

Recognising such concerns, we tread lightly when referring to what has been learnt to date and whether other researchers' practices and observations are encouraging. However, we would be remiss if we did not acknowledge what is now part of the scientific record. Accordingly, consider an early randomised control trial of HAES by Bacon et al. (2005). Their research, undertaken with 78 women, aged 30 to 45 years, reported better psychological, cardiometabolic and behavioural outcomes in the HAES group compared to a dieting control group. These benefits were sustained after two years, outlasting the control groups' often transient weight-loss. The HAES intervention did not generate negative outcomes and over 90 per cent of participants stayed with the six-month programme, whilst 41 per cent dropped out from the diet group. Thereafter, Bacon (2006) urged the medical community to 'end the war on obesity' and 'make peace with your patients'. They also subsequently wrote the following endorsement of HAES with Aphramor (Bacon and Aphramor, 2014: 85):

> The HAES research clearly shows that it is possible to dump the obsession with food and weight, and the self-hatred and shame about your body. You can reclaim the joy in eating – and it can improve your health and how you feel!

More recent interventions have been assessed. Drawing from data from Health and Social Service Centers in Québec, Canada, Bégin et al. (2019) report the outcomes of a 14-week HAES intervention where women 'struggling with weight and body image' (p. 248) met weekly with health professionals. The authors state that HAES participants (216 women, BMI: 35.76 kg/m^2) showed greater improvements on various measures (i.e. for eating behaviours and psychological correlates) relative to a comparison group (110 women, BMI: 34.56 kg/m^2). Improved measures, in the short term and during a one-year follow-up, were reported for, inter alia, susceptibility to hunger, intuitive eating, obsessive-compulsive eating, body-esteem, depression and self-esteem. Elsewhere, a HAES general education course with college students found that, compared to standard dieting control and comparison groups, HAES produced greater body esteem and intuitive eating, less dieting behaviours and reduced anti-fat bias (Humphrey et al., 2015). Another non-dieting intervention was conducted mostly with Caucasian women categorised as 'morbidly obese' (Borkoles et al., 2016). The intervention produced increased physical activity and better psychological function for at least 12 months. Emphasising the sometimes ambivalent positioning of HAES, Borkoles et al. reference the potential of this intervention to produce weight outcomes (although these outcomes were ultimately not produced).

Mensinger et al. (2016) identify literature on the effectiveness of 'weight-neutral' approaches that explicitly draw from, or are aligned with, HAES. For reviews, they point to Cadena-Schlam and Lopez-Guimera (2014), Clifford et al. (2015) and Schaefer and Magnuson (2014). Summarising main observations, Mensinger et al. (2016: 33) write:

> studies that have tested weight-neutral programs demonstrated improvements (compared to baseline values) in many physical health, eating, and well-being indices such as: lower total cholesterol, low density lipoprotein cholesterol, triglycerides, systolic blood pressure, disinhibited eating, bulimic symptomatology, drive for thinness, body dissatisfaction, poor interoceptive awareness, and depression.

However, what is unclear from these studies is 'whether there are moderators that strengthen or weaken their effectiveness. Moderators answer the question of *when* or *for whom* a given relationship exists or an effect occurs' (p. 33, emphasis in original). Critically, as part of their own randomised control trial with 80 'community women' with a BMI >30 kg/m^2, Mensinger et al. (2016) found that the beneficial effects on eating behaviours produced in a non-dieting healthy living program were mediated by internalised weight stigma, which they define as 'the adoption and personal endorsement of negative weight-based societal stereotypes' (p. 33). The sustained benefits produced by the intervention, as compared to a conventional dieting program, were evident only in those with low internalised weight stigma. Comparable results were found for physical activity (Mensinger and Meadows, 2017). Similarly, among women labelled obese and living with depression who participated in a healthy living intervention – incorporating HAES principles and Acceptance and Commitment Therapy – participants emphasised the value of self-acceptance and learning methods of coping with psychosocial issues (Berman et al., 2016). Therefore, even when HAES programs are conceptualised primarily as individual lifestyle interventions, it is the size acceptance component that may be the most critical aspect or moderator of their effectiveness. This remains challenging. Note the mediated public pedagogies and stigmatising experiences of fat embodiment (or fear of becoming fat), discussed earlier in our book, in contradistinction to the delimited focus in psychological research on cognition (Williams and Annandale, 2019; Chapter 2). Moreover, 'the weaponising of stigma in neoliberalism' (Scambler, 2018: 141) indicates that whilst self-acceptance or love might be necessary as a means of challenging fat hatred it is insufficient.

Societal fat acceptance: resonance and challenges

Despite challenges, HAES and its underlying principles have received broader recognition in high-income nations wherein health is widely (incorrectly) assumed to be within everybody's reach. For instance, alongside recent writings in paediatrics (Raffoul and Williams, 2021), researchers cite HAES when discussing larger women's ability to relate to health promotion images (Lawson and Wardle, 2013) and body size diversity/inclusivity among yoga enthusiasts, as promoted through 'digital media activism' (Webb et al., 2019: 156; see also Chapter 2). Temporal shifts in ideal sizes and the possible influence of HAES are also referenced (Roberts and Muta, 2017; Webb et al., 2013, 2017), and weight stigma interventions and positive body image are emerging areas of exploration (Alberga et al., 2016; Lee et al., 2014; Robertson and Thomson, 2014). The latter include researchers' reflections on the policy and practice relevance of HAES in stigmatising environments. For instance, drawing from a study of men recruited from a weight management group, Lozano-Sufrategui et al. (2016: 21) deem HAES worthy of consideration because 'camaraderie' or solidarity 'was often more meaningful for participants than weight loss itself' (p. 21).

Lee and Pausé (2016) justifiably critique aspects of HAES in a global context (e.g. the impossibility of supporting all bodies in nations marred by poverty and war) and question whether *too much is being asked of the movement*. Written before the COVID-19 pandemic, their words have increased relevance as time progresses, not least amidst concerns from the United Nations about mass starvation with particular reference to the Global South (Anthem, 2020). Additionally, even if restricting oneself to affluent nations, one cannot ignore recent reports that millions of Americans are experiencing hunger and other problems related to mass homelessness, incarceration, lack of medical insurance, racial prejudice and inequality (Berwick, 2020). Nonetheless, writing from a position of relative security, Lee and Pausé (2016) assert that HAES principles are 'very useful' (p. 11) for health professionals. Accordingly, they counterbalance the biased biomedical view that weight-loss should be pursued at any cost.

Elsewhere, NAAFA has supported HAES over the past decade, hosting its first 'HAES International Summit' in 2010 (Kwan and Graves, 2013: 62). HAES has also been discussed at large mainstream health and obesity conferences (Bacon, 2014a, 2014b). Andrea has spoken on HAES-relevant content at standard public health and obesity conferences such as the American Public Health Association Annual Meetings and the Canadian Obesity Network Congress. Furthermore, numerous examples of HAES have emerged in teaching practices that challenge the WCHP in health pedagogy, health professions (Ward et al., 2016) and (in)formal educational settings (Cameron and Russell, 2016; Chapter 5). The *Canadian Journal of Public Health* also recently featured a commentary on the value of combing HAES with Indigenous perspectives (Cyr and Riediger, 2021).

Besides resonating with certain fat activist groups, researchers, clinicians and educators, Kwan and Graves (2013: 68) explain that 'there is some indication that the [HAES] perspective has some public support'. They cite an online 'HAES Pledge' that received support from 4,261 individuals in March 2012 (the figure in January 2022 exceeded 21,000) and Lee's UK-based research on men's orientations to physical activity and public health anti-obesity campaigns (see Monaghan, 2008). We would add that whilst the men in Lee's research reported no prior knowledge of HAES, some of their critical views were compatible with size acceptance tenets. The gendered aspects of this finding – specifically the everyday association of robust masculinity with physical presence and fitness rather than thinness – are worth underscoring since they cast a different hue on the following statement by a HAES practitioner: 'Letting go of the goal of weight loss has made HAES controversial in a society where the pursuit of thinness is an unquestioned prescription for health and happiness' (Burgard, 2009: 42). We also remain cognisant of ongoing resistances to the obesity offensive by laity, including via social media (Lupton, 2018; Chapter 2). Preliminary findings from Australia suggest that criticism around 'fat shaming' is growing online (Cain et al., 2017). Even the popular site Buzzfeed featured an article on community members' reasoning behind quitting dieting and adopting self-acceptance (Tamarkin, 2016).

As reported in Chapter 4, with reference to Andrea's research, Canadian women identifying as (formerly) obese referenced HAES. Again, this suggests growing public awareness of, and/or alignment with, health-based alternatives to dieting. However, even when invoking HAES, some participants continually referenced an ongoing impetus to engage in particular health behaviours as part of their ambivalent relationship with weight (loss), patriarchal norms of feminine beauty (the aesthetics of slenderness) and wish to avoid anticipated health problems in older age. This internalisation of health moralism (which is evidently entangled with sizeism, ageism, sexism, healthism, stigma and biomedicalisation) suggests HAES may be taken up in everyday life as a less radical and more assimilative approach to size acceptance (LeBesco, 2004). To return to LeBesco's (2010) experience of facilitating a HAES group at college, some participants 'admitted a desire for weight loss' and 'some members fell away, presumably because they wanted to reach for the standard brass ring of health eschewed by our [size acceptance] group' (pp. 79–80).

Such ambivalence is indicative of the degree to which 'thin' may be 'in' not only as a standardised measure of biomedical health but also of social fitness in Western culture, incorporating 'conventionally' defined images of feminine beauty (Greenhalgh, 2015; Kwan and Graves, 2013; Monaghan and Malson, 2013). Despite the seeming growth in size acceptance, advocating for the widespread adoption of HAES within the current public health environment may be difficult for a whole raft of social, cultural, political and economic reasons (Monaghan, 2008, 2017). Within academia and policymaking contexts, support is higher for adopting 'weight-neu-tral' language and guidelines that ensure potential confounders and side effects are incorporated in research reports than for funding HAES research. Yet, as suggested by O'Reilly and Sixsmith (2012), the latter could more profoundly influence policy that is based on scientific evidence and ethical claims to do more good than harm.

There are, of course, multiple domains wherein weight-inclusive approaches could be promoted. Well-evaluated HAES teacher resources, which encourage healthy behaviours without triggering body-image issues or eating disorders, have been produced and may be used instead of weight-centric school health programs (McVey et al., 2009). However, challenges persist in broadly disseminating size acceptance. This was observed in Emma's research on fat pedagogy among school-girls in England (Chapter 5), notably with reference to relational and institutional constraints (e.g. the social distance between students and staff, the contradictory content of health education). Elsewhere, some teachers in Canada have expressed resistance to teaching body acceptance, so as not to 'excuse' fatness, especially in classes with larger students (Robertson and Thomson, 2014), whilst the palatabil-ity of HAES for undergraduate psychology students in Australia was constrained by their assumptions about the controllability of weight and the obligatory nature of health (Cain and Donaghue, 2018). Similar scepticism is seen among Australian fitness trainers, who viewed HAES as only acceptable as a last resort for their clients when all attempts to lose weight through behaviour had failed (Donaghue and Allen, 2016). In Ireland, whilst undertaking ethnography in a commercial slimming club, O'Toole (2019: 18) mentioned HAES to a class leader but received an incredulous response: 'No one could ever think it is okay to be fat. No one is ever happy to be fat. No one'. In the USA, recent Latino immigrants viewed HAES as an intriguing concept but one that did not align with cultural norms of 'cleaning one's plate' or of women's familial roles (Greaney et al., 2012). Thus, whilst HAES is making inroads within public discourse around health and size, it continues to grapple with, inter alia: existing educational policy and practice, entrenched notions of the mutability of the body, gendered body aesthetics, ethnic cultural norms (shaped, in part, by a history of poverty and economic marginalisa-tion) and the ideology of personal responsibility for health.

Controversies, fractures and inconsistencies within and beyond HAES

In recent years, lively debate, tensions and disruptions have appeared among the various camps supportive of fat acceptance. For example, recently after ASDAH trademarked HAES® in America (avowedly to protect it from 'misappropria-tion' by the dieting industry), Gingras and Cooper (2013) raised concerns about the negative effects of this in a (corporatised) field that lacks transparency. In their view, trademarking HAES may lead to exclusionary, protectionist and com-modifying practices. They contend that trademarking may collapse and foreclose complexities that have long shaped body acceptance work, or even erase the rich history of fat activism(s) as lived by participants with diverse biographies and priorities. There are additional elements in this critique, especially from the viewpoint of those immersed in radical fat activism and queer theory who contest the relationship between professionalised organisations and grassroots activism. Cooper is ambivalent about HAES in general given, for instance, its concern for academic respectability and producing a sanitised account that reduces 'fat iden-tity and fat culture ... to a question of health' (Gingras and Cooper, 2013: 2–3). Cooper (2016a) subsequently added to this critique. Focusing on access, profes-sionalisation and class, she lambasts the 'gentrification' of fat activism (pp. 175–6). For Cooper, 'hierarchies and elites' are produced at the expense of a 'grassroots affair' (p. 176) that was presumably more accessible when practiced by amateurs.

The processual nature of HAES and ASDAH's move to trademark the name mean that it will likely continue to witness internal strains and dissent. However, certain core principles of HAES appear to have filtered into the broader healthcare and research community, albeit in an inconsistent manner. For instance, a cursory review of articles identified by the search term 'Health-at-Every-Size' reveals numerous articles that ostensibly state their focus to be on HAES, but continue to frame inter-ventions as potentially beneficial in terms of weight-loss or preventing weight-gain (e.g. Borkoles et al., 2016; Greaney et al., 2012). This framing is inconsistent with a legitimately 'weight-inclusive' approach to health, and it may suggest the strategic positioning required to obtain funding and get published in the health field, or find acceptance within neoliberal contexts. Such problems go beyond LeBesco's (2010: 80) fears about HAES researchers 'buying into conventional [scientific] modes of resistance' and would likely bolster her preference for 'a playful approach that desta-bilizes traditional understandings of health' (also Cooper, 2011, 2016a).

Mainstream biomedical 'stakeholders', such as those at the University of Connecticut's Rudd Center for Food Policy & Obesity, have positioned themselves as opponents to obesity stigma and have made considerable strides in advancing this agenda. This work tends to focus on ensuring treatment in clinical contexts is respectful (Bombak et al., 2016), which is important because anti-fat bias in the health professions influences health outcomes and patients' uptake of care (Mensinger et al., 2018; Phelan et al., 2015; Schwartz et al., 2003). However, authors such as those at the Rudd Center rarely critically situate their work within existing social theory. Nor are they interested in interrogating the problematisation of body size per se (Bombak et al., 2016). Hence, their approach retrenches existing problems in clinical practice, for instance, the offen-siveness of labelling somebody obese (Aphramor, 2009).

Conceptual models have also been developed that explore the multiple pathways through which weight stigma may affect health (Brewis, 2014; Hunger et al., 2015).

These models seek to explicate some of the associations found between weight stigma and cardiovascular reactivity, activation of the 'fight or flight' responses, lower self-acceptance, mood and anxiety disorders, and attempts to avoid and escape stigma. At the same time, the inclusion of overeating, refusal to diet, self-control and decreased physical activity in their models, and the persistence of weight-gain as an adverse consequence of weight stigma, illustrate the uncertainty and tensions in adopting a size acceptance approach (Brewis, 2014; Hunger et al., 2015; Tomiyama, 2014) in contexts dominated by the WCHP.

There is a surprising paucity in the literature on attempting to accept life in a larger size and adopt a fat acceptance or HAES perspective. This paucity is not absolute (Lee and Pausé, 2016), but most literature in the area explores individuals' induction into the Fatosphere (the online size acceptance community, introduced in Chapter 2) (e.g. Hynnä and Kyrölä, 2019), or auto-ethnographic discussions from scholars who encounter ambivalence for personally desiring altered bodies whilst critiquing weight-centrism (Heyes, 2006, 2007; Longhurst, 2012; Murray, 2005a, 2008; Sheach Leith, 2015; Throsby and Gimlin, 2010). For instance, Murray (2008: 109, emphasis in original) rejects what she sees as fat activism's proposal that 'fat persons' can 'simply *chang[e] [their] mind[s] about [their] bod[ies]*'. This critique is taken up by Lupton (2012), who states the focus of HAES on natural set-points and internal cues ignores the socio-cultural contexts within which people live and experience their bodies. These contexts, she explains, shape both eating practices and individuals' capacity for self-acceptance (see also Lupton, 2018: 92–3). Current literature would suggest the focus of HAES on individualistic behaviour change and self-love does little to alter societal attitudes, and, without such shifts, advising individuals to be more size accepting may be futile. Lupton's (2012) blog motivated a response from then-prominent HAES proponents Bacon and Aphramor. Their response focused on the value, including political value, of individual size acceptance and reiterated the HAES movement's commitment to encouraging societal size acceptance.

The HAES movement's perceived uncritical neoliberal concentration on individual behaviour change or 'healthy lifestyles', as hinted at above, has subsequently been challenged from within. In response to their growing sense of dissonance at the differences between HAES and their more politicised vision, Aphramor (2016) argues for a greater focus on inequity, body respect and the psychosocial determinants of health. Aphramor, along with several colleagues, has continually sought to reframe the tenets of the HAES movement in a more political, equity-centric direction (Aphramor and Gingras, 2011; Brady et al., 2013). For example, Brady et al. state:

> HAES cannot be offered up as an emancipatory alternative to today's prevailing weight-centered, healthist discourse if it is understood and practiced as if it were simply another, albeit weight neutral, choice for individuals to fulfil a duty to be healthy.
>
> *(p. 347)*

Over time, Aphramor sought to further politicise HAES and extend its impact beyond individual non-dieting approaches via what they called Health In Every Respect. This approach entailed challenging healthism and pushed for criticality, which exceeds the narrow, non-reflexive, critical appraisal endorsed by positivism (Aphramor, 2017). Eventually, however, Aphramor left the HAES movement to develop Well Now, a more radical 'social action approach' that places social justice centre stage (Aphramor, 2016, 2019b). Well Now promotes 'compassionate self-care' and 'emancipatory learning' in a broader context, emphasising embodied power relations and working with people to 'respond more effectively to social factors affecting health and health behaviours' (Aphramor, personal communication, 2018). Well Now courses are aimed at 'professionals and students working in nutrition, counselling, coaching and public health ... anyone working around intersectionality and trauma, and for those who are simply curious about what a "health-gain and body respect approach" might look like' (personal communication, 2018). Aphramor has since written much more when advancing Well Now, critiquing foundational ideas such as 'intuitive eating' and foregrounding issues such as trauma during the COVID-19 pandemic (Aphramor, 2019b, 2020a, 2020b, 2020c).

ASDAH appears to have recognised at least *some* of Aphramor's early critique of HAES (notably, the charge that it reproduces healthism and individual responsibilisation for health), and has responded by adding the following statement to its website (emphasis in original):

> ASDAH's HAES Principles reject judgments about health and any discourse of individual *responsibility* around health, in favour of a discourse of individualized health *needs* ... ASDAH also recognizes that many of the factors that determine our health are not individual in nature. Social, political, and cultural factors ... may have an even greater impact on health outcomes than individual choices. On a collective level, we support creating health-promoting environments and removing barriers to access. On an individual level, we seek to empower people to engage in those personal practices that best support health and wellbeing for the individual. There should be no judgment about what people choose to do (or not do) to enhance their well-being.
>
> *(ASDAH, 2013)*

These distinctions fail to resonate with critics of the HAES movement who otherwise support size acceptance. Certainly, Aphramor (2016) remains dissatisfied with efforts to modify the architecture of HAES ultimately as a *lifestyle intervention* rather than radically redraw its plans by *integrating* concepts such as 'allostasis, metabolic inheritance, somatophobia, power, silences, gender and nutrition justice, critical pedagogy, trauma and shame alongside critical appraisal of weight science and the need to challenge fat stigma' (p. 1). More recently, Aphramor (2020a) contends that HAES reproduces White supremacy, which is ubiquitous even in practices 'that we imagine are anti-oppressive'. Suggestions for action range from 'wising up' to Orwellian 'doublethink' (saying things that are mutually incompatible and/or known to be untrue) to rejecting the HAES phrase 'Health is not a moral obligation' given 'the fact that racism harms health' and requires a moral response at a collective, political level. Arguably, these responses reflect the ways in which the size acceptance movement is growing or maturing, resulting in different emphases, epistemic assumptions and politicised concerns that are unashamedly 'biased' towards supporting social justice and dissent rather than 'in-group' orthodoxy and the status quo. Size acceptance and its various camps generate sufficient self-reflexivity to now host, albeit sometimes uneasily, multiple divergent viewpoints. Yet, the degree to which more radical arguments are acknowledged, digested or rejected by size acceptance leaders remains inseparable from the broader neoliberal context within which health policies are framed, debated and funded. The need for radical alternatives is a theme to which we will return in our epilogue when rethinking obesity, health and society.

Summary

This chapter has drawn from relevant literature within and beyond the social sciences, focusing on dieting, alternative interventions and some limitations with a commonly proposed 'size acceptance' paradigm, HAES. Whilst not without critique (e.g. Aphramor, 2016, 2020a; Lupton, 2018) and even vociferous opposition (Sainsbury and Hay, 2014), HAES deserves broader recognition in (social) scientific and policy debates. Of course, this is with the proviso that societies are able to meet basic human requirements, ensuring that the infrastructure and economic conditions are in place to nourish and care for populations that may be traumatised. Advocates of HAES writing in the Global North prior to COVID-19 have nonetheless usefully opened up this alternative health movement to expansion, diversification, internal reflection and the potential to imagine strategies for advancing body equity in multiple domains. Thus, it could be argued that despite various limitations, HAES remains an invaluable launching point to challenge individuals, educators, practitioners and trainees embedded in health disciplines wherein striving to be responsible, healthier citizens is an entrenched goal. To extend Gard's (2016: 244) point about 'intellectually ethical fat pedagogies' and becoming 'scientifically literate', HAES literature provides these groups the opportunity 'to work through the *very discursive substance* of the "obesity epidemic" itself' (p. 244, emphasis in original) through its deployment of positivist science and clinical, measurable outcomes. By relying upon, but challenging, what is familiar territory for many audiences, HAES allows us to take the requisite time to answer the question, 'what does this mean for me as a practitioner, researcher or educator?' before aiming for more critical, and indeed, more crucial, stakes. With regard to Aphramor's more recent work, which has served as a notable point of reference in this chapter and to which we will return in our epilogue, we are reminded of what Scambler (2013b, 2018), following

Archer (2007), terms 'dedicated meta-reflexives'. Such actors, in an ideal-typical sense, exercise resistance and seek to make a difference via therapeutic, community-oriented action. Concerns for more 'rounded' knowledge and collective action underpin the remainder of our book, which is also attuned to the declared COVID-19 pandemic and controversial efforts to control its spread and impact.

8

RETHINKING OBESITY IN THE (POST) COVID SOCIETY

Paving the way for more 'rounded' knowledge and collective action

As we were close to completing this book and thinking about the future directions of public health and obesity discourse, the COVID-19 pandemic erupted. This global event complicated and amplified concerns about public health, weight/fatness and, indeed, the future of society. As outlined in Chapter 6, the pandemic was accompanied by mass lockdowns that were having a significant impact, transforming 'the social, economic and political landscape across the globe' (Bell and Green, 2020: 379). During this period of heightened uncertainty – fear and panic even (Žižek, 2020) that continued into 2021 – the news media was dominated by reports of developments and effects, for instance, the daily rising global death toll and control measures taken (or being reintroduced) in different nations and regions. Exceeding the reductionist foci of biology and virology, the pandemic invoked issues of power, politics and economics but so too of particular forms of citizenship and governance. For example, power and politics infused mundane actions and items, such as attempts to access public space and the wearing of face masks. The spectre of mass unemployment also quickly ensued as global financial markets, which already appeared to be veering towards 'systemic collapse' (Vighi, 2021), exhibited extreme volatility. The urgency of the declared pandemic brought into sharp relief models of intervention, policies and practices, raising questions about public health both in the short term and, importantly for the focus of this chapter, thereafter. As will be discussed below, it is within this tumultuous landscape that various authorities, notably public health doctors and politicians, reiterated the fat as fatal frame and WCHP as if they provided unequivocal knowledge and safe, effective remedies. In so doing, they presented intentional weight-loss as an effective and thus sensible means of preparing for subsequent 'waves' of COVID-19. To cite one newspaper headline, four months into the pandemic: 'Britain is told to lose weight for the winter as deputy chief medical officer admits she is "very concerned" about a second

DOI: 10.4324/9781315658087-12

wave [of COVID-19] and urges people to slim down to cut their risk of dying' (Blanchard, 2020).

Preceding chapters, especially Chapter 7, should give readers pause for thought. Just as the war on obesity cannot be 'black boxed' as ever more urgent and necessary, COVID-19 (or, perhaps more accurately, societal responses to this) rapidly became a contested and divisive issue (Caduff, 2020; Ioannidis, 2020b; Monaghan, 2020). To borrow from Strong (1990), COVID-19 quickly became steeped in 'plagues' of moral controversy and suspicion, even intensifying hostility towards 'outsiders' – a contingent construct but one that typically reproduces existing prejudices and inequalities tied to nationhood, ethnicity, social class, stigma, embodiment, etc. The COVID-19 pandemic is – and will likely remain for some time – a polarising issue in already 'fractured societies' such as the UK and kindred nations (Scambler, 2020b). To avoid misunderstanding and counter possible misrecognition (Chapter 2), then, we will stress that whilst we agree with Dingwall (2020a) that 'a sense of proportion' is required when considering the risks represented by SARS-CoV-2, we do not dismiss legitimate concerns about public health, safety and well-being. We do not deny the potentially devastating physical impact of COVID-19 alongside the negative consequences of mitigation measures, notably mass lockdowns, especially for the most vulnerable in society. To do so would mean denying the materiality of the human body alongside broader socio-economic determinants of health. Moreover, we have little interest in feeding suspect dichotomies, such as lives versus livelihoods, which stymie nuanced debate. Rather, we approach what has been framed as the dual obesity and COVID-19 pandemics (e.g. Ryan et al., 2020; Rychter et al., 2020) through a different analytical lens that foregrounds society and embodied relations. In so doing, and in view of the pervasive sense of 'dis-ease' intimated by French and Monahan (2020), public opinion polls (Asmundson and Taylor, 2020) and others (e.g. Barnes et al., 2020; Žižek, 2020) early in the pandemic, we pose some critical questions and signpost potential areas for future research. Wherever possible we also cite subsequent writings on the social aspects of the pandemic (response), work published shortly before *Rethinking Obesity* went to press (e.g. Armstrong, 2021; Dingwall, 2022; Lupton and Willis, 2021; O'Connell et al., 2021; Pausé et al., 2021).

Alongside suggesting agendas for social research this chapter could inform alternative approaches to public health and, indeed, social organisation more generally – themes to which we return in the epilogue. Before considering these more rounded or expansive concerns, we need to cover some ground regarding the 'meeting' or 'layering' of epidemics, pandemics and crises. As noted early in our book, mass media and policy responses quickly evoked a relationship between overweight/obesity and COVID-19 (increased risk of infection, of being hospitalised in intensive care and death) (e.g. CDC, 2020; Donnelly and Newey, 2020; WOF, 2020). These concerns were, in turn, dramatised and amplified in the UK during the summer of 2020, as seen with the headline, above, from the *MailOnline*, and the accompanying report where citizens were instructed by England's Deputy Chief Medical Officer to '[m]ake yourself as fit as possible' (cited by Blanchard, 2020). In this chapter we consider the myriad issues this 'dual crisis frame' has raised for public health. No doubt, the 'critical situation' (Giddens, 1979) confronting the world has raised questions and potential lines of investigation that exceed the constraints of our text. However, certain matters demand attention insofar as they were explored earlier in our book and have resurfaced in 'the global COVID society' (Lupton and Willis, 2021). For example, recent events have thrown into relief how shared understandings of health risk are mediated by socially constructed frames, discourses, affects and practices. As collective events, pandemics implicate communicative, political matters (Bjørkdahl and Carlsen, 2019) and thus policy formations and public pedagogy.

Just as sociologists advised against premature evaluation and rushing to formulate conclusions during the relatively early days of the COVID-19 pandemic (Bell and Green, 2020; Will, 2020), we exercise caution. Throughout our discussion we are interested in posing questions just as much as delving into earlier and emerging scholarship that could provide a basis for future work. Some relevant questions include: How should we analyse stigma relations in this 'changed' world (Lupton, 2020), wherein the psychologising of health problems has continued apace (Drury et al., 2020)? How are (dis)trust and anxiety materialising amidst uncertain science and suspicions surrounding early government, media and public health responses to the pandemic (Calnan et al., 2020; Ioannidis, 2020b; Loke and Heneghan, 2020; Rebughini, 2021)? What of the limits of science, especially when dealing with matters pertaining to social values and ethics? What might critical weight studies and cognate approaches, such as fat studies, have to offer in this context of risk, fear, uncertainty, controversy, contestation and proposed solutions (Strong, 1990)? What about inequality and its impact on health, including the consequences of social class during the outbreak (Arber and Meadows, 2020)? Will public health crises and responses to them fuel a legitimation crisis in capitalism (Scambler, 2020b)? Our basic premise here is that we cannot proffer alternatives to the WCHP, or even approaches such as HAES, without making sense of a larger social world riddled with tensions and declared crises, including the meeting of obesity and COVID-19. We surmise others would agree, as recently evidenced among critics seeking 'to explore the problematisation of fatness in contemporary responses to the COVID-19 pandemic' (Pausé et al., 2021: 1).

This chapter is structured into four main sections. First, we broach what the social sciences and humanities teach us about emerging infectious diseases and pandemics, noting some core insights for the current era plus the need for further research. Second, drawing from Strong's (1990) classic essay and our previous work that utilises his model on 'infectious' psychosocial forms (Monaghan et al., 2018), we offer critical reflections on what might be called 'pandemic psychology' (Monaghan, 2020) in the context of COVID-19 and obesity. Third, we examine the relationship between contested science and policymaking processes, revealing how the complexity of obesity scholarship is largely absent in this risk landscape. Finally, we discuss the obfuscation and reproduction of extant inequalities via the articulation of a dual crisis frame that positions weight/obesity as a continuing problem to be fixed by responsible individuals.

Pandemics and infectious diseases in social context: some insights for the current era

Confusion surrounds terms such as 'pandemics' and 'epidemics', with authorities such as the WHO (1998, 2021) also muddying the waters by repeatedly referring to obesity as a 'global epidemic'. However, as explained by Dingwall (2022: 3), the word 'pandemic' denotes an outbreak of an infectious disease on 'a global scale', whereas an 'epidemic' is confined to a specific country or region. He adds that such phenomena are 'just as much cultural as biomedical' (p. 3). Indeed, large-scale outbreaks of infectious disease emerge from and (re)shape social conditions and relations that are irreducible to biology, incorporating matters such as: historically transmitted ideologies and practices (e.g. racism within public health), governance, culture, (dis)trust, power, emotions, stigma, violence, media communications, the economy, geopolitics and collective social psychology (Bjørkdahl and Carlsen, 2019; David and Le Dévédec, 2019; Dingwall et al., 2013; MacGregor et al., 2020; Monaghan, 2020; Strong, 1990). The social sciences and humanities therefore matter (Lupton and Willis, 2021), proffering valuable insights and ways of thinking in challenging, if not traumatic, times (Thoune, 2020; Chapter 6).

Whilst we will outline some sociological insights below, contributions from other disciplines should also be signposted. This furthers our aim to traverse boundaries whilst also informing efforts to rethink authoritative medicalised understandings of obesity as a 'big' health problem that is now entangled with infectious disease (risk) and other crises. Anthropology, for instance, demonstrates how people, at a collective and experiential level, have already confronted major disease outbreaks in recent years (MacGregor et al., 2020). Others show how media and 'medical scapegoating' of 'outsiders' (such as Chinese Americans) is hardly new, as evidenced during the 2003 SARS epidemic (Eichelberger, 2007: 1286). Historical literature on earlier plagues and public health responses is also noteworthy. Among the many readings recommended by Barnes et al. (2020), crucial insights are offered on issues such as theological explanations (disease related to 'moral transgression' and 'divine retribution') and colonising tendencies within public health that pathologise Black bodies (for related arguments about the social sciences and 'Northern theory', see Connell, 2007).

Such critical insights could advance more expansive knowledge of obesity, health and society, which is necessary when encountering relatively privileged (typically White, middle-class) groups who might otherwise enact symbolic violence and control. (In the case of COVID risk and overweight/obesity, those targeted for moralising 'advice' are the undisciplined masses whose failings are manifest in their abject flesh, or, more 'objectively', their BMI.) Indeed, the social sciences and humanities are well placed to analyse how responses to a novel coronavirus are inseparable from pernicious ideologies, discriminatory value judgements and injurious ways of feeling and acting that are patterned according to relatively enduring social structures (such as class, gender and ethnicity). Why might any of this matter? For those benefitting from the status quo, the short answer is that none of this may matter much, or at all! However, whilst the privileged tend to forget that humans have always been susceptible to communicable disease, the spectre of contagion – and thus disorder at a personal and macrosocial level – is never far away.

Relatively recent outbreaks of measles in North America (Sanyaolu et al., 2019), and, since then, COVID-19 globally, reveal that rapidly spreading viruses are always imminent, scientific *and* social facts. Whilst imagined divisions between 'the West and the rest' might mitigate effective responses to emerging infectious disease in high-income nations, anthropologists and historians remind us of the importance of broadening our lenses, especially when certain scientists advise on policy. For instance, MacGregor et al.'s (2020) ethnographic research on the West African Ebola outbreak contradicts the blinkered, yet influential, report from UK epidemiologists that claimed highly socially disruptive public health interventions had not been previously attempted (Ferguson et al., 2020). In a related vein, Barnes et al. (2020) indicate that the entrusting of exclusive authority to medical science and laboratories during disease outbreaks is untenable as people seek to make sense of shared fears and anxieties (for additional critique of what is termed iatrocracy, or rule by the medical elite, see Dingwall, 2022; Smith, 2020). In the time of COVID-19, these unsettling emotions are entangled with everyday interpretations of contradictory lockdown policies, scientific uncertainty, risk and the quest for ontological security via technical control (Rebughini, 2021).

Whilst every medically categorised illness or disease is different and contexts matter a unifying theme within the social sciences and humanities is that 'medical phenomena' are also 'communicative and political phenomena' (Bjørkdahl and Carlsen, 2019: 6). Such reasoning is perhaps easily appreciated following earlier chapters in *Rethinking Obesity*, especially our discussion on media, body pedagogy, stigma, meta-critique (Chapter 2), public health policy (Chapter 3) and the politics of cruelty (Chapter 6). Analysing declared public health crises as communicative and political events, critical public health scholars observe how international bodies, including the WHO, have recently been emphasising *preparedness*. David and Le Dévédec (2019: 365) argue that in this new paradigm, 'preparedness replaces the risk universe with a horizon of plausible but unpredictable biological threat that requires adaptation beyond all probability'. Similar themes emerge in Dingwall et al.'s (2013) edited collection.

In view of such work, outlined further below, we suggest that the recent dual emphasis on the COVID-19 and obesity crises potentially reconfigures the biopolitical framing of 'excess' weight/fatness to models which make 'an uncertain future available to intervention in the present' (Lakoff, 2007: 253). Again, such a response is not completely novel, especially post-9/11 when threats to 'domestic security' came to the fore in the USA and beyond. Rather, the declared COVID-19 emergency appears to have amplified and accelerated trends previously scrutinised within critical weight and fat studies (see Evans and Colls, 2011; Chapter 3). Mindful of such literature, our basic argument here is that the emergent

COVID-19 and obesity dual crisis frame could have significant implications for the future of public health policy and pedagogy, accelerating and deepening all that is problematic vis-à-vis what we and others have already observed in social studies of epidemics and weight. Problems include an 'epidemic' of 'moralisation' (Strong, 1990: 254) and 'truncated theorising' (Aphramor, 2005: 334), compounded by behavioural explanations and policy prescriptions that hold (groups of) individuals responsible and which are hardly mitigated by environmental accounts (Chapter 2).

Turning to Dingwall et al. (2013), they state that 'the shadow cast by HIV' plus other outbreaks and bio-threats has meant that 'actor-networks' have emerged with the goal of countering 'possibilities for future disorder' via 'stabilisation in advance' (p. 3). They explain that living, as we now do, in an 'intensely globalised arena, marked by supra-national as well as national and local actors' (p. 6), underscores the need for sociological insights on social contexts, organisational practices and processes. Substantive topics in their collection range from the use of 'model-based evidence in the governing of pandemics' (Mansnerus, 2013) to how international media framed the 2009 H1N1 influenza pandemic (Staniland and Smith, 2013). Foregrounding organisational networks (e.g. the WHO), global and local politics and policy implementation (e.g. the production of authoritative, yet questionable, narratives via quantification; the problems with public–private collaborations), their text offers many insights that could also inform social research on the COVID-19 pandemic (response) in the months and years ahead. Staniland and Smith's (2013) work on media framing of the 2009 H1N1 influenza outbreak, for instance, notes how classic literature on moral panics and epidemic psychology has utility but it may also require further critical reflection. Consider, by way of example, how ideas are now rapidly shared globally via digital media (similarly, see our discussion on media in Chapter 2). Mansnerus (2013) is also germane, focusing on statistical modelling as a presumably precise and authoritative means of stabilising the future within policy fields but which has the effect of black boxing many issues and uncertainties. Accordingly, Dingwall et al. (2013: 171) state that modelling is 'a latter day version of oracles, divination or clairvoyance, deriving their societal licence from science rather than religion'. Of course, to reconnect with our extension of Bernstein (2000) to obesity policy in Chapter 3, scientific and state-mandated health knowledge is structurally comparable to religion, distinguishing authoritatively between the sacred and profane. Within this cosmology, when a novel and highly contagious virus threatens populations, economies and social order, the 'sins' of 'gluttony and sloth' must be renounced by the overweight masses hoping for salvation.

Within modernity such processes are, of course, framed as eminently rational rather than theological, with the aim of anticipating and minimising future problems. In a similar vein to Dingwall et al.'s (2013) point about organisational efforts to ensure stability in advance of an outbreak and accepting 'known unknowns' (e.g. the question of when, not if, a novel and highly infectious disease will strike), David and Le Dévédec (2019: 363) state 'preparing for the next epidemic' has been a recurrent theme in global health in recent years. Beginning with SARS and 'intensifying after the 2013–2016 Ebola outbreak', their article flags the promotion of largely privatised technological fixes, notably vaccines as discussed at pro-business events such as Davos (for critical reflections on 'the spirit of Davos', see our epilogue). In such a context, critical public health scholars have considered the scientific base/knowledge production that informs various decisions, particularly those related to propagation of epidemics and immunity control. David and Le Dévédec write that the 'urgency of preparing for the next health disaster has been recommended by numerous global health stakeholders' such that 'preparedness' is now a newly emerging health paradigm, alongside prevention (p. 363). Reading their work with an eye on the COVID-19/obesity dual crisis frame, we think it is necessary to scrutinise what the (arguably truncated) preparedness paradigm means for social relations, including those mediated by 'insider' experts and policy enactments. Through such work we may better understand how calls for prevention and preparedness – relatively early in the pandemic but also with likely implications for inequalities thereafter – typically individualise risk for citizens who are expected to behave 'responsibly' (e.g. lose weight under doctors' orders, as if this was a prophylactic).

A key issue here, building on Part 1 of our book on contested obesity science (Bombak, 2014b; O'Hara and Taylor, 2018; Chapter 2), concerns knowledge or epistemology. Knowledge, however fallible or imperfect, is consequential. As with the now 'infamous' Imperial College epidemiological report (Caduff, 2020; MacGregor et al., 2020), which precipitated mass lockdowns, policymakers invoke 'the science' (*sic*) in order to legitimate all manner of interventions without broad-based scrutiny and democratic deliberation (Martin et al., 2020a). Pertinent questions here might include: what is known about a disease and ways of responding to it, what is the form and status of that knowledge, how is knowledge selected, what assumptions are being made and by whom, what is being excluded and silenced, is mathematical modelling the only 'credible' way of knowing the world, what do we think we know, what is known to be unknown, how is knowledge recontextualised as public pedagogy, and, relatedly, what are the implications of enacted knowledge for social relations and consciousness in scientifically and state mandated fields of power, control and inequality?

Such epistemological concerns and, by extension, recognition of profound uncertainty, run through social scientific scholarship on pandemics as political enactments. Bjørkdahl and Carlsen (2019) observe that pandemics in general are surrounded by uncertainty and, given their nature and how quickly they can develop, are often 'sites of contestation and conflict' (p. 1). They add that uncertainty 'is not the same as a *threat*, nor is it equal to *fear*, though it is intimately connected with both. We can think of uncertainty as a mental and emotional space that we cannot fill using reliable methods' (p. 3, emphasis in original). Yet, pandemics must be urgently managed on a large scale, often without complete or unambiguous scientific evidence or consensus. This, in turn, raises further questions about how people interpret and experience events that blur or threaten boundaries such as nature and culture, reason and emotion, public and private, freedom and constraint, order and disorder, expertise and laity. Within this messy terrain, authoritative actors also capitalise upon widespread shock and confusion (Klein, 2007, 2020; Monaghan, 2020), fuelling it even for their own ends (Vighi, 2021). As we will go on to observe, and with reference to other recent critical scholarship, the COVID-19 pandemic subsequently became an easily exploited space wherein politicians and their allies furthered 'simplistic and stigmatising ideas about bodyweight and health' (O'Connell et al., 2021: 143), detracting attention from much bigger matters.

In sum, when discussing pandemics in broader contexts it is necessary to draw from multiple disciplines, including the social sciences and humanities. Writings noted above and much besides (e.g. Abeysinghe, 2019; Davis, 2019; Dodsworth, 2021; Foucault, 1995 [1975]; Lupton and Willis, 2021; Pickersgill, 2020; Rhodes et al., 2020; Sandberg and Fondevila, 2020; Sherlaw and Raude, 2013; Williams, 2008) proffer critical insights on socially embedded practices that deserve attention now and for the foreseeable future. However, insofar as we began writing this chapter shortly after the declaration of the COVID-19 pandemic, we will return to a classic sociological model for making sense of *initial* collective psychosocial responses to large-scale, infectious disease (Strong, 1990). We will also tease out some of the implications of Strong's heuristic when scrutinising layered crises. As part of that task, we aim to build upon our earlier critique of the designation of obesity as one of several 'neoliberal epidemics' (Schrecker and Bambra, 2015). Through this discussion, we flag some core insights pertaining to fear, panic, moralising action, intense stigma and conversion to various causes (Strong, 1990). Intentionally selective, these insights also run through the remainder of this chapter as we offer a critical perspective on matters of concern.

Pandemic psychology in the context of the COVID-19 and obesity crises

What Strong (1990) terms 'epidemic psychology' denotes a collective sensibility rooted in language and interaction. Strong proffers an ideal typical model for interrogating social psychological responses to potential or actual threats – especially a new disease, *or* if there are unusual and persistent trends. We have previously drawn from Strong when responding to the designation of obesity as a 'neoliberal epidemic' (Schrecker and Bambra, 2015), wherein 'excess' weight/fatness is pathologised and attributed to a toxic mode of political economic organisation (Monaghan et al., 2018). Such critique seemed apt to us not least given medical and media discourses regarding the spread of obesity within social networks – discourses invoking notions of 'contagion' and 'infectious bodies' (Brown, 2014: 117) that have also 'informed' public health anti-obesity campaigns (Dukelow, 2017; Chapter 3).

Although Strong's (1990) essay has served as a useful point of reference prior to COVID-19 (Dingwall et al., 2013; Eichelberger, 2007; Monaghan et al., 2018;

Staniland and Smith, 2013), a case could be made for revisiting his work and underscoring its continued value (similarly, see Dingwall, 2022; Pickersgill, 2020). For example, Bjørkdahl and Carlsen's (2019) edited collection on pandemics, publics and politics makes no reference to epidemic psychology. Subsequently, in the context of COVID-19, Strong (1990) is ignored in an otherwise insightful critical contribution that asks: 'How did we end up in a space of thinking, feeling and acting that has normalized extremes and is based on the assumption that biological life is an absolute value separate from politics?' (Caduff, 2020: 467). Yet, Strong (1990: 249) explicitly refers to 'political response' (see the next section on the politics of uncertainty). In short, Strong's reasoning retains fecundity and it could be extended to the COVID-19/obesity dual crisis frame, our primary substantive focus. First, however, we will summarise Strong's 'general sociological statement on the striking problems that large, fatal epidemics seem to present to social order' (p. 249). He explains:

> A major outbreak of novel, fatal epidemic disease can quickly be followed both by plagues of fear, panic, suspicion and stigma; and by mass outbreaks of moral controversy, of potential solutions and of personal conversion to the many different causes which spring up. This distinctive collective social psychology has its own epidemic form, can be activated by other crises besides those of disease and is rooted in the fundamental properties of language and human interaction.
>
> *(p. 249)*

As well as citing European folk memories of the Black Death, Strong refers to reactions to AIDS in the 1980s when proposing a conceptual scheme for exploring the 'initial social impact' of a 'major epidemic' (p. 250). Utilising a microsociological approach to interaction and meaning making, derived, in part, from the Chicago School's pragmatist focus on 'collective behaviour' (Dingwall et al., 2013: 168), Strong (1990) sketches an ideal typical model that inevitably contains oversimplifications but which seeks to establish the core dynamics of how individuals and groups respond to socially defined threats. Such responses, which can vary independently of the biological reality of a disease, may also be potentially infectious and corrosive. In short, Strong's model aims to discern patterns of action amidst chaos and disruption to social order. Furthermore, if Strong's model pertains to *epidemics* in regionalised contexts and national jurisdictions then it potentially has even greater relevance when an emerging infectious disease is classified as a global *pandemic* (Dingwall, 2022).

Importantly, and given early concerns about 'psychologizing disasters' (Drury et al., 2020: 686) in the context of COVID-19, it should be stressed that Strong's (1990) position differs from 'atavistic psychologies which assume that disorder results from primitive emotions unleashed by such threats' (Dingwall et al., 2013: 2). Rather, behaviours that might seem bizarre and indicative of 'psychological frailty' (Drury et al., 2020: 686) are intelligible once understood in the context of a profound shock that ruptures everyday routines and a previously known topography of risk. As Belousov et al. (2007: 162) explain, 'of central importance here is the logic of situations in which people are placed by the context in which they find themselves'. Drawing from Strong (1990: 258), they add that 'the origin of the social pathology of what he terms "epidemic psychology" lies "not so much in our unruly passions as in the threat of epidemic disease to our everyday assumptions"' (Belousov et al., 2007: 162). Additionally, this social form is not confined to laity. It extends to experts who may similarly struggle with a new, frightening reality that demands interpretation and action.

Strong's (1990) model contains at 'least three types of psycho-social epidemic' which, in practice, overlap: (i) 'fear', (ii) 'explanation and moralisation', and (iii) 'action, and proposed action' (p. 251). In brief, Strong describes how previously innocuous objects and actions evoke fear (e.g. touching door handles, people and animals); how initial explanations reflect disorientation and are followed by an 'epidemic of interpretation'; and how 'control measures' emerge that 'may cut across and threaten our conventional codes and practices' (e.g. disruptions to trade, travel and invading personal liberties) (p. 254). Such responses have a history: whilst Strong refers to the Black Death in the fourteenth century, Foucault (1995 [1975]) describes proposed measures to control the plague in seventeenth-century Europe.

Insofar as Strong (1990) offers a heuristic, whether such responses correspond with social reality is an empirical question. As observed from March 2020 onwards, the declaration of the pandemic and mass quarantining of otherwise healthy populations appeared to be quickly followed by many of the collective psychosocial responses outlined by Strong – waves of fear, anxiety, moralising action, intense stigma, conversion to various causes, etc. Writing in the *Journal of Anxiety Disorders*, Asmundson and Taylor (2020) cite early public opinion polls from North America indicating widespread fear. They call this 'coronaphobia' and raise concerns about mental health. Initial responses to government mitigation measures, and not simply SARS-CoV-2, also became layered onto and complicated already existing global public issues and private troubles. For instance, following the research reported in Chapter 6, the initial COVID-19 lockdown inflamed anxieties about weight gain, fatness, food, eating, physical (in)activity and the moral imperative of health. Responses to the pandemic and the need to avoid burdening hospitals, in turn, provided further basis for framing 'fat people' as a potential drain and problem to be 'fixed' – the 'weaponising of stigma' (Scambler, 2018: 141) *and* fear (Dodsworth, 2021). Amidst concerns that lockdown/quarantine leads to depression and people consuming 'high-sugar foods', Mediouni et al. (2020: 1) also warned that 'countries should be prepared for the upcoming epidemic' of what they call 'depreobesity'. As per David and Le Dévédec's (2019) work, such pronouncements evidence the paradigm of preparedness. We will return to this point later in this chapter, drawing from others, such as Davis (2019: 34) on 'choice immunity' and managing one's body and those of dependent others.

In line with Strong's (1990) point about 'activating crises', early psychosocial responses to COVID-19 not only emerged amidst a failed war on obesity and pre-existing concerns about mental health but also other 'big' societal and planetary issues. These problems include: the 2008 crash that cascaded into a crisis in the economy, government finances (austerity) and politics (Dinerstein et al., 2014; Walby, 2015), (bio)terrorism, migrant crises, global trade wars, 'renewed threat of nuclear holocaust' (Lown et al., 2021) and the 'declared climate emergency' (MacBride-Stewart, 2022). Elements of COVID-19 pandemic psychology have ranged from scapegoating outsiders and xenophobic explanations about disease origins (e.g. eating wild animals, which is hardly unique to China), to the fear that everybody is a potential vector who could infect others if failing to behave 'responsibly'. Echoing the type of response that has long framed fat bodies as irresponsible, people 'flouting' so-called social distancing rules have been labelled 'Covidiots' (Maidment, 2020b) – an ugly neologism and headline grabber for dramatising mass media which, as explained in Chapter 2, fuel 'moral panics' (Cohen, 2002 [1972]; on how the media quickly amplified the COVID-19 crisis, see Ioannidis, 2020b). Besides being labelled idiotic, these types were deemed selfish and dangerous. Indeed, they quickly became the antithesis of 'heroic' frontline clinicians facing the 'horrors' of a 'war' on COVID-19, a fight that was reportedly leaving many panic-stricken, 'suicidal and afraid to hug their kids' (McKelvie, 2020) – though, given the infectiousness of pandemic psychology, clinicians have also been typified as 'contagious' and attacked (Sandberg and Fondevila, 2020). Early media reports of 'financial contagion' and 'panic' (Tooze, 2020) also stoked fears about economic catastrophe, a probable outcome that existed prior to COVID-19 given financialised capitalism's crisis tendencies (Streeck, 2016; Vighi, 2021). The initial panic even led (or, arguably, provided cover for) the US Federal Reserve to inject $1.5 trillion into financial markets, prompting concerns about policies likely to benefit Wall Street more so than Main Street (Klein, 2020; for subsequent evidence of and a critical response to growing inequality, see Avanceña et al., 2021; Chancel et al., 2022).

As noted, Strong's (1990) essay refers to control measures and contestation. During the early lockdown in the UK, concerns were expressed about the rise of the police state with reference to contradictory actions that appeared to both undermine and support healthist tenets and 'choice immunity' (Davis, 2019). In England, Derbyshire constabulary faced harsh criticism after deploying surveillance drones and social media to track and attempt to shame people for taking physical activity in the open country (at a time when restrictions on mobility was a ministerial preference, not a law) (see Monaghan, 2020). A Chief Constable also 'threatened to start checking shopping trolleys for "unnecessary" items' during the lockdown (Bienkov, 2020). Outside of subsequently retracted threats from those policing the pandemic, there have been ongoing antagonisms and challenges to authority, extending to the legitimacy of governments and their advisors who contravened lockdown restrictions. Given the rapid exchange of ideas in an increasingly digital society, relevant questions here might include:

How have populations responded with and to social media that provide *critically informed* space to learn from each other, including COVID contrarians in fields such as medicine, epidemiology and population health? Might parallels be drawn with the contestation of obesity discourse, especially in digital environments that provide alternative critical pedagogies? In the context of what Flinders (2020) terms 'crisis fatigue' – itself a consequence of repeated declarations of 'impending doom' and reported distrust of politicians, mass media and declining deference to other authorities – have different elements of pandemic psychology been more or less likely to manifest among various groups? Just as French citizens did not panic during the 2009 influenza pandemic (which proved to be relatively mild and was, of course, not entirely new) (Sherlaw and Raude, 2013), one cannot assume people will necessarily act in line with Strong's (1990) model. Rather than 'epidemics' of fear and panic, other responses might include: frustration, anger, disbelief, resignation, boredom, guilt, disappointment and disdain towards authorities acting in a draconian, possibly ill-advised and inconsistent manner. Elsewhere, as explained by Williams (2004: 75), who also draws from Strong (1990) when reflecting on bioterrorism, it would be incorrect 'to suggest that everyone is running around scared stiff or panic stricken'.

Constituting an important field for sociological and not just psychological research, we would make three further points here. In presenting these we are not only mindful of an agenda for future studies but also orientations to health(care) that are unencumbered by the tenets of the WCHP and war on obesity. First, as with critical readings on moral panic theory in obesity debates (e.g. Fraser et al., 2010; Raisborough, 2016), it would be a mistake to dismiss emotions or 'affects' as polluting, unwelcome and antithetical to reason; indeed, these might be informative and productive of social collectivities. For instance, how might clinicians' fears mobilise collective action and 'radicalisation'? How might such experiences, amidst stigma and inequality, inform or undermine future clinical education intended to promote 'structural competency' comprising humility and grass-roots advocacy for social justice (see Metzl and Hansen, 2014)? Second, to adapt Raisborough (2016) on media and fatness (Chapter 2), to what extent is society witnessing the emergence of a COVID sensibility that constitutes subjects as socially responsible, regulating and disciplined biocitizens, the virtuous antithesis of 'Covidiots' (e.g. 'conspiracy theorists', 'granny killers')? What might such sensibilities mean for social relations, identities and practices in myriad contexts that are crosscut by already existing modalities for judging, degrading and punishing people? Third, insofar as the theoretical traditions informing Strong's (1990) model are derived from interpretivists (notably G.H. Mead and A. Schutz), different approaches will foreground other matters that warrant investigation. For instance, critical or corporeal realists would likely pose questions about and seek to investigate ontological matters and mechanisms, which have broader political economic salience for bodies differentially located in society. Here we might consider the significance of social class vis-à-vis everyday actions and life-chances (e.g. the need to spend time in public space and risk viral exposure) (see Arber and

Meadows, 2020), and possible future macro-social scenarios (Scambler, 2020b). Other entangled concerns, likely of interest to advocates of 'new materialist' perspectives within critical obesity studies (Fullagar et al., 2022), might include how *particular bodies come to matter* in pandemic times (as immoral, fat, abject, requiring intervention). Such points are worth bearing in mind in our ensuing discussion, going from contested science to pandemic inequalities. Again, amidst uncertainty, we will pose additional research questions, with the ultimate aim of informing alternative approaches to obesity, health and society.

Contested science, urgency and the politics of uncertainty

In response to COVID-19, governments and other actors quickly recruited bio-medical and life sciences for clinical and epidemiological information and guidance. Our focus here is the relationship between contested science, politics and publics as policymakers and authorities attempted to control the spread of SARS-CoV-2 and how particular knowledges have been communicated within a dual crisis frame comprising a reinvigorated war on obesity. Our discussion also relates to preparedness and immunity. In the face of emerging and incomplete evidence, public health, medical, government and media attention turned to the alleged relationship between COVID-19 and obesity in two significant ways: first, questions were raised about the impact that obesity has in terms of worsening coronavirus outcomes; second, fears around COVID-19 were politicised in such a way that weight/fatness and lifestyles once again became prominent within the OFR and PRF of anti-obesity policy (Chapter 3). Such matters were salient in Britain during 2020. As part of our discussion we will also draw further insights from Strong's (1990) model, particularly on 'conversion' and 'proposed solutions' that appeared in UK Government policy during this period (DHSC, 2020).

First some caveats and general observations. An obvious difference between the declared COVID-19 and obesity crises is their respective temporal dimensions. We are now over 20 years into the putative 'global obesity epidemic' (WHO, 1998), and, despite campaigners' calls for urgent government action, this issue has been 'slow burning' (Raisborough, 2016) (Chapters 1 and 2). In contrast, global responses to COVID-19 have been swift and dramatic, due, in part, to the new and highly infectious nature of this disease – a novel coronavirus that is literally contagious, rather than metaphorically so as seen with certain representations of obesity spreading within social networks (Brown, 2014; Dukelow, 2017). Yet, as with obesity, official responses to COVID-19 have been problematic. Loke and Heneghan (2020), for instance, critique Public Health England (PHE) for over-exaggeration and regularly communicating misleading information to the public (for similar early objections in a global context, see Caduff, 2020; Ioannidis, 2020b). After explaining that the dramatically higher daily death toll, and thus public concern, in England (relative to Scotland, Wales and Northern Ireland) were due to a 'statistical flaw' in how PHE compiled data, Loke and Heneghan (2020) add:

Anyone who has tested COVID positive but subsequently died at a later date of any cause will be included on the PHE COVID death figures. By this definition, no one with COVID in England is allowed to ever recover from their illness. A patient who has tested positive, but successfully discharged from hospital, will still be counted as a COVID death even if they had a heart attack or were run over by a bus three months later.

There are precedents here, as reported in critical obesity scholarship. Referring to a highly cited medical article on possible declining life expectancy in the US population (Olshansky et al., 2005), Gard (2016) states the authors *assume* that deaths among people with a BMI ≥30 kg/m^2 were due to obesity. Estimated deaths could thus include mortality caused by road accidents, for instance, or anything else not causally related to a higher body mass. More generally, it is known within the sociology of official statistics and Death Certification that establishing the cause of mortality for individuals and populations has never been an exact science; rather, it is a social and thus interpretive practice that is open to contestation (Armstrong, 2021).

Of course, at a time when the COVID-19 pandemic was relatively new and (dubious) assumptions underpinned quickly devised statistical models (oracles) (cf. Dingwall et al., 2013; Mansnerus, 2013), mistakes were likely inevitable. Moreover, these problems and spaces for contestation, among and with different experts, became visible as science intersected with politics and public communication. Again, earlier work is informative. Drawing from Collins and Evans (2002), Williams (2008: 80) comments, 'it has been noted that the speed at which political decisions need to be made is greater than the speed at which scientists can produce consensual solutions to technical problems'. This has been the case with previous pandemics, such as the 2009 swine flu, described by Abeysinghe (2019: 14) as an 'evolving and uncertain risk' where the scientific evidence unfolded at 'a timescale that [was] slower than that of policymakers' needs'. Such factors pose challenges for pandemic management and the public communication of responses by governments and health organisations. Problems have been particularly visible with COVID-19 given 'the exceptionally widespread media coverage of the viral outbreak', potentially fostering 'a new expression of anxiety, reflexively oriented towards constant examination of practices in the light of incoming, and often contradictory, information' (Rebughini, 2021: 564). Nonetheless, such contradiction did not stop the UK Government and its senior medical advisors from focusing on obesity and dispensing lifestyle prescriptions in mid-2020, claiming, without conclusive supporting evidence (Chapters 2 and 7), that weight-loss will save money, lives and the NHS.

The state of knowledge on COVID-19 at this time, as with the WCHP critiqued throughout our book, hardly provided a credible basis for renewing the war on obesity. Reflecting the drive for a rapid response from research funders, governments and health organisations, a perhaps unprecedented proliferation of published research and public commentary quickly emerged on the COVID-19 pandemic. However, critical public health scholars questioned whether the speed at which academic/scientific knowledge was being produced was ironically contributing to further ambiguity or misinformation. Bell and Green (2020: 379) refer to 'an avalanche of preprints' posted online and an accompanying 'concern that weak, or even wrong, findings' could 'enter into scientific and popular discourse'. Arguably, in the race to produce evidence for policy (Rhodes et al., 2020), the COVID-19 pandemic led to 'an epidemic of interpretation' (Strong, 1990: 254) that 'infected' scholarly publications. For instance, prestigious medical journals hastily published flawed articles, only to subsequently retract these (Ioannidis, 2020b). Caduff (2020: 477) bemoans how the COVID emergency 'displaced a reliance' on 'basic' scientific procedures, with speed appearing to take precedence over 'the quality, rigor, and integrity' of research outputs. Furthermore, as with PHE, as described above, state-sanctioned bodies became vectors for pandemic psychology rather than stalwart 'representatives of social order' (Dingwall et al., 2013: 171). Elsewhere, when critically appraising 'fear-based public health campaigns', Brown (2020: 15) writes: 'Sampling bias in coronavirus mortality calculations led to a ten-fold increased mortality overestimation in March 11, 2020 U.S. Congressional testimony'. Such mistakes might be forgiven by those who moralise COVID-19 interventions and elevate them to a sacred value, but they are consequential. Notably, there has been a disconcerting tendency to ignore or grant 'less moral weight' to the human costs that have accrued beyond the direct health effects of the disease (Graso et al., 2021), such as those associated with lockdowns, an eviscerated economy and ill-fated weight-loss advice.

It is not our intention to single out specific public health actors as incompetent, especially when funding has been limited, pressures are high and neoliberal governments are disposed to axing public health bodies that expose health *inequalities* (as distinct from the politically neutered focus on health 'variations' or 'disparities'; see Scally, 2021). Furthermore, it should be stressed that consensus does not exist in times of 'post-normal science' where stakes are high, urgent action is required and there is input from many disciplines (Martin et al., 2020a). Inevitably, space for contestation and controversy is further heightened because scientists are dealing with social values, ethics and deeply entangled bodily matters that evoke questions about what is (un)acceptable to various publics. In short, there has been no pure scientific basis upon which policy decisions could be made (see also Williams, 2008). Indeed, such issues are entangled with affect and publics, underscoring the value of past research when orienting to COVID-19/obesity and posing questions that could be addressed in future social studies.

Earlier research suggests that the relationship between publics and experts is complex and potentially ambivalent (Wynne, 1998). For instance, the sociology of lay knowledge demonstrates how 'ordinary people' may justifiably resist 'the enormous condescension of professional experts' – especially when scientific knowledge is uncertain or flawed (Williams et al., 2022: 220). What might we learn from such literature today amidst uncertain, rushed and contested science and ethically dubious fear-based government and media responses to COVID-19

(Brown, 2020; Calnan et al., 2020; Dodsworth, 2021; Ioannidis, 2020b)? How have different publics interpreted the cacophony of authoritative claims, proposed and actual action? Whilst some people – especially those with 'authoritarian longings' (Caduff, 2020) – might express moral outrage when others, including researchers, merely question COVID-19 interventions (Graso et al., 2021; see also the epilogue), how is that response justified? Do others find it difficult to 'listen to the experts' (Kearnes et al., 2020) when public health messages have been inconsistent and have changed rapidly? As became quickly apparent in 2020, such advice was also differentially embraced and enacted in policy and law. Within the PRF, the COVID-19 pandemic resulted in what Strong (1990: 254) terms 'converts' who seek 'to warn, educate and convert other people' and who promote actions for 'containing and controlling the disease'. Strategies for 'salvation' (p. 255) have even exceeded what was legally mandated in the ORF (to return to the example of a police chief in England who threatened to inspect people's shopping trolleys, or, as reported elsewhere, much worse; see Caduff, 2020).

In short, COVID-19 communications, as with those already encircling obesity, have been 'deeply moral in nature', inviting moralising actions (Strong, 1990: 254) that extend to the control, regulation and even destruction of life (Caduff, 2020). For Strong (1990), the mass outbreak of a novel infectious disease 'presents such an immediate threat, actual or potential, to public order, it can also powerfully influence the size, timing and shape of the social and political response in many other areas affected by the epidemic' (p. 249). To return to Bernstein (1996, 2000, Chapter 3) on the pedagogising and recontextualising of knowledge, we might ask: how has COVID-19 been presenting such a moment within the OFR and PRF of obesity science, public health policymaking and campaigning?

Building on Chapter 3, and to draw parallels with earlier studies of anti-obesity policy, numerous avenues warrant analytic attention. For instance, researchers might explore the distributive rules that have defined, first, who can transmit this knowledge (relations of power) and, second, which knowledges (relations of control) are deemed 'legitimate'. The role of mathematical experts and modelling is an obvious topic here, discussed by social scientists early in the pandemic, albeit without a focus on obesity discourse (Caduff, 2020; Rhodes et al., 2020). What also interests us is how such knowledges impact the conditions of life; how they circulate through complex material-discursive relations that affect people (similarly, with reference to leisure and COVID-19, see Fullagar and Pavlidis, 2021). In all of this, social research could usefully explore 'controversies in scientific evidence and more obviously how evidence is mediated through particular political regimes' (Halford, 2020). However, as per Kearnes et al.'s (2020) commentary, we were reminded early in the pandemic that expert judgements are value-laden and emerge from 'specific social and political acknowledgements' as articulated by various actors. Mindful of those 'converts' (Strong, 1990) noted above, and their positioning within relations of power and control, future analyses will be important in understanding how and why different governments and state agencies implemented particular strategies (for emerging studies on related matters, see Lupton and Willis, 2021; Will and Bendelow, 2020). For our purposes, however, we will reflect upon the consequences of these (re)contextualising practices via a focus on the early articulation of the dual COVID-19/obesity crisis frame.

As the virus spread during 2020 and before the mass rollout of vaccines, governments, scientists and health authorities turned their attention to the putative relationship between COVID-19 and obesity in managing risks and immunity. Despite uncertain science and evidence, debates around 'excess' fatness/weight and health were again (re)contextualised through policy discourses as settled scientific 'truths'. Earlier in our book, we discussed how, despite the contradictions, uncertainties and ambiguities associated with the WCHP, obesity discourse is constructed through narratives of certainty (Chapter 2). Furthermore, as elaborated in Chapters 3 and 7, such narratives extend to the putative efficacy of behavioural interventions. Researchers and journal editors quickly emphasised the dual threats of obesity and COVID-19 and the need to tackle these, with varying emphasis given to T2 factors (e.g. the food industry, an obesogenic environment) whilst ultimately drifting towards lifestyles (T1 explanations) in policy. Such interpretation and (proposed) action proceeded through a 'pedagogic device' and forms of 'symbolic control' (Bernstein, 1996, 2000) emphasising individual 'empowerment', 'behaviour change' and 'healthier choices' (DHSC, 2020). In their editorial, Ryan et al. (2020: 847) comment

> the COVID-19 pandemic is challenging the world in unprecedented ways. We at *Obesity* have been sounding the alarm about the obesity epidemic and now must take up the cause for our patients with obesity in the face of this dual pandemic threat.

Elsewhere, Tan et al. (2020) suggest 'the covid-19 outbreak seems to be yet one more health problem exacerbated by the obesity pandemic' and 'the viral pandemic makes tackling the obesity pandemic even more urgent' (p. 1). Rychter et al. (2020) added to such concerns, albeit in a 'nonsystematic review' (p. 1). Although reproducing a dual crisis frame, they also admit the evidence-base is limited and uncertain and mention the possibility of 'obesity paradoxes' that might confer protective effects (for a later article, indicating the need for a 'balanced' approach, see Ioannidis, 2020a). Unsurprisingly, as per Chapter 2 on media and public pedagogy, news outlets recontextualised biomedical discourses about obesity and viral risks with alarmist stories and weight-loss injunctions (Pausé et al., 2021; Walker, 2020a).

In the UK, the framing of obesity and COVID-19 as a 'dual threat' featured strongly in government, public health and related media communications. In May 2020, the Secretary of State for Health and Social Care, Matt Hancock, declared a 'new' (*sic*) 'obesity war' (Sheldrick, 2020) on the heels of a NHS England study that claimed 7,466 people who died in hospital with COVID-19 also had type 2 diabetes (Barron et al., 2020; though, on the problematic conflation of obesity with type 2 diabetes, see Bombak et al., 2020; McNaughton, 2013; Riediger et al., 2018;

Chapters 2 and 7). Voicing depoliticising malevolent assumptions and commitment to an ineffective, if not harmful, weight-centred strategy, Hancock announced:

> We are determined to tackle the problem of obesity, and I am looking very closely at evidence it can worsen the effects of coronavirus. I'm convinced we need to reverse obesity rates to make our NHS fit for the future, and I look forward to working with the Prime Minister to meet our goal.
>
> *(cited by Sheldrick, 2020)*

This commitment to 'tackle obesity' also came after the British PM, Boris Johnson, was hospitalised with COVID-19 with him 'blaming his intensive care stint on excess weight' (Stewart and Walker, 2020). Johnson's public confession, in turn, prompted further political engagement as captured in the headline 'Labour welcomes PM's "conversion" on obesity after coronavirus scare' (Stewart and Walker, 2020, emphasis added). The issue of public responsibility invoked in these communications is not simply about preventing obesity, as advocated by those 'converts' anticipated by Strong (1990). Emphasis is also given to getting ready for a potentially catastrophic impact on the NHS as reconfigured through the preparedness paradigm and choice immunity, noted above. Of course, such concerns preceded COVID-19 but were subsequently amplified by fear-based social psychologies surrounding viral infection and the possible collapse of the health system.

The above 'emotional maelstrom' (Strong, 1990: 249) was mounting when we were first drafting this chapter. In July 2020, PHE published a report that suggested 'excess weight is associated with an increased risk of the following for COVID-19: a positive test, hospitalisation, advanced levels of treatment (including mechanical ventilation or admission to intensive or critical care) and death' (Blackshaw et al., 2020: 6). Dr Alison Tedstone, Chief Nutritionist at PHE and one of the report's authors, stated: 'The case for action on obesity has never been stronger' (cited by Courtney-Guy, 2020). Later that month, PM Johnson announced a new policy paper, *Tackling Obesity: Empowering Adults and Children to Live Healthier Lives* (DHSC, 2020). The paper proposes various measures but also clearly reinstates previous policy approaches that emphasise individual responsibility with 'a call to action for everyone who is overweight to take steps to move towards a healthier weight, with evidence-based tools and apps with advice on how to lose weight and keep it off' (DHSC, 2020). The continued attempt to 'nudge' people into particular behaviours is again reflected in policy, such as the requirement for menus to include calories to 'help people' make 'healthier choices' when eating out.

Whilst Britain's PM and mass media framed the new policy as 'helpful' – the new 'obesity drive will not be "bossy or nannying" according to the PM' (Walker, 2020b) – this reiteration of the WCHP remains deeply problematic. In particular, weight-loss prescriptions are stripped of the uncertainties and complexities that we outlined in earlier chapters. Codified in these recontextualised policy responses to a 'dual crisis' are retreats back to positions of assumed cohesion of obesity science and efficacy plus safety of weight-centric interventions (Chapters 2, 4 and 7; see also O'Connell et al., 2021). Yet, in the run-up to this new policy, England's Deputy Chief Medical Officer, as quoted at the start of this chapter, lent her support via the mass media to a renewed war on obesity. Her advice to the public to get fit and lose weight was also expressed on the College of Medicine and Integrated Health's (2020) website. Similarly, NHS England's chief executive – on the basis of a diabetes intervention that only lasted 9 to 12 months and resulted in participants losing 'an average of 3.6 kg' – announced that 'the evidence is in … this pandemic is a call to arms to adopt medically proven changes in what we eat and how we exercise' (cited by Helm and Campbell, 2020). Given the evidence reviewed in *Rethinking Obesity*, we would simply ask: really? In our view such claims, expressed with authority and certainty, are unhelpful and even unethical not least given the well-documented history of failed weight-centric interventions (for a critical response in the British mass media, see Orbach, 2020). Sociologically speaking, what we observe here is a paradigmatic case of 'strategic ignorance' among so-called smarts (McGoey, 2019).

Other objections have also been raised, such as the 'ill-defined' depiction of COVID-19 striking in 'waves' – a view expressed by a WHO spokesperson in the mass media during this time (Beaumont and Graham-Harrison, 2020). We would add that for England's Deputy Chief Medical Officer to moralise about weight (loss), whilst also lambasting young people for allegedly 'ignoring social distancing rules' (Blanchard, 2020), mandates the already well-worn media trope that 'fat people' are immature and selfish (Raisborough, 2016). Something else to consider, given the greater vulnerability of minority ethnic groups and working classes to COVID-19 (see below), is how 'the recontextualising rules' (Bernstein, 2000) of anti-obesity policy and attendant lifestyle drift (Chapter 3) reproduce an invisible pedagogy that is deeply racist and classist (to echo what is known by historians writing about earlier public health responses to plagues [Barnes et al., 2020]). COVID-19 may be associated with certain types of body. However, the crucial issue, we would contend, is their location on embodied social hierarchies plus the structuring and accumulation of (dis)advantages that are not amenable to individual change. Furthermore, how might chief medics and policymakers respond here to subsequent evidence indicating that whilst a BMI >30 kg/m^2 was associated with hospital admission with COVID-19, 'amongst minority ethnic individuals, a greater proportion were admitted to the ICU with a lower BMI than White British' and '[t]hose with lower BMIs were more likely to die in critical care' (Mitha et al., 2020)?

In sum, contested science, urgency and the politics of uncertainty have saturated UK Government, medical and mass media responses to COVID-19. Within this context, weight/fatness continues to be rendered highly problematic (Chapters 1 and 6), with the dual crisis frame providing a state-mandated (legitimised) opportunity to reinstate failed and possibly harmful public health policies and prescriptions that have already been extensively critiqued (Chapters

3 and 7). As with *Tackling Obesity: Empowering Adults and Children to Live Healthier Lives* (DHSC, 2020), this 'body project' (Shilling, 2012) acquires a novel appeal for various entrepreneurs (or recontextualising agents) in the midst of a corrosive pandemic psychology that has the potential to 'infect' various domains of social life. In addition to PM Johnson's so-called conversion (actually a reiteration of his weight-related concerns that were enacted before Brexit; see Knibbs, 2019), England's Deputy Chief Medical Officer and NHS England's Chief Executive publicly expressed commitment to fighting COVID-19 by urging the overweight masses (read: virtually everybody) to lose weight and get fit (a sizist injunction that prejudicially assumes, among other things, people with a BMI ≥25 kg/m^2 are not already healthy and/or fit). Similarly, the Secretary of State for Health and Social Care further legitimated the WCHP via the problematic conflation of diabetes with obesity. Rooted in language and interaction (Strong, 1990), pandemic psychology appears to have reinforced a pathology focused, individualising frame comprising ugly neologisms, such as 'depreobesity' (Mediouni et al., 2020). The entanglement of COVID-19 with obesity and 'related' crises (e.g. in mental health and healthcare funding) frames the 'problem' and 'management' of weight/fatness in such a way as to emphasise readiness. This future-oriented 'problem frame' (Saguy, 2013) incites vigilance and technological assistance (use of modelling in the absence of evidence, promotion of m-health apps), evoking a sense of urgency and the need for dutiful biocitizenship. According to the logics of anticipatory medicine, biomedicalisation and oracular powers, additional problems are on the horizon and the overweight majority must take control to avoid death and/or burdening others. The 2020 UK obesity strategy (DHSC, 2020) enacts such thinking via the pedagogic device and recontextualising rules of anti-obesity policy that serve as a symbolic ruler for consciousness (Bernstein, 2000; Chapter 3). Basically, the public ought to be losing weight (or become dedicated converts), through diet and physical activity, to prepare for further 'waves' of COVID-19. Yet, what about those inequalities that are framed as the outcome of lifestyle choices and reproduced through public pedagogy?

Reproducing pandemic inequalities through an affective pedagogic device

Opportunities exist for more expansive knowledge in (post-)pandemic times. Halford (2020) wrote early in the COVID-19 crisis that 'we have the opportunity to learn more about social divisions, social cohesion and social change'. Initial commentary from others is also salutary. Within the context of disaster response, Drury et al. (2020: 687) explain: 'Disasters do not affect everyone in the same way; those already disadvantaged suffer disproportionately'. Whilst we have undertaken some research on such matters (Chapter 6) and contributions are emerging as *Rethinking Obesity* went to press (e.g. Lupton and Willis, 2021), more social studies are needed. Accordingly, we will be better able to understand the impact of this critical situation on people, now and as part of the aftermath period as habits are disrupted and measures are taken to re-establish or invent new routines (Shilling, 2008; Chapter 4). We lack space to examine these social issues in depth here, including calls to build 'fairer' societies (Marmot et al., 2020b) and, most starkly, tackle global inequalities (as noted in Chapter 7) at a time when the billionaire class have done extremely well (Chancel et al., 2022). Rather, we merely draw critical attention to, and pose questions about, the consequences of the dual crisis frame and pandemic politics described earlier. Following our policy analysis in Chapter 3, we can see how such ideas in nations such as the UK and USA are again mediated by an affective 'pedagogic device' (Bernstein, 2000) that reproduces inequalities and problematic communications on 'lifestyle choices' (diet, physical activity).

Our concern here is not only with the tendency to fill spaces of uncertainty with sacred health knowledges, but so too embodied affects comprising fears, moral views and expectations. Negative affects evidently infuse class-based sensibilities, including those embodied by some clinicians, further compounding intolerance and weight-related stigma. Early evidence of this could be observed, for example, in the 'Twitter storm' that occurred in April 2020 when Royal Free London posted a picture of a delivery of 1,500 Krispy Kreme doughnuts to staff at one NHS hospital. Various medics were appalled. A debate ensued after cardiologist Dr Aseem Malhotra (2020) tweeted:

> absolutely disgraceful. Feeding junk food to already overweight and obese #NHS staff? I will forward this to CEO of @NHSEngland Simon Stevens personally and I can assure you he won't be impressed especially as THESE foods a (*sic*) root cause of increased death rates from #COVID19.

An affective economy (Ahmed, 2004) of anger, abhorrence, blame and 'social abjection' (Tyler, 2013) circulated in this, and the accompanying, social media commentary as 'pedagogies of disgust' (Lupton, 2015; Chapter 3).

To be clear, our response here would not simply be a dismissive 'let them eat cake'. After all, the UK is embedded in a capitalist world-system wherein myriad for-profit enterprises have sought to 'leverage' the pandemic and have been lambasted for 'signalling virtue [whilst] promoting harm' (Collin et al., 2020). However, what we find most problematic here is the moral outrage directed at eating for pleasure and the conflation of overweight and obesity with increased health risk in ways that eclipse crucial structural matters, notably in this case social divisions in formal healthcare. After all, those frontline NHS clinicians at greatest risk from COVID-19 have been women and minority ethnic groups whose general subordination in society is reproduced in the healthcare division of labour (Theodosius, 2022). Indeed, subsequent evidence of systemic racial bias towards minority ethnic health *and* social care workers in the UK indicates that social structures (not eating behaviours) placed them at greater risk of COVID-19 infection relative to White carers (Kapilashrami et al., 2021). In that respect, the moral disgust over the giving and consuming of 'profane' foodstuffs, what might otherwise be interpreted as an act of gratitude and affective practice that brings comfort and pleasure to beleaguered NHS staff, misrecognises and reproduces inequity. What we observe here is the further enactment of pandemic psychology that could intensify weight-related stigma, 'medical scapegoating' (Eichelberger, 2007) and other corrosive responses that undermine health justice. Inseparable from insider/outsider dynamics and pre-existing sizist tendencies, such problems deserve wider recognition by medics aiming to become politically engaged in these crisis times. Misrecognising such matters could not only reinforce unethical healthcare (Aphramor, 2005) but it could also have a boomerang effect that hurts clinicians who are typified as fat or fear becoming so (Chapter 4; Monaghan, 2010a, 2010b). On the latter point, see Pausé et al. (2021) on the unavailability of personal protective equipment for essential workers who come in various shapes and sizes, especially women and 'fat people'.

As fear and blame continue to be inflamed in this period of crisis (e.g. with the 'unvaccinated' [sic] coming to represent the new scapegoats for governments' failures), it will be important to track the circulation and trajectory of such affects. If, as David and Le Dévédec (2019: 365) suggest, 'epidemics are seen in the preparedness model as separate from both their social and historical contexts' then there could be serious implications in the (post) COVID society in terms of exacerbating extant divisions and health inequalities. Issues of social class inequality, foregrounded by sociologists from the outset of the pandemic (Arber and Meadows, 2020), could also be a key area of future research within critical weight and fat studies. This point is worth underscoring given what is already known about relations between weight, health and class gradients (Ernsberger, 2009) and 'the weaponising of stigma in neoliberalism' (Scambler, 2018: 141). All of this is consequential and disconcerting. Flows of affect, the guilt and shame associated with 'over-burdening' healthcare systems, circulate in the public discourse around healthy lifestyles as prudent, precautionary action. Such talk positions 'choices' as individual and population concerns rather than structurally indebted practices tied to material security, (dis)advantage and histories of oppression that fuel distrust of authorities.

Such issues are not unique to the COVID-19 pandemic but have intensified the sort of weight-centric public health paradigms that frame obesity as a self-imposed state, which can be modified through physical activity and diet (Bombak, 2014b). These policies not only ignore the moral dimensions of body size by failing to consider the impacts of racism, sexism and social inequalities beyond a 'thin' (methodologically individualising) understanding of society (Chapter 3). Such policies, as public pedagogies, reproduce corrosive weight-centric meanings and practices which also operate as social determinants of (ill) health. People experience (suffer from) these determinants, possibly precluding opportunities for equitable healthcare that is respectful, supportive and non-judgemental. As explored in earlier chapters, weight-related stigma and poor treatment in healthcare systems mean that many people feel uncomfortable seeking essential care and may even avoid it – a problem likely to be compounded given fears of viral infection and being shamed and blamed for allegedly overburdening hospitals.

Others have not been blind to this. Relatively early in the COVID-19 pandemic, numerous organisations in different nations (see below) issued guidelines and 'calls to action' in response to the heightened stigmatisation of weight. Yet, we would maintain that such calls cannot be taken at face value irrespective of advocates' good intentions and credentials.

Following the COVID-19 outbreak, several organisations condemned the intensification of obesity stigma and discrimination. For instance, Obesity Canada's EveryBODY Matters Collaborative issued a call to action in May 2020 titled *Weight Bias – Obesity Stigma and COVID-19* (Salas et al., 2020). Their contribution sought to advise healthcare providers, policymakers and researchers in the midst of the pandemic. The report contains relevant commentary (e.g. the risks of COVID-19 might be increased for 'people with obesity' who fear poor treatment in clinical settings). Critically, though, this organisation still engages in 'obgobbing' (Aphramor, 2018), reproducing pathologising biomedical labels that often offend laity (Aphramor, 2009; Monaghan, 2008). Elsewhere, the Association for the Study of Obesity on the Island of Ireland et al. (2020) write: 'people living with obesity and their families are very concerned and worried about Covid-19. Unfortunately, many recent media reports have added to that concern, by including unreliable and misleading information'. A representative from the Irish Coalition for People Living with Obesity, adding to this joint statement, complains that such information 'can only directly lead to increased stigma shown towards people living with obesity'. Yet, these organisations reproduce the WCHP; hence, it could be objected that their calls amount to 'coronawashing' (Rickett, 2020). This performance is analogous to 'greenwashing', i.e. when polluting industries promote environmentally friendly actions as part of a public relations exercise that ostensibly purifies them of their sins. Understood as a performance, what is important here is 'being seen to be supportive in the face of a national or global tragedy'. Coronawashing entails projecting 'an image of public-spirited compassion' by actors who co-create the problems they seek to redress (Rickett, 2020).

The fact that certain organisations are charities does not exempt them from our critique. These and other modes of obesity epidemic entrepreneurship, alongside obgobbing and coronawashing, cannot be extricated from widely circulating (state-legitimated and media-amplified) fears about viral infection, lockdown weight-gain, preparedness and choice immunity. Such fears have reinvigorated tropes about weight-loss as a simple matter of lifestyle choices, with little consideration of the affective dimensions of obesity discourse and socio-economic inequalities which lead to differential infection and mortality outcomes. Rather, throughout the pandemic recurrent emphasis has been placed on avoiding 'sinful' behaviours. For instance, early in the pandemic the UK's Centre for Perioperative Care endorsed the type of health behaviours that individuals should do before surgery to increase immunity and avoid becoming an 'unnecessary burden'. As reported by the BBC News, in a report with a picture of people exercising outdoors in what appears to be a public park (ironic given the ways in which such spaces were policed early in the pandemic), medics were:

[E]ncouraging people to take brisk exercise, stop smoking, maintain good nutrition and mental health and have alcohol free days to reduce their chances of becoming severely ill from the virus and over-burdening the NHS.

(Connor, 2020)

Amidst such moralising advice, other voices within the global ORF quickly raised 'dual crisis' concerns about physical inactivity and calorific diets among children. Obesity scholars in the USA opined that COVID-related 'school closures, may exacerbate the epidemic of childhood obesity' adding that whilst 'stocking up' on long-life food is necessary in terms of 'preparedness' and reducing visits to shops (fine for those with disposable income), they anticipated 'many children will experience higher-calorie diets' (Rundle et al., 2020: 1008). These early class-based fears and predictions appear to be contradicted by subsequent reports of 'child hunger' during school closure, when '[r]ecord numbers of Americans, including one in four families with school-age children, don't have reliable access to food' (Poole et al., 2021: 1; for the UK, see Walker et al., 2020). However, middle-class moralising, which also misrecognises how food insecurity is especially pronounced among minority ethnic groups (Gupta et al., 2020), undergirds those biopedagogies and inequalities described in Part 1 of our book. Such communications 'instruct' populations, particularly mothers, to undertake 'responsible' parenting in response to decreased availability of services (leisure, physical activity, formal schooling). Again, the imperative for individuals to cultivate their own and others' protection via nutrition and exercise reflects the 'choice immunity' (Davis, 2019) response to COVID-19. The responsibilisation of parenting circulating through such biopedagogies is also seen in early calls for schools to send physical activity plans home to be delivered by families (Rundle et al., 2020).

Within the PRF, celebrities also quickly emerged as pedagogues who were closely aligned with the ORF. These individuals were delivering online lessons either to replace or supplement children's learning during school closures, with a Sport England (2020) survey naming Joe Wicks, a 'fitness expert', as being particularly influential. Wicks even 'declared himself "The Nation's PE teacher"' (O'Connell et al., 2021: 147) as he delivered online 'PE lessons' to millions of viewers during lockdown. Wicks commented: 'When things started to get bad, I had lots of parents asking me how they could keep their children active while they were home schooling, or if they were self-isolating. I started to feel quite emotional' (cited by Bakare, 2020). The effects of these adaptations to learning are significant. For B. Williamson et al. (2020a), emergency distance education is a widespread matter of concern as 'pandemic pedagogies' become a distinctive, normative approach to teaching. Such educational practices, representing significant business prospects for 'opportunists' (Monaghan et al., 2010), may have negative long-term implications for education systems and, by extension, inequity (B. Williamson et al., 2020a). These are not abstract matters. Personal testimonials offered by O'Connell et al. (2021), for instance, describe the collateral damage associated with, inter alia, the message that one must 'earn' food by first undertaking physical activity.

As pandemic pedagogies leave their mark and new types of powerful pedagogues intervene in and perhaps profit from citizens' health concerns, we require a better understanding of such practices. Elsewhere, and prior to the manufacturing of the COVID-19/obesity dual crisis frame, research had begun to highlight how celebrities function as powerful pedagogues who offer 'particular visions of health, consumption and citizenship' (Gray et al., 2018: 16), notably pertaining to food (see also Rich, 2011). Further research might critically explore the educative impact of the growth of these types of celebrity health pedagogues, particularly in moments of crisis. Following our discussion on coronawashing, our intention is not to denigrate individuals. Rather, we wish to express caution about the way in which pandemic politics and psychology in the ORF can exert inequitable affects/effect within the PRF, mediated via the pedagogic device (Chapter 3). In the case of physical activity, scholars are scrutinising how fitness sessions, which are narrow in scope, are being mistaken for PE. Yet, PE is a pedagogical practice with much broader educative intent; for Harris (2018), PE ought to provide the educative basis for lifelong participation in physical activity. For Stirrup et al. (2020), 'the "one-size-fits-all" approach adopted by Wicks and others fails to provide an inclusive experience, as seemingly little (or no) consideration is given to students' ages, abilities or backgrounds'. Such standardisation is, of course, already well established in the commercialised anti-obesity terrain via the McDonaldization of bodies (Monaghan, 2007a).

The above instructional discourses emerged in response to circulating uncertainties, fears and anxieties about lockdown, at a time when sport and leisure facilities remained closed. Whilst 'patrician policymakers' (Dingwall, 2020b) routinely expected dutiful citizens to make the 'right' decisions, these have been impossible for many people. Socio-economic inequalities plus the specifics of lockdown policies (e.g. not being able to venture far from home) have eroded people's abilities to enact 'obvious' health practices, such as 'appropriate' food consumption, exercising outdoors and following online physical activity lessons. On the latter point, it is worth highlighting Arber and Meadow's (2020) observation on the 'digital divide' and gradients in 'digital literacy' that might exacerbate class inequalities in the time of COVID-19. It is hardly surprising that diet has also come under such scrutiny given claims that it can help maintain immunity (Jayawardena et al., 2020), and, by extension, profit a food industry that has often been vilified as a source of illness and obesity (risk). Yet, even in relatively affluent nations, the 'healthy diets' encouraged to 'protect' against COVID-19 remain unaffordable to many people living on limited/insecure incomes (Barosh et al., 2014) – an issue that will likely be compounded given accelerating food price inflation (Food and Agriculture Organization, 2021) and disrupted global supply chains. Moreover, during this time many workers lost their incomes whilst others had to remain in jobs where employers could not provide support or protection to comply with 'physical distancing' measures and hygiene practices – factors that are implicated in COVID-19 risk. None of this is remotely touched upon by the UK Government and their medical advisors when prescribing weight-loss and physical fitness in order to 'prepare' for further 'waves' of COVID-19. Obesity discourse, pandemic psychology and strategic ignorance evidently make good bedfellows, taking social problems from the political to the private sphere where the onus is placed on individuals and families to 'do the right thing'.

Such problems, recognised as *social* problems (French and Monahan, 2020), fuel growing inequalities and violence (structural, symbolic and physical). Consider not only the demonisation of specific racialised groups (notably Chinese people) who are framed as destabilising and threatening to the White body politic (Chapter 6) but also evidence on how COVID-19 mortality has disproportionately impacted subordinated groups. Whilst urgently compiled data need to be interpreted with caution, the UK's Office for National Statistics (2020: 2) reported early in the pandemic that 'Black males are 4.2 times more likely to die from a COVID-19-related death and Black females are 4.3 times more likely than White ethnicity males and females' (see also Platt and Warwick, 2020). Alongside the (increasingly difficult to hide) injuries of race and class, domestic violence against women and children during lockdowns is generating concern plus gender inequalities within the household division of labour and caring responsibilities (Annandale, 2022; United Nations, 2020). There will be much research to undertake to fully understand the consequences of these inequalities. Emerging feminist scholarship is beginning to signpost future directions and underscore the significance of these unavoidably political, embodied issues (e.g. Fullagar and Pavlidis, 2021). Despite the jettisoning of gender equality when 'real problems arise', there is a need to examine the impacts of the pandemic and governmental responses after schools and most workplaces closed and many people were confined to their homes (Stephenson and Harris-Rimmer, 2020).

These are just some examples of the social and thus affective issues that warrant critical exploration. It will be crucial to further investigate how pandemic policies, biopedagogies and recontextualisation reproduce extant inequalities. We need to ask how particular social groups are differently affected not only by (non-)communicable diseases but also by crisis responses, including oppressive forms of 'care and control' (French and Monahan, 2020: 6). How, for example, during periods of lockdown do people typified as fat experience further (intensified) stigma, in and through various media as they seek to maintain or extend social connections? What about the experiences of neglect, even, especially when inequalities intersect? To what extent might such experiences underpin short-sighted 'conversion' (Strong, 1990) to elements of pandemic psychology wherein the anxious scold other perceived 'miscreants' who putatively threaten public health (e.g. disabled people who are unable to wear a face mask in public)? What violence is also done to Black Lives when obesity discourse, rather than structural racism and eugenical logics, positions minority ethnic frontline workers (including health and social carers) as ill-prepared and unfit to survive pandemics? It will be important not only to consider these matters during the COVID-19 pandemic, but also to investigate how issues such as the heaping of blame onto shame (Scambler, 2018) continue (intensify even) thereafter. In so doing, it would be useful to bear in mind Strong's (1990: 249) warnings about the possibility of a medicalised 'nightmare' or 'war of all against all' when societies confront a large-scale novel, infectious disease - outcomes that could benefit elites who divide, rule (Friedman et al., 2022) and seek to accumulate ever more profits via a 'shock doctrine' response (Klein, 2007, 2020; Monaghan, 2020).

In sum, the continued reification of the WCHP and weight-centric policies, albeit through 'novel covid responses', may continue to contribute to 'the obfuscation of the policy failures and underlying structural issues that are responsible for many of today's problems' (Caduff, 2020: 480). In this perhaps watershed moment, the need for alternative approaches to public health is thrown into stark relief, extending, we might venture, to much bigger concerns about social organisation and the very future of society. We reflect further on such matters in our epilogue, going from critique with others to collective hope and possible action.

EPILOGUE

Resist TINA, recognise TARA

This book has invited readers to rethink what biomedicine terms obesity and its precursor, overweight. Such a task cannot be divorced from broader health concerns and society. This fact, in turn, prompts questions such as, 'what sort of society do we want to share and where are we heading?' These questions extend beyond fatness and are especially pertinent following the declaration of the COVID-19 pandemic that has thrown into relief public health concerns, collective modes of living and possible future trajectories. Are there better ways of thinking about and responding to 'the global obesity epidemic' (WHO, 1998, 2021; Chapter 1), health and society in these crisis times? *Rethinking Obesity* foregrounds matters that will likely rouse concerns for some time to come. Accordingly, we draw this book to a close with an epilogue, to avoid the finality implied by the word 'conclusion' at a time when much in society remains uncertain, chaotic and in flux. Our basic message, though, drawing from what we have learnt and navigated when undertaking critical weight studies, can be summed up as such: 'resist TINA, recognise TARA' (see Table E.1).

TINA and TARA are acronyms. TINA refers to the oft-expressed neo-liberal mantra, associated with the likes of former UK Conservative PM Margaret Thatcher, on the capitalist political economy – 'There Is No Alternative' (see Harvey, 2005). According to such thinking, the existing world-system might be polarising, inequitable and hierarchical, but that is the order of things. Capitalism is the best way to get societies lean, fit, productive and geared to tackling any problems that humanity faces – including pandemics of non-communicable and infectious diseases (Chapters 6 and 8). TARA indicates 'There Are Reasonable Alternatives'. According to such thinking, another world is possible that is more egalitarian and conducive to social and health justice. Other sociologists discern similar orientations to a world that has been in deep structural crisis since at least the 1970s. Note, for example,

DOI: 10.4324/9781315658087-13

TABLE E.1 From TINA to TARA – Ideal Typical Approaches to Obesity, Health and Society*

	APPROACHES TO OBESITY, HEALTH AND SOCIETY	
	Type 1: TINA – *There Is No Alternative*	*Type 2: TARA –* *There Are Reasonable Alternatives*
FRAMES OR DISCOURSES	Fat as fatal, frightful and a costly 'global epidemic' – obesity discourse, or the WCHP, entangled with a gendered aesthetic frame that (dis)credits bodies Current, escalating and entwined public health crises that demand urgent solutions (e.g. a syndemic, the dual obesity and COVID-19 pandemics) Healthism, personal choice and responsibility Making neoliberal societies efficient, lean and mean, i.e. conducive to the ongoing accumulation of capital	Weight inclusive approaches to health Fat acceptance/admiration and body positivity Civil/human rights Social (health, gender, etc.) justice Calls for 'more rounded' knowledge and praxis that are ethically defensible – rethinking obesity, health and society
KEY ACTORS	Obesity epidemic entrepreneurs Converts and allied professional experts whose interests/practices are not confined to obesity and who support the Biomedical TechnoService Complex Inc. (e.g. biomedical researchers and patrician policymakers who promote health as sacred, productive capacity) Focused autonomous reflexives (the governing oligarchy)	Practitioners/clinicians/educators who reject obesity discourse and the WCHP Critical weight studies scholars and those working in cognate fields (fat studies and critical obesity research) Fat activists, admirers and organisations/media such as ASDAH, NAAFA and the Fatosphere The oppressed struggling against global neoliberalisation, patriarchy and a history of colonialism Certain social sciences (e.g. critical, foresight and action sociologies) Dedicated meta-reflexives (e.g. the radical dietician and political activist seeking a fairer world)

KNOWLEDGES	Hegemonic, (bio)medicalised and often expressed with (unjustified) certainty	Counter-hegemonic, transdisciplinary and reflexive about uncertainty
	The dominant WCHP as a form of state-backed 'sacred health knowledge'	HAES, Well Now and fat pedagogy – diverse and subordinated but becoming more visible within the mainstream
	Methodological individualism, life and behavioural sciences (a preference for medicine, psychology, epidemiology, behavioural economics)	Receptive to cultural (anthropological) and social structural (sociological) analyses that foreground relationality
	Derived from and buttressing neoliberal logics and practices that are ultimately individualising and self-responsibilising	Ideally attuned to the reciprocal and consequential relationship between individuals and society
	Rationalised or McDonaldized, with an emphasis on calculability, efficiency, predictability and technological control	Partly rationalised but, as seen with weight-inclusive health paradigms, practitioners reject cheap/efficient measures such as the BMI or waist circumference (e.g. preferring to measure metabolic health)
	Ostensibly objective and detached though, in practice, ideology and values may be more important than evidence	More-or-less 'biased' towards supporting social justice and critically engaging with multiple forms of evidence
	Elitist and closed: patriarchal, sexist, classist, colonising and entwined with White supremacist thinking	Egalitarian and open: gender equitable, queer, intersectional, non-colonising and reasonably inclusive (extending to non-Western scientific, Indigenous and grassroots or 'lay' knowledges)
	Reductionist (e.g. the womb as an obesogenic environment, emphasising specific proximate risk factors, preparedness as a technical matter, statistics/statistical modelling that also serve as oracles)	Holistic (e.g. not reducing understandings of health and well-being to common risk factors and numbers)
	Conceptualising the human body as a machine and image, to be continuously worked upon, corrected and enhanced; future-oriented biomedical knowledge aspires to vanquish disease and suffering	Appreciating that mechanical metaphors and dominant images betray socially located bodies, which remain more-or-less vulnerable in unequal societies
	Health as an outcome	Health as a process
	Pathogenic	Salutogenic
	Reproduce/fortify existing power relations	Challenge/mock existing power relations

(continued)

TABLE E.1. (Continued)

	Type 1: TINA – There Is No Alternative	Type 2: TARA – There Are Reasonable Alternatives
TENDENCIES AND PRACTICES	Biomedical labelling, denoting disease (risk) and the need for bodily surveillance, improvement and even transformation	Rejecting, rethinking and politicising labels (e.g. replacing 'obese' with 'fat')
	'Top down' regulation and disciplining of 'targets' – going from specific 'problem populations' to practically everybody	'Bottom up' or grounded collaborations that tend towards humility, criticality and solidarity with the oppressed
	Susceptible to (the exploitation of) epidemic or pandemic psychologies	Resistant to epidemic or pandemic psychologies, understood as pathological social forms
	Alarmist, dramatising and prone to making exaggerated claims (e.g. 'excess' *weight* is an increasingly prevalent disease that will result in children dying before their parents and will bankrupt economies)	Scrutinising non-evidence-based claims and interventions; non-conformist vis-à-vis hegemonic/sacred interests and practices that rely upon authority, faith and oracular power – asserting that obesity knowledges, pedagogies and policies are not God-given truths
	Esurient, anticipatory and pre-emptive (prosecuted in the name of public health, biosecurity and averting the apocalypse)	Incessantly curious and questioning, asking, for instance, 'who benefits' and 'what is obscured or hidden'?
	Quantifying, standardising, technocratic and instrumental (e.g. physical activity as outcome focused)	Quality-driven, attuned to diversity and expressive; values meanings, rich experiences and inclusive opportunities (e.g. physical activity at every size)
	Visualising inside and outside of the objectified body (e.g. images of visceral fat, slim ideals); treating the body as an accumulation strategy	Relating to lived bodies as multi-dimensional (e.g. objective and subjective, biological and social), not 'things' serving a capitalist economy
	Fearful or suspicious of sensuous bodies, their freely shared pleasures and appetites (tends towards somatophobia)	Embraces shared embodied pleasures and appetites, which sustain and enrich life
	In line with the distributive rules in the ORF, attacking the 'profane' and censoring 'the unthinkable' – dichotomising, moralising and purifying (e.g. thin = good, fat = bad; insiders = healthy; outsiders = diseased)	

Responding to proximate causes of morbidity and mortality with various technologies (e.g. apps and other digital media, pharmaceuticals, surgery)	Constructive critique *with* others who demonstrate 'goodwill' (underlabouring but also building bridges)
Prescriptive/proscriptive about health – 'do this and don't do that!' – in accord with meddlesome, puritanical, patronising, prejudicial, authoritarian, intolerant and exclusionary tendencies	Emphasising distal (fundamental) causes of morbidity and mortality, which demand an ambitious macro-social or political economic response
(Un)intentionally harmful (e.g. contribute to an adipophobicogenic environment, disordered eating, body dissatisfaction)	Non-prescriptive/proscriptive about personal health decisions (suggestive and advisory)
Combative, ostensibly competitive and comparative (e.g. waging a world war on obesity, constructing international league tables)	Calling on clinicians to 'Do No *More* Harm' whilst also extending health ethics beyond healthcare systems
Misleading, deceptive, corrupt (e.g. perpetuating myths, presumptions, strategic ignorance, erasing uncertainty and history, obscuring lack of evidence with numbers, neoliberal corporate bias)	Tends to be co-operative and peaceful but also challenges injustices and harms (e.g. a moral duty to fight racism)
Weaponising stigma – appending deviance and blame to shame (notably 'mother blame' and scapegoating; weaponising fear to obtain compliance	Honest and committed (e.g. admits to making mistakes, learns from history, identifies gaps in the knowledge base and undertakes/promotes further research)
Conservative, austere and even cruel (penchant for health fascism)	Rejects stigma as a public health strategy and critiques the broader system that profits from creating shame and embarrassment
Disregards the larger public as deficient, deviant and/or dangerous (e.g. sick, pitiful, ignorant, childish, apathetic, lazy, gluttonous, reviled folk devils or even domestic terrorists to be neutralised)	Liberal, kind and caring (tending towards therapeutic, community-oriented action)
	Regards the larger public as capable and creative agents of social change (whilst they are a potential threat to the governing oligarchy, the real danger comes from a bifurcating capitalist world-system, bureaucratic state power, authoritarian longings and militarised modes of social organisation)

(continued)

TABLE E.1. (Continued)

	Type 1: TINA – There Is No Alternative	Type 2: TARA – There Are Reasonable Alternatives
BODY AND PUBLIC PEDAGOGIES	Sizist, fatphobic biopedagogies instructing individuals to make the 'right' choices	Size acceptance, compassionate self-care, body equity and diversity – promoting fat and critical health pedagogies
	Simplistic (e.g. energy-in, energy-out, eat less, move more), reflecting tendencies to infantilise the public	Mature relationship with various publics in order to grapple with complex matters of concern (e.g. discredited eating, the 'big' causes of disease in the population)
	The moral obligation/imperative to 'choose' health and slenderness	Learning that the 'correctness' and (in)effectiveness of choices are variable and are influenced by embodied social structures, culture and power
	Promoting common sense, manufacturing consent (e.g. the meritocratic mantra that hard-working people are rewarded, bad things happen to bad people, the body is an index of moral worth or failure)	Promoting good sense or structural competency (e.g. explaining that 'lifestyle choices' are patterned, and life chances are unequally distributed; exploring what promotes and prevents health development in broader contexts)
	State-backed agencies within the PRF issuing blunt warnings (e.g. schools sending letters to parents of children deemed overweight or obese; public health organisations evoking negative affects, or feelings of dis-ease: shock, disgust, fear, anxiety, panic)	Debunking authoritative 'fat fabrications' and becoming 'wise' to Orwellian 'doublethink' within systems of (thin) privilege and disenfranchisement
	The makeover paradigm within popular culture and media, especially aimed at women as desiring/desirable bodies	Critical media analyses (e.g. on 'moral panic' or the cultivation of 'bodily sensibilities' that discredit fat)
	Entwined with civilising processes, middle-class perfection codes and the pedagogic device that regulates consciousness	Deconstructing civilising processes, which further classicism, (colonial) violence, exploitation of Indigenous people and their lands
	Behaviourist body pedagogies that are correctional, promissory and profit from misplaced hope (e.g. longing for redemption from the sins of gluttony and sloth)	Foresight and imagining new pedagogic possibilities in the public sphere, geared towards sociality and collective hope
	Disrespectful towards and ignorant about the working class, women, young people, racialised groups, the marginalised and others who are especially vulnerable or traumatised	Respectful and supportive towards, and open to learning from, the oppressed
	Targets must learn their proper place in society: to become docile, disciplined, compliant, productive bodies	Emancipatory learning, possibly geared towards radical social action and liberation in traumatic times

POLITICS AND POLICIES	Neoliberal, patrician policymaking in an age of austerity and post-welfarism, ultimately serving (financialised) capitalism and dominant class interests	Varied, context-specific and emergent but radically democratic and intimating 'another politics of life' – likely post-capitalist, post-neoliberal
	Nominally yet hardly democratic, favouring iatrocracy and biopolitics – governance and regulation of life by targeting/changing the body (e.g. instructions to lose weight to 'save' healthcare systems and the economy)	Prioritising systems change with a well-informed demos in order to improve well-being and life chances, exceeding the common emphasis on personal bodily change (e.g. debating the case for socialising finance, a debt jubilee, tackling inequity, a Green New Deal)
	Health and social care as commodities (privatisation and insurance, state-backed opportunities for debt-leveraged speculation and profiteering)	Health and social care as collectively funded and valued public goods
	Marketised 'solutions' to the 'epidemic' of chronic and communicable diseases, generating not only opportunities to make money but also shift costs from the state to individuals – lifestyle drift and citizen shift (downstream, de-collectivised health interventions for 'redressing' inequalities)	Socially supportive and protective: for people, as valued human beings, rather than for private profiteering; addressing upstream social determinants of health inequalities and power-related diseases
	Postfeminist, which might be seductive but is also de-politicising; policies that advance and legitimise individualism and healthism for personal resilience, alongside the construction of (bio)citizens and 'the totally pedagogised self' as responsible consumers or even disciplined patriots	Feminist; advancing gender justice for intergenerational, societal and even planetary resilience/health/flourishing
	Going from 'soft' to 'hard' power – if 'expert' advice, persuasion and education fail then resort to coercive and punitive measures (e.g. going from behavioural nudges to shoves)	Explicitly against behavioural manipulation, coercion and threats, especially when enacted and legitimised through government policy (rejecting symbolic violence and other assaults on the life world)
		Genuinely supporting Indigenous communities (e.g. by advancing their land rights politics)
		Conducive to local, national and international co-operation and mutual aid

(continued)

TABLE E.1. (Continued)

Type 1: TINA – There Is No Alternative	Type 2: TARA – There Are Reasonable Alternatives
Treating Indigenous people as just another 'problem population' to be targeted and monitored by the state bureaucracy Conducive to local, national and international competition/rivalry/conflict Contradictory and fomenting further crises (e.g. consumers challenging medicine, exploitative global markets paving the way for reactionary nationalism or proto-fascistic populism) Misrecognition, enabling certain elites (the 0.1 per cent) to deflect criticism and profit massively from real, exaggerated or manufactured crises (the shock doctrine, accumulation by dispossession) Following the declared COVID-19 crisis, issuing calls to 'build back better' (read: 'better' for the governing oligarchy and their supporters who seek state-backed revenue streams and control of potentially recalcitrant populations) Politics of distrust, indifference and cruel optimism (hardly tempered by displays of charity and philanthropy in a context of extreme/increasing wealth inequality) Spirit of Davos	Seeking constructively to work with and through tensions and contradictions in order to limit, overcome and learn from crises and associated societal responses Recognition and redistribution in order to benefit the majority who suffer, or who cannot realise their full potential, under current (highly unstable, crisis prone) political economic conditions Following the declared COVID-19 crisis, calls to 'build back fairer' by advancing social (gender, health, nutrition, etc.) justice, in alignment with anti-systemic movements that protest against 'the social organisation of misery' Politics of trust, (self-)acceptance, kindness and collective hope – negating the need for charity and philanthropy by ending extreme/increasing wealth inequality Sprit of Porto Alegre

* N.B. This is an ideal type. Elements in this model may share an elective affinity but social reality is more complex and contradictory.

Wallerstein's (2011) reference to what he calls 'the spirit of Davos' and 'the spirit of Porto Alegre' (for an interview with Wallerstein on this, see Curty, 2017). These contrasting spirits exceed any specific group or event. However, the former is evidenced annually at the Davos World Economic Forum (comprising the world's elites and pro-business interests), whilst the latter is embodied at the World Social Forum's parallel event, which first met at Porto Alegre to counter the World Economic Forum's visions of 'an inegalitarian system' (Wallerstein, in Curty, 2017: 333). We believe TINA and Davos might find allegiance whereas TARA would favour Porto Alegre.

TINA and TARA refer to discernible configurations, comprising embodied modes of being, practices, relations and logics. As typifications they are irreducible to specific individuals and organisations but, to follow Wallerstein (2011), incorporate contrasting spirits and ultimately proposed solutions to a world-system in structural crisis. If we personify TINA and TARA for illustrative purposes, with the caveat that these are not actual people in a morality play comprising villains and heroines, we might be better placed to appreciate why it is important to rethink not only the putative obesity epidemic but also health and society more generally. We start with a description of TINA's signature elements, before moving to TARA. The remainder of the epilogue then discusses the importance of constructive critique with others, the need for collective hope, public pedagogy and calls for 'another politics of life' (Caduff, 2020: 479). Our text draws from various contributors, such as Scambler (2018) on the importance of sociological critique, foresight and action, and Aphramor (2019b, 2020a, 2020b, 2020c), a maverick within the health professions with whom we have had the privilege of working with in the past (Monaghan, 2014b; Monaghan et al., 2014; Rich et al., 2011).

Two contrasting ideal typical spirits

TINA is calculating, moralising and profits (not just financially) from (bio) medicalising weight or fatness via recontextualised expert risk knowledges. Everything and everyone, for TINA, should be colonised and subjected to her rationalised class project wherein the commodified body is an 'accumulation strategy' (Harvey, 1998). She is, as with public health, 'esurient' meaning she 'has a voracious appetite for consuming the social world' in an attempt to render 'all that is around [her] part of' herself (Dew, 2014: 141). Capitalising on 'strategic ignorance' (McGoey, 2019), pervasive anxiety and alarmism, she erases scientific uncertainty whilst also enacting stigmatising body and public pedagogies of disgust, fear, panic, shame and guilt for the overweight 'deviant' majority. Deemed an unenviable mass within TINA's worldview, these individuals must be educated about and prepared for the ills and risks that they allegedly face (Lupton, 2015; Chapter 3). TINA sees value in measuring and labelling the larger public, especially children, who need to be 'saved' (Evans et al., 2008; Chapter 1). If her targets are not considered pathetic victims (e.g. overwhelmed by the obesogenic environment or harmed by irresponsible mothers who are akin to 'domestic terrorists' [Rail et al., 2010]), they are blamed for being indolent, greedy and their own worst enemies. Fat, after all, is not only frightful but also fatal, a global public health crisis, demanding an ongoing/intensified war on obesity (Kwan and Graves, 2013; Saguy, 2013; Chapter 1). For TINA, the larger public cannot be trusted and are infantilised. They need to be given simple messages (eat less, exercise more) to fix the body as a machine, subjected to surveillance and, if necessary, disciplined and punished via symbolic and economic mechanisms of control (Bernstein, 1996; Chapter 3).

TINA turns to the market for services and goods to 'solve' the global obesity crisis. Saleable items purportedly mitigate early death and disease and improve the health of citizens qua consumers. Popular technologies include diets that promise to 'help' consumers help themselves via behavioural or lifestyle change. This project is thus entangled with healthism, nutritionism, postfeminism and health fascism that not only fuel intolerance and divisions but also constitute subjectivities. Some might say TINA profits from propagating 'cruel optimism', involving 'an impasse shaped by crisis in which people find themselves developing skills for adjusting to newly proliferating pressures to scramble for modes of living on' (Berlant, 2011: 8). Many people are seduced by the promise of making their own and/or others' bodies slim and trim, especially women and girls, though dissatisfaction and other costs often ensue (as explored empirically in Part 2 of *Rethinking Obesity*).

TINA tends to be unsympathetic to the plight of those who are less privileged and unable or unwilling to heed 'sacred health knowledge' (Evans et al., 2008). As per Dingwall's (2020b) discussion on 'patrician policymaking' in the context of COVID-19, TINA ignores the (dis)advantages people experience within extant hierarchal power relations that 'fundamentally cause' social, economic and thus health inequalities (McCartney et al., 2021). Because TINA supports a neoliberal capitalist system that is also structurally racist and sizist – she has White 'skin in the game' so to speak, intersecting with her middle-class 'thin privilege' – she rewards those biocitizens who demonstrate the ostensible 'will' and choice to adhere to the social order. Pro status quo, TINA benefits from an extensive apparatus that includes but is not limited to obesity epidemic entrepreneurs (Monaghan et al., 2010; Chapter 1) (e.g. governments, celebrities, journalists, obesity researchers, charities, transnational health organisations). These actors (unwittingly) advance TINA's symbolically violent project and would likely endorse the spirit of Davos. This spirit cannot be divorced from the interests of the 'governing oligarchy' or 'focused autonomous reflexives' (Scambler, 2018) who profit from an inequitable, crisis-prone capitalist society that needs scapegoats (Friedman et al., 2022; O'Flynn et al., 2014).

TARA tries to resist TINA's ideological declarations (deceptions or fat fabrications), structured interests and pedagogies. TARA's interests range from improving clinical practice at the micro- and meso-levels of society to fighting for social justice in solidarity with a broader community, including activists, clinicians and scholars. She listens respectfully to others with alternative or counter-hegemonic views on how to 'be' in the world, rather than censoring or attacking them for deviating from TINA's 'advice'. TARA hungers for 'more rounded and expansive' knowledge. She understands that evidence takes many forms and much litters the pathway to a fairer world; 'underlabouring' is necessary (Williams, 2003; see also Monaghan, 2013). She has no time for healthism, nutritionism and other reductionist approaches to public health that are depoliticising and obscure the upstream (fundamental) causes of inequalities. Reflexive, TARA is aware that her knowledge is always partial and in a process of becoming. This awareness motivates her to not only continually learn from and critically engage with the sciences, including 'inconvenient' social sciences (Connell, 2020), but also develop insights with the oppressed who struggle against social injustice in a global context.

Although 'against health' (Metzl and Kirkland, 2010) as constituted via reductive, neoliberal modes of governance, TARA seeks to better understand what promotes and prevents health development (or, more generally, well-being and human flourishing). When ambitious, TARA looks beyond formal healthcare (often privatised and unfairly distributed), hoping to transform the exploitative status quo. She believes another world is possible, one that could benefit the majority regardless of their weight/fatness. She respects embodied difference and the need for identity politics (whilst conceding these are exercises in damage limitation), favouring body pedagogies and knowledges that are supportive, kind, holistic and non-stigmatising. Her salutogenic approach views lived bodies as relational, multidimensional sources of connection, mutual aid and embodied expertise. Lived bodies are not deficient objects to be commodified and 'fixed' by capitalism and the Biomedical TechnoService Complex Inc.

TARA aspires to build and maintain a mature and empathetic relationship with the larger public. She knows they have value by virtue of being human rather than 'McDonaldized' (Ritzer, 2010) consumers in the neoliberal marketplace. Of course, many people, quite understandably, express health-related anxieties, fears and dissatisfaction with their 'looking-glass bodies/selves' (Waskul and Vannini, 2006; Chapter 4). People are often seduced by colonising, biomedicalised, yet largely ineffective, individualised 'solutions' to their problems. Rather than promising redemption through ill-fated purification rituals, which are also the mainstay of reality weight-loss media (Raisborough, 2016), TARA seeks to build trust. She does this by admitting uncertainty on contested matters that have not been settled by science and are entangled with social values (Chapters 2 and 8). At the same time, she advises on possible (unintended) harms associated with existing social arrangements, discourses, knowledges, pedagogies and practices (Chapters 3 and 7).

TARA, especially in fat activist contexts, can be playful and mocks those in power with whom she disagrees, but, overall, tends towards democratic inclusion. Her approach steers the polity away from iatrocracy, with some influential medics perhaps agreeing with TARA's stance because they recognise that a world administered by doctors (and those who would hide behind them, notably politicians) is not necessarily a better one (Smith, 2020). TARA not only accepts but also embraces and identifies with people who are marginalised, exploited, oppressed, silenced and traumatised by privileged actors who exercise power over their lives. Even if such power takes the form of gentle 'nudging' or communications calling for greater public 'empowerment' (e.g. OECD, 2017; Chapter 3), TARA remains unimpressed. She refutes TINA's prescriptions and proscriptions not least because they assume the efficacy and ethics of interventions that position folk as either pathetic victims or a pathologised mass of deficient/deviant/sick/ugly/lazy/costly/irresponsible individuals. TARA understands that the majority live under constraining material conditions that pattern health outcomes in a structured (unequal) manner. In short, TARA is a 'dedicated meta-reflexive' (Scambler, 2018) who strives to help bring forth another politics of life that serve broader community interests, much in line with the spirit of Porto Alegre, outlined above.

Some readers might object that TINA and TARA lack substance. Indeed, it could be asserted that TINA, in particular, is simply a 'straw woman' or crude caricature, fabricated by us so as to destroy what is in fact an artefact of our own imagination and confer superiority on her antithesis, TARA, with whom we would align. Hence, it is important to qualify the above depiction and clarify our intentions before commenting in further detail on certain aspects captured in Table E.1 that strike us as particularly important.

Crucially, we are not presenting concrete reality when describing TINA and TARA; rather, we are re-presenting aspects of reality. We have done this via the deliberately provocative construction of an ideal typical model, or heuristic device, which serves as a means for studying society and perhaps informing action to change it. For the purposes of this epilogue, what we have presented above provides a neat way of capturing the problem field that we have sought to navigate and rethink throughout our book. This field comprises not only the WCHP that is dominant within neoliberal health domains and policymaking but also alternative approaches. The latter range from clinically relevant practices and pedagogies that challenge obesity discourse to more ambitious calls to rethink society wherein designated biomedicalised public health problems are reduced to unwanted bodyweight and/or presumed 'bad' behaviours. When referring to TINA and TARA we are not discussing actual people (though some may embody these ideal typical orientations). Rather, we are discerning and mapping complexes of social meanings (including master frames, discourses), organisational practices, knowledges, tendencies, pedagogies, politics and policies. We, of course, recognise that these elements may be assembled in other ways, with various components of each of the types enacted in different times and places. In short, reality is far messier than our 'second-order' sociological construct which, we should stress, is not exhaustive. Other readers may even wish to add to or expand upon this model given their priorities and proposed alternatives to biomedicalisation and 'healthisms' (Overend et al., 2020). 'Indigenous food sovereignty', recently emphasised within critical dietetics, might be one such concern (Dennis and Robin, 2020). Following Connell's (2007) exposition of 'Southern

Theory', there are certainly good grounds for advancing such a project within and beyond the global metropole.

There are also nuances and contradictions in the real world, which our heuristic does not capture or glosses over. As per Clarke et al.'s (2010) reflections on biomedicalisation, complications abound. For example, elements associated with TARA emerge within modes of obesity epidemic entrepreneurship, which are also stylised performances (Monaghan et al., 2010). This 'deviation' was observed during ethnography in a commercial slimming club when participants 'expressed distance' from or 'secondary adjustment' (Goffman, 1961) to the rationalised culture of weight-loss (e.g. rejecting and scoffing at the BMI) (Monaghan, 2007b). That orientation, however, was also compatible with neoliberal logics as enacted in an organisation seeking to accommodate customers' preferences. This observation fits with more general processes reported in studies of social movements that challenge biomedicine (Crossley, 2022), possibly extending to a 'crisis' in medical malpractice litigation that doctors attribute to the growth of consumerism (Gabe, 2022). Conversely, elements of TINA run through TARA as seen when HAES insiders champion behavioural approaches to health (inequalities) whilst also ignoring or erasing subsequent input from former advocates who express dissenting views (see next section). Furthermore, because some fat activists and critical obesity researchers misrecognise critical weight studies, alternatives to the WCHP are not unified and harmonious (Monaghan, 2013; Chapter 2). As per Wallerstein's (2011) description of contrasting social movements, there are different intra-group perspectives, moral preferences and strategies for responding to crisis. This is a crucial point. It is worth underscoring in view of various actors' responses to entwined societal and public health problems that are also gaining wider recognition within medicine, such as structural racism and threats to Black Lives. On the latter issue, see *The Lancet*'s (2020) editorial which admits to the journal's historical support of colonialism and the need for social change.

At the same time, given the softer or gentler forms of power noted in Table E.1, vigilance is required. Within recontextualised health policy and pedagogy, apparent recognition of upstream determinants of disease and death tends to drift downwards towards lifestyles and behavioural prescriptions (Chapter 3). Yet, 'healthy lifestyles' do not redress inequalities in power-related diseases; in fact, they may increase them insofar as people enjoying secure material conditions of existence are better able to follow prescriptions and proscriptions that are conducive to health. Furthermore, as per Chapters 2 and 8, it is disingenuous for transnational health organisations, charities and other obesity epidemic entrepreneurs to lament weight stigma whilst enacting it through 'obgobbing' (Aphramor, 2018), 'coronawashing' (Rickett, 2020) and related practices. Somewhat disturbingly, such trends are apace, in a similar vein to how factions of the World Economic Forum and the Davos crowd co-opt 'the slogans that have emerged from the antisystemic movements' whilst enacting the opposite (Wallerstein, 2011: 86). For instance, Obesity Canada (2020), which is wedded to the idea of obesity prevention and treatment, markets itself as a leading voice championing the rights of 'people with obesity' (*sic*) (cf. Meadows and Daníelsdóttir, 2016) by advancing anti-discrimination and policy change. However, there is something quite insidious about ostensible anti-stigma campaigners and opportunists who market themselves as experts in this area whilst enacting the very problems they purport to tackle. As per pandemic psychologies, such responses are potentially infectious. Why would a disinterested layperson not assume they were engaging in helpful anti-stigma strategies when echoing Obesity Canada talking points (for a recent critical realist analysis of 'ethical tensions' in Obesity Canada's website, see Kanagasingam et al., 2021)?

Two last points are worth making here before endorsing constructive critique with others. First, none of the above detracts from the value of presenting an ideal typical model. Insofar as social reality is complex, there is scope for detailed research to discern how different elements in our model may or may not manifest in the empirical world and with what effects/affects. Second, contradictions and tensions emerging within alternative paradigms should not give cause for concern and despair. If the general spirit of TARA is recognised and prevails then we take faith in democratic deliberation and debate, the very lifeblood of a healthy society. Spaces, including pedagogical sites ranging from the inclusive university to the street corner, could enable the demos to enter into deliberative and participatory dialogue. In so doing, they may air concerns, respond to each another without fear and advance ways of relating, being and knowing geared towards solidarity and bringing about a fairer world. Of course, there are obstacles. The constellation of ideas, interests and practices associated with TINA remain antithetical to such a project. This problem is especially acute not only in the neoliberal university or populist right-wing social media (Chapter 6) but also in public health circles wherein the enactment of a dual obesity and COVID-19 crisis frame (Chapter 8) has reinvigorated the WCHP and war on obesity. Accordingly, we need to underscore TARA's tendency towards offering constructive critique in a world riddled with tensions, corrosive tendencies and forms of violence that are (hardly) justified in the name of health. Given our disciplinary backgrounds we continue to foreground sociology and other social sciences without obviating the need to go beyond disciplinary silos, noted in Table E.1 and to which we will return in the final section.

Towards constructive critique: critical social science *with* others?

Rethinking Obesity has documented difficulties when critiquing the WCHP and associated policies and pedagogies, ranging from lifestyle drift to fear-based public health campaigns. Such difficulties are ongoing and relate to health matters more generally. For instance, Warin and Moore (2021) explain how tensions and conflict go beyond state-sponsored social studies of obesity, with health researchers reporting problems ranging from funders attacking their interpretations to censorship. Yet, sociology helps to make sense of this animosity. Analytically, we argued that 'the pedagogic device' (field of forces implicated in symbolic control) delimits the thinkable from the unthinkable, the sacred from the pro-fane (Bernstein, 2000; Chapters 2, 3 and 8). Such processes have consequences within neoliberal policymaking and societies wherein dutiful citizens are morally obliged to 'choose health'.

As discussed throughout our text, the pedagogic device operates in multiple social domains, ranging from formal schooling to mass media that amplify and dramatise 'fat panic' (LeBesco, 2010). This field of rule-bound forces transmits body pedagogies that potentially regulate consciousness and shape lives (Evans et al., 2008; Evans and Davies, 2020). However, insofar as pedagogic practices/ outcomes are inescapably political they remain unstable. Disruption is possible. To return to a key argument in Chapter 3, we have sought to interrupt authorita-tive claims that 'communication policies to tackle obesity are advancing' (OECD, 2017: 8). We are not alone in this endeavour. Indeed, following the WHO's (1998) report decrying the 'global epidemic' and licensing a world war on obe-sity (Chapter 1), critical perspectives have burgeoned (Chapter 2; Monaghan, 2014b). Furthermore, alternative approaches to health – notably HAES and fat pedagogy – are filtering into the mainstream (Chapters 4, 5, 7).

At the same time, we do not shy away from challenging 'in-group' arguments directed at critical weight studies and cognate approaches (fat studies, critical obesity research). Meta-critique affords opportunities to further clarify and, if necessary, revise fallible scholarship (Fraser et al., 2010; Chapter 2). Our argu-ment extends to individualising health movements that challenge the WCHP (Chapter 7). Aphramor's (2020a) meta-reflexive critique of their earlier influen-tial contributions to HAES is worth noting, incorporating issues such as White supremacy. Yet, even here, debate is difficult. Aphramor reports being omitted from the HAES lineage when advocates refer to a celebrated co-authored text (Bacon and Aphramor, 2014), prompting speculation about intent, morals, con-trol and leadership of the movement.

At least two questions strike us as important here. First, what are the condi-tions under which greater legitimacy is afforded to ultimately individualising, pathologising, self-responsibilising and de-politicising understandings of health and prescriptions that drift towards lifestyles (and body composition as a proxy for risk behaviours)? Second, how might critics and sceptics of the WCHP pro-mote positive critique in the interests of health and social justice? By responding to such questions, broader communities of learning and praxis may be better able to cultivate and enact progressive visions for change. Such work includes efforts to get at the root causes of power-related diseases – defined as an 'epidemic' by Aphramor (2019a: 39; Chapter 3) with reference to oppression – rather than treat-ing population weight and presumed poor behaviours as reliable health proxies and targets for change.

In response to the first question, above, current social conditions are ren-dering already marginalised critique especially difficult. Following the declara-tion of the COVID-19 crisis, Caduff (2020) cogently explains how societies have entered 'a difficult place for critique' by sidestepping democratic deliberation;

indeed, 'critical analysis has become almost impossible' because it is associated with 'right-wing politicians' who 'seem unconcerned with public health and the staggering inequalities that afflict our world' (p. 481). In the midst of a declared public health emergency and the possible influence of pandemic psychologies (Chapter 8), social actors (notably, patrician policymakers) tend to reinforce familiar tropes, idioms and orthodoxies – worldviews comprising prejudicial prescriptions/proscriptions and already-existing tendencies to ignore or attack critical social science. Those who seek to defend critical public health scholarship are noteworthy here. Four months into the COVID-19 pandemic, Green (2020) asks rhetorically: 'Who needs critical social science in a crisis?' She adds:

> For those working overtime to save lives and keep society going in extremis, critical scrutiny and debate appear as unhelpful carping from the sidelines … When all hands should be on deck for the common good, voicing dissent risks being frivolous – or worse. The anxiety is that questioning the science will feed into public uncertainty, foster fake news and undermine clear, evidence-informed messaging.

Green cites Martin et al.'s (2020b) rapid response to contested science and possible unintended harms after the public were instructed to wear face coverings (e.g. impacting supply for healthcare workers, potential for 'risk compensation'). Attuned to power and exclusionary practices that rest on shaky scientific grounds, Green (2020) calls on her peers to be 'brave enough' to 'subject the knowledge claims of public health to critique' even at the risk of getting things wrong. Disciplinary insights and expertise extend to cultural (rather than behavioural) matters, which are hardly the preserve of native 'others' studied by anthropologists. 'Social impacts of the pandemic' requiring further research range from the meanings and (im)practicalities of working from home to expressions of 'so-called conspiracy theory' that manifest shared anxieties that might otherwise be difficult to express individually. Yet, despite leading medical sociologists' valuable interventions in media and policymaking, such action has its costs. In a statement that would likely resonate with those challenging the war on obesity, Dingwall (2020c) writes: 'trying to be a voice for sociology in [COVID-19] pandemic policy-making can be a bruising experience'.

In short, existing societal conditions disfavour critical social science, amplifying entrenched neoliberal tendencies to 'assault' such scholarship (Connell, 2007: 230). As described in our book, other academics have recently been encountering intense hostility – especially minorities confronting systemic racial injustice or women challenging weight-centric discourses (Hamera, 2019; Kamola, 2019; Chapter 6). One might add to this mix earlier evidence on how organisational and interactional dynamics may even hinder clinicians from 'speaking up' about potentially harmful practices, despite policies and practices intended to redress such problems (Szymczak, 2016). Yet, if informed critique is currently encountering strong headwinds – including fears fuelled by, inter alia, 'neoliberal health policies, nervous media reporting and authoritarian longings' (Caduff, 2020: 467) – then it is necessary, following the second question posed above, to engage with recent calls for more effective critique *with* others. We briefly reflect on this below, drawing from Mykhalovskiy et al. (2019), albeit with the caveat that their propositions are modest and imperfect.

Mykhalovskiy et al. (2019) seek to overcome polarising positions and strictures, such as the in/of kind observed with reference to sociology and medicine. In so doing, they endorse critical social science *with* others in the health field. After explaining how medical sociologists have sought to overcome the binaries associated with their relative attachment to – or detachment from – the medical profession (institutionalised, enacted and emplaced relations, as seen when sociologists are located inside or outside of medical schools), Mykhalovskiy et al. focus on relations with public health. Their discussion flags opportunities and dangers. For example, whilst there may be institutional incentives and access to research sites they express concern about 'the epistemic vulnerability of social science' or, more problematically, social science taking on a 'service relation' (p. 524). Such a relation means that its 'theories, concepts and methods are used to support public health aims, while the scholarly autonomy of the social sciences is subordinated to applied public health reasoning and objectives' (p. 524). How to get people to comply with weight-loss advice might be one instance of this.

Understandably, then, there are sound reasons to favour a sociology *of* public health as 'a form of normative power' (p. 526), with Mykhalovskiy et al. citing scholars presenting Foucauldian analyses and those critical of obesity discourse (e.g. LeBesco, 2011). Desiring alternatives to the in/of trope, Mykhalovskiy et al. (2019: 526) add:

> While this work is important, we have become concerned about its ossification and overwhelmingly negative style of critique. By negative critique we mean a tendency to take pleasure in pointing out the failings of public health, while remaining relatively unencumbered by an obligation to help produce something that might work differently.

Whilst it is inadvisable, in the absence of empirical evidence or the caveat of ideal types, to attribute motivations and feelings (such as pleasure) to others, we understand Mykhalovskiy et al.'s concerns. If we preside over 'ruins' (Latour, 2004: 228; Chapter 2) then, besides underlabouring, there is a need to rebuild *with* others within and across disparate fields. As stated in our introduction, *building bridges* is laudable, whether engaging public health actors or fat activists. And, to return to sociological analyses of 'framing contests' (Kwan and Graves, 2013; Saguy, 2013; Chapter 1), we remain open to the possibility of inter-frame dialogue and connections. In so doing, we may arrive at a shared understanding of how health interventions are inseparable from – and may (unwittingly) reproduce – structured social processes and relations that are exploitative, corrosive, stigmatising and a profound source of ill-health in ways that exceed the world war on obesity

(Brewis and Wutich, 2019). This project does not mean denying tensions and political or epistemological differences; rather, it implies engaging productively across divides by, for example, encouraging reflexivity and eschewing a coercive/threatening approach to lived bodies, discourse and action.

One of Mykhalovskiy et al.'s (2019) suggestions involves 'bringing the experience' of those people targeted for behaviour change into public health workers' 'phenomenal universe' (p. 525). We concur, albeit in a qualified sense, as evidenced in Part 2 where we explored the experiences of women who also happened to be clinicians who desired thinner futures plus schoolgirls negotiating postfeminist sensibilities and healthism (Chapters 4 and 5). Experiential accounts are valuable but in themselves do not trump the need for a critical, evaluative stance (Williams, 2003). For instance, organisations reproducing the WCHP and fatphobia may draw from 'the lived experience of people with obesity' (*sic*) by recruiting their own (often treatment-seeking) patients and sending them to conferences paid for by pharmaceutical companies. Hence, we need to be critical of how, even when working with others, 'patient-centred research' in particular contexts may be tokenistic white washing (Bombak and Hanson, 2017). We need an ethically defensible approach that is more ambitious than mere damage control. Rather than simply engaging in 'collaborative research' and 'seeking to lessen the harmful effects of public health practice' (Mykhalovskiy et al., 2019: 522), we favour the cultivation of collective hope and debating visions for macro-social change that are salutogenic and independent of *neoliberal corporate* interests.

The latter point is worth underscoring given the problem of 'neoliberal corporate bias', as described in studies of pharmaceuticals development and regulation (Abraham, 2008), or the manipulation of obesity science and policy by the soda industry (Greenhalgh, 2019; Chapter 2). Vigilance is especially crucial following the COVID-19 outbreak, with ongoing turmoil providing fertile conditions for 'the shock doctrine' (Klein, 2007) and the channelling of wealth to elites. Whilst evidence of this emerged from the outset of the COVID-19 pandemic (French and Monahan, 2020; Klein, 2020), this redistributive (extractive, corrosive) process continues. When we were drafting this epilogue in November 2020 the *British Medical Journal*'s executive editor lambasted the 'medico-political complex' for 'corruption' and suppressing 'good science' (Abassi, 2020). Working with others in medicine, public health and elsewhere thus necessitates not only goodwill but also political acumen. Much needs to be scrutinised. Working with others is not a simple, straightforward panacea in the health field.

Supplanting individual with collective hope: towards another politics of life

Aspects of our text might be depressing, especially at a time when 'coronavirus capitalism' has enabled some elites to profit from 'cascading shocks' and 'widespread panic' (Klein, 2020). In the wake of possible 'pandemic psychologies' (Monaghan, 2020) described in Chapter 8, we might even worry about 'a medical version of the Hobbesian nightmare: the war of all against all' (Strong, 1990: 249) alongside a pathogenic world war on obesity (O'Hara and Taylor, 2018; Chapter 1). However, in seeking better approaches to health and society, we will finish this book by underscoring three interconnected themes, discussed separately for heuristic purposes: (i) promoting collective hope, (ii) advancing critical public pedagogy and (iii) incorporating alternative forms of knowledge. These are 'lines of emphasis' rather than 'formulaic agenda of action' (Wallerstein, 2011: 87), but they could have practical value.

First, similar to those interrogating the 2008 crash (e.g. Dinerstein et al., 2014), we remain *hopeful*. Hope provides space for foresight and imagining different futures. Of course, we need to explain what we mean by 'hope' – a seemingly straightforward term that has nonetheless been subject to competing definitions. Like others (e.g. Berlant, 2011; Petersen and Wilkinson, 2015) we view hope in *collective* terms. In so doing, we resist the potential injustices of evoking psychosocial notions of resilience (Ward, 2020), which instruct individuals to find positives in the wake of crises and social inequalities and instead we orient our understanding towards a sociology of hope focused on 'collective practice' (Pedersen, 2012). In the contexts of health, medicine and healthcare, Petersen and Wilkinson note we 'live in an era saturated with the language and imagery of hope' but in ways that 'fit' with our earlier discussion of lifestyle drift (p. 114):

> In healthcare and medical practice, moreover, 'hope', advocated as a life orientation, personal attribute, or as an acquired set of values, is understood to provide the basis for 'resilience' and the strength of will required to promote healing. It is not only the case that an 'attitude of hopefulness' is deemed to hold therapeutic value, but further that the 'instilling of hope' is viewed as the overriding goal of effective healthcare in practice.

At the current juncture, pandemic policies and pedagogies have reinvigorated individualised understandings wherein biocitizens are urged to find 'positive' and 'hopeful' ways to exist. However, as noted when discussing TINA, cruel optimism reduces issues of social change and justice to individual responsibility. Here the imperative is for the public to learn various techniques or self-management 'skills', build resilience and find happiness in moments of adversity or significant rupture. Such thinking fits with the political economy of health and biomedicalisation wherein 'future-oriented hopefulness and hypefulness' serve as legitimating discourses (Clarke et al., 2010: 8). This reasoning might offer some buoyancy for individuals who may otherwise feel like they are drowning, but what of the macro-social conditions that produce suffering whilst promising (marketing, selling) thin (superficial, suspect) 'solutions'?

Eschewing 'negative critique' (Mykhalovskiy et al., 2019: 526), we are inclined to positively rethink hope and what it 'does'. Rather than, for instance, reifying and celebrating 'individualistic and psychotherapeutic orientation to managing health and illness' (Petersen and Wilkinson, 2015: 114) – an approach that aims to personally empower individuals and develop literacy to make 'better' lifestyles choices – we 'hope' for social transformation that might benefit most of humanity. To be sure, there are many ideas 'lying around' that intimate a brighter, more hopeful, future (e.g. socialising the financial system, a debt jubilee, universal basic income, a Green New Deal). However, our aim here is not to present a blueprint for social action and change. Rather, we are supporting calls to explore such matters with myriad actors, not just clinicians, who oppose ideas 'designed to further enrich the already unimaginably wealthy while leaving the most vulnerable further exposed' (Klein, 2020).

Crucially, unveiling opportunities for hope is not a linear process unfolding in a social vacuum (Friere, 2014 [1992]). What might come is entwined with (representations of) what has been, including entrenched structured interests/tendencies/biases that are playing out as we write. Hope might even seem quite fanciful given the durability of neoliberalism, evidenced after the 2008 crash, and progressive academics' perhaps unfounded faith in the possibility of institutionally embedding socially protective policies 'within the apparatuses of the state' (Cahill, 2011: 479). Nonetheless, in the aftermath of crises, scholars note how political unrest *could* provide opportunity for potentially egalitarian social transformation (Lipman, 2011; Martínez-Rodríguez and Fernández-Herrería, 2017), including extensive spontaneous localised life-supportive action within the 'shell' of the existing system (Preston and Firth, 2020: 67). Projects for change, even if mired by setbacks and the state's cruel indifference – evidenced in the aftermath of the Grenfell Tower fire and ongoing activism – instantiate 'a caring world' wherein communities 'value human life and solidarity and keep fighting for them' (Cornish, 2021: 293). That point, from a nuanced analysis that befuddles the hope/despair dichotomy, is worth underscoring, especially given the 'ugly' reactions reported in Chapter 6. Elsewhere, Walby (2015) states progressive political resistance has occurred in recent years (notably in response to fiscal crisis and austerity) but history teaches us that minorities tend to be scapegoated. Alternatively, collective hope might be more easily enacted when most of the public are scapegoated by political elites and mass media for myriad ills that can be traced to the basic structure of society, rather than weight/fatness and 'irresponsible' behaviours.

This brings us to our second point about *critical public pedagogies*, incorporating efforts to ascertain how certain meanings are legitimised as common sense within the dominant social order (see Rich, 2011). This line of emphasis fits well with the conceptualisation of 'pedagogy writ large as bridges, or rather as multiple crossing points' (Hickey-Moody et al., 2010: 234). When interrogating the WCHP and world war on obesity, such pedagogy entails expanding 'health education' not just for scholars but also teachers, researchers, cultural workers, practitioners, students, activists and others desiring broader social transformation. Avoiding fear-based pedagogy and manufactured disgust (Lupton, 2015), we contend that knowledge production, action and publicness (Biesta, 2012) necessitate a shared journey of learning, creativity, humility and openness. In view of the conditions and responses described above, public space must exist for ethically defensible debate with people demonstrating *'goodwill'* (Wallerstein, 2011: 87, emphasis added). In so doing, much may be gained by exploring proposed actions that are believed to be 'sensible and fair, designed to keep as many people as possible safe, secure and healthy' (Klein, 2020). To be sure, life is never completely safe (Dingwall, 2021) and 'safety' could be invoked to justify almost anything (e.g. state-enforced curtailment of civil rights and basic freedoms). However, we are also reminded here of Harvey's (2005: 39) point, noted in Chapter 1 and listed in Table E.1, on the necessity of 'good sense' that is critical of neoliberal mantras and processes that disproportionately benefit the 0.1 per cent (Chancel et al., 2022).

Other scholars have recently highlighted related concerns when 'reimagining new pedagogical possibilities' (Peters et al., 2020). For these authors the COVID-19 pandemic has foregrounded 'issues of sociality' or the importance of reflecting on how 'people within and across communities' could relate to one another in ways that give rise to 'new cultural and social formations' (pp. 1–2). As with conceptualisations of hope, sociality should not be framed simply as a matter of helping individuals to be resilient to social problems. Rather, what is crucial is the formation of relationalities that promote critically and democratically informed (grounded or bottom-up, rather than authoritarian or top-down) actions that challenge classism, racism, gender inequality and other intersecting structures. Arguably, such actions are necessary, in part, to reclaim the public sphere and duties that have been threatened and devolved by processes of neoliberalisation that extract value from the public body (see Giroux, 2020). When responding to what might be regarded as highly deceptive, parasitic processes (Monaghan and O'Flynn, 2017), pedagogy needs to be rooted in and for society comprising solidarity, recognition of interconnectedness and interdependency. *Rethinking Obesity* supports critical public pedagogy so that collective action for change is widely informed and the world has a chance to heal and flourish. In short, such pedagogy must be focused on the quality of human relationships and togetherness, on events becoming public (Biesta, 2012), not the recontextualisation of 'protection' as an atomising, 'socially distanced' (*sic*) practice as recently enacted/enforced in 'the COVID society' (Lupton and Willis, 2021).

Third, we underscore the importance of *incorporating alternative forms of knowledge* when, to return to a point made in Chapter 1, seeking to 'dismantle the old ordinances and draw new maps' (Aphramor, 2005: 317). For instance, we are not alone in proposing an embodied perspective that challenges Cartesian dualistic legacies of the mind/body, reason/emotion, nature/culture, society/biology, public/private, us/them kind (e.g. Williams and Bendelow, 1998; Williams and Monaghan, 2022). Alongside embodied sociology, which disabuses us of the notion that the lived body can be adequately conceptualised and treated as a machine, there is scope to learn from alternative cosmologies so as to rethink health and society. In particular, we need an alternative to hierarchical, colonising, technoscientific tendencies that manifest as power over or domination of lived bodies, as if biology existed outside of society, culture, history and politics

(Caduff, 2020; Chapters 1 and 8). Elsewhere, we have incorporated Indigenous understandings of relational bodies when responding to the framing of obesity as a 'neoliberal epidemic' and proposing alternative ways of knowing (Monaghan et al., 2018). Although not explicitly referring to Connell (2007), such work might be advanced with reference to the global dynamics of knowledge production vis-à-vis colonialism, imperialism, violence and calls for the metropole to learn from the Global South. Subsequent scholarship in critical dietetics and public health also underscores Indigenous knowledge (Cyr and Riediger, 2021; Dennis and Robin, 2020) plus anthropological work that recognises traumatic histories of colonialism, damaging biomedical practices and hope as an 'ambiguous space' (Warin et al., 2020: 102). In a similar vein, Aphramor (2020a, 2020b) endorses reflexive and respectful engagement with Indigenous and non-Western scientific knowledges as well as writings on futurity. Such reasoning offers a useful antidote to the neoliberal mantra, TINA, undergirding forward-looking practices with a global awareness of what has been and currently is the case.

Of course, other alternative approaches foreground relationality and are gaining traction among social scientists exploring obesity and health-related matters. For instance, 'new materialist' theories and methodologies (e.g. Fox and Powell, 2021; Fullagar et al., 2022) raise questions about how bodies come to *matter*. Fullagar et al. (2022: 95, emphasis in original) promote these approaches for advancing 'a *relational ontology* concerning what the matter of fat bodies "does" and how such agentic capacities are produced through entangled biopolitical relations (biological, cultural, economic and ecological)'. For these authors new materialist approaches open up potentially novel ways of thinking, doing and being across obesity research, policy and health practice (see also Lupton, 2018: 24–5). Whether or not one is swayed by such arguments (and there may be grounds for evaluating the professed 'newness' of such work via a critical realist approach), they certainly deserve to be debated. Such work might also be read alongside other literature on transdisciplinarity, especially since health matters 'span biology, social positionality, place and generation' (Yoshizawa, 2012: 348). Going beyond disciplinary silos is crucial as scholars grapple with external and internal (biosocial) environments that shape health – or, more broadly, the conditions under which humans flourish, merely survive or perish.

In building upon the previous point and underscoring the need for debate, we would note two further contributions. First, MacBride-Stewart (2022) calls on medical sociologists to develop new materialist perspectives in order to better explain how intersecting societal-biophysical processes contribute to human and planetary health. Her call is worth engaging amidst emerging concerns about the so-called global syndemic (Swinburn et al., 2019) which, in its current formulation, contains various red flags (e.g. endorsement of the World Economic Forum) (for additional critique directed at this and other examples of 'political epidemiology', see Schorb, 2021). Second, foregrounding in utero environments and possible associations with obesity in gendered relational contexts, Warin (2015) endorses material feminism when grappling with the interplay and connectedness of biology and society. Although justifiably critical of some strands of social science that reduce the body to text or discourse, her reasoning is compatible with embodied sociology, which foregrounds 'the multi-dimensional body' (Shilling, 2012; Watson, 2000), and calls to redress upstream social determinants of health. This thinking reminds us of earlier commentary from Aphramor (2005) on, inter alia, the foetal origins of disease in contexts of global power, inequality and border crossings. It potentially offers a welcome alternative to blaming mothers for an obesity crisis. Crucially, when making this point we resist reductionist and stigmatising elements associated with TINA (Table E.1) that frame higher-weight women's wombs as another 'obesogenic environment' (Bombak et al., 2016; McPhail et al., 2016; Chapter 2).

There is much we could signpost when underscoring the need for alternative or counter-hegemonic knowledges and ways of living in the context of real, manufactured or exaggerated crises. Another example is Preston and Firth's (2020) recent synthesis of Marxian and anarchist perspectives when exploring COVID-19, class and mutual aid. Such thinking could acquire increased significance in 'Western liberal democracies' amidst the ominous intensification of state authoritarianism that has largely been unchallenged (embraced even) by 'the Academic Left' (Simandan et al., in press). However, in returning to a continued source of inspiration from the coalface of healthcare and community praxis, we are particularly moved by Aphramor's (2020c) recent intervention on reframing health ethics. Issuing a meta-reflexive call for liberation within and beyond healthcare, Aphramor asserts that we need to be more ambitious than relying on reductionist science (approaches dominated by methodological individualism, Chapter 3). Rather, the aim is to understand 'phenomena through interconnection' and a 'relational shift' that 'opens up widely different scientific and ethical imagination sparking the radical break we need for liberation'. Aphramor comments here on the Hippocratic Oath 'Do No Harm' that is located in 'clinician–patient interaction'. They suggest this phrase 'wipes out social dimensions of health ethics. In other words, it perpetuates a healthist view of health where health ethics [are] limited to the healthcare system'. Their alternative call to 'Do No *More* Harm' (emphasis in original) instead foregrounds the body politic, recognising 'harm has already been done' within broader systems of oppression and privilege, including White privilege. Aphramor is basically arguing for health ethics that recognise myriad harms through 'connection' and, 'by inscribing relationships', such thinking 'surfaces hidden histories, breaks culturally proscribed silences and better serves the global majority'. Through this relationality and togetherness we may recognise that for many the 'catastrophe has already happened' – be that displacement, battling disaffection because of weight stigma, hunger due to food poverty (exacerbated during and in the aftermath of the COVID-19 pandemic response), racial inequality and other injustices that harm public health.

We finish *Rethinking Obesity* by returning to the 'big' questions that we posed at the start of this epilogue: 'what sort of society are we heading towards and what sort of world do we want to share?' With our eyes on the past, present and possible future we are not naive to the fact that there is much to do, but we also remain optimistic about productive opportunities for building alterative visions and projects. Such a sentiment hopefully resonates with others in our discipline and the society it studies, as suggested by the theme for the British Sociological Association's 70th Anniversary Conference, 'Remaking the Future' – a theme formulated in response not only to COVID-19 but also to other crises related to the environment, employment, racial injustice and threats to critical social science. Of course, in these crisis times, which are amplifying pre-existing anxieties within modernity (Rebughini, 2021), it is easy to despair and/or perhaps retreat into privatised pursuits for those fortunate enough to have that option. Besides despondency or focusing on 'problems' that *seem* to be more immediately under individual control (e.g. unwanted weight/fatness and efforts to reshape the commodified body), waves of pandemic psychology could fuel increased distrust or mistrust and smash the already 'fractured society' (Scambler, 2018). At the current juncture there is much to digest, with publics and academics alike seeking to 'process the [COVID-19] pandemic' (Will and Bendelow, 2020) and entangled problems such as mass unemployment, social isolation, censorship, corruption, threats and penalties issued in the name of public health. Unfortunately, under such conditions a new system could emerge that is as bad or worse than what we currently have (Wallerstein, 2011), amplifying populist proto-fascistic tendencies and authoritarian longings (Caduff, 2020; Scambler, 2020b). Whilst Wallerstein (2011: 88) might add to this pessimism when advising 'we must run like the plague from any sense that history is on our side, that the good society is certain to come' he also offers counsel that buttresses our call to supplant individual with collective hope. Indeed, we are encouraged by his historicised point that human agency could tilt an unstable world-system in particular directions. Actions can make a difference, especially if a bifurcating system in structural crisis has drastically veered from equilibrium. Drawing from Lorenz on 'the butterfly effect', Wallerstein explains that even small actions 'affect the climate at the other end of the world a little bit' (cited in Curty, 2017: 334). The results cannot be predicted. However, stating there is a 50/50 chance that we could help develop a more equal, less hierarchical and polarising system, he urges people to 'go forth and be effective little butterflies!' (p. 334). Accordingly, what messages might these butterflies convey? Going from the substantive focus of our text to bigger matters, we have some suggestions: Obesity is no more than a crude proxy for power-related diseases. Every*body* deserves respect. Solidarity with the oppressed. Reject authoritarianism and the weaponisation of fear. Dismantle the machinery of inequality. Recognise TARA. Another politics of life is possible.

REFERENCES

Abassi, K. (2020) Covid-19: politicisation, 'corruption', and suppression of science, *BMJ*, 371: m4425.

Abeysinghe, S. (2019) Global health governance and pandemics: uncertainty and institutional decision-making. In K. Bjørkdahl and B. Carlsen (eds), *Pandemics, Publics and Politics: Staging Responses to Public Health Crises*. Gateway East, Singapore: Palgrave Macmillan.

Abraham, J. (2008) Sociology of pharmaceuticals development and regulation: a realist empirical research programme, *Sociology of Health & Illness*, 30(6): 869–885.

Academy of Medical Royal Colleges (2013) *Measuring Up: The Medical Profession's Prescription for the Nation's Obesity Crisis*. Online: <www.aomrc.org.uk/wp-content/uploads/2016/05/Measuring_Up_0213.pdf> Accessed 9 August 2016.

Ahmed, S. (2004) *The Cultural Politics of Emotion*. New York: Routledge.

Alberga, A.S., Pickering, B.J., Alix Hayden, K. et al. (2016) Weight bias reduction in health professionals: a systematic review, *Clinical Obesity*, 6(3): 175–188

Allison, D.B., Bown, A.W., George, B.J. and Kaiser, K.A. (2016) Reproducibility: a tragedy of errors, *Nature*, 530: 27–29.

Almond, D., Lee, A. and Schwartz, A.E. (2016) Impacts of classifying New York City students as overweight, *Proceedings of the National Academy of Sciences of the United States of America*, 113(13): 3488–3491.

Andrejevic, M. (2002a) The kinder, gentler gaze of Big Brother, *New Media & Society*, 4(2): 251–270.

Andrejevic, M. (2002b) The work of being watched: interactive media and the exploitation of self-disclosure, *Critical Studies in Media Communication*, 19(2): 230–248.

Annandale, E. (2022) Gender. In L.F. Monaghan and J. Gabe (eds), *Key Concepts in Medical Sociology*, 3rd edn. London: SAGE.

Anthem, P. (2020) Risk of hunger pandemic as coronavirus set to almost double acute hunger by end of 2020. *World Food Programme Insight*. Online: <https://insight.wfp.org/covid-19-will-almost-double-people-in-acute-hunger-by-end-of-2020-59df-0c4a8072> Accessed 3 November 2020.

Aphramor, L. (2005) Is a weight-centred health framework salutogenic? Some thoughts on unhinging certain dietary ideologies, *Social Theory & Health*, 3(4): 315–340.

Aphramor, L. (2006) Scales before our eyes: fatness as if social justice mattered, paper presented at *Expanding the Obesity Debate*, Limerick University, Ireland, 9 January.

Aphramor, L. (2009) Disability and the anti-obesity offensive, *Disability & Society*, 24(7): 897–909.

Aphramor, L. (2010) Validity of claims made in weight management research: a narrative review of dietetic articles, *Nutrition Journal*, 9(30): 1–9.

Aphramor, L. (2016) *The Well Now Way and HAES Theory: A Think Paper*. Shropshire: Benbella.

Aphramor, L. (2017) Effecting change in public health, *NHD-Extra: Public Health*, 126: 55–59.

Aphramor, L. (2018) Preventing fat stigma and repairing harm: a practical, pragmatic, radical response for advancing weight justice through public health policy and everyday conversation. Keynote talk. *6th Annual Weight Stigma Conference*, Leeds, June 18.

Aphramor, L. (2019a) Creating knowledge for transformation: understanding healthism in nutrition discourse, *Network Health Digest*, 140: 38–40.

Aphramor, L. (2019b) Does your approach to treating eating disorders aim at prison abolition? *Medium*, 13 May. Online: <https://medium.com/@lucy.aphramor/does-your-approach-to-treating-eating-disorders-aim-at-prison-abolition-d27e64fcef0d> Accessed 6 March 2020.

Aphramor, L. (2020a) Eight signs of white supremacy in HAES (Health at Every Size) and ideas for action, *Medium*, 9 June. Online: <https://medium.com/@lucy.aphramor/eight-signs-of-supremacy-in-haes-health-at-every-size-and-ideas-for-action-e04b7f5c86fb> Accessed 9 August 2020.

Aphramor, L. (2020b) Talking of fat rights, is your citation ethical? *Medium*, 29 January. Online: <https://medium.com/@lucy.aphramor/talking-of-fat-people-is-your-citation-ethical-c62bca67f894> Accessed 1 February 2020.

Aphramor, L. (2020c) Reframing health ethics to support liberation, *Medium*, 12 May. Online: <https://medium.com/@lucy.aphramor/reframing-health-ethics-to-support-liberation11063da4e46> Accessed 13 September 2020.

Aphramor, L. and Gingras, J. (2011) Helping people change: promoting politicised practice in the healthcare professions. In E. Rich, L.F. Monaghan and L. Aphramor (eds), *Debating Obesity: Critical Perspectives*. Basingstoke: Palgrave Macmillan.

Arber, S. and Meadows, R. (2020) Class inequalities in health and the coronavirus: a cruel irony? *The Blog of the Department of Sociology at the University of Surrey*, 23 March. Online: <https://blogs.surrey.ac.uk/sociology/2020/03/23/class-inequalities-in-health-and-the-coronavirus-a-cruel-irony/> Accessed 6 April 2020.

Archer, M. (2007) *Making Our Way through the World*. Cambridge: Cambridge University Press.

Armstrong, D. (1995) The rise of surveillance medicine, *Sociology of Health & Illness*, 17(3): 393–404.

Armstrong, D. (2021) The COVID-19 pandemic and cause of death, *Sociology of Health & Illness*, 43 (7): 1614–1626.

Aronovitch, H. (2012) Interpreting Weber's ideal-types, *Philosophy of the Social Sciences*, 42(3): 356–369.

ASDAH (2013) *Association for Size Diversity and Health*. HAES® Principles. Online: <www.sizediversityandhealth.org/content.asp?id=152> Accessed 10 March 2019.

Asmundson, G.J.G. and Taylor, S. (2020) Coronaphobia: fear and the 2019-nCoV outbreak, *Journal of Anxiety Disorders*, 70: 102196.

Association for the Study of Obesity on the Island of Ireland et al. (2020) Statement from the Association for the Study of Obesity in Ireland, The National Obesity Management Clinical Programme and the Irish Coalition for People Living with Obesity. Online: <https://asoi.info/wp-content/uploads/2020/05/Obesity-and-COVID-19-Statement-from-ASOI-ICPO-Obesity-Mgt-NCP.pdf>Accessed 10 August 2020.

Atanasova, D. (2018) 'Keep moving forward. LEFT RIGHT LEFT': a critical metaphor analysis and addressivity analysis of personal and professional obesity blogs, *Discourse, Context & Media*, 25: 5–12.

Atkinson, M. (2014) Schoolboys, physical education and bullying: 'Hey, leave those kids alone!' In L.F. Monaghan and M. Atkinson, *Challenging Myths of Masculinity: Understanding Physical Cultures*. Aldershot: Ashgate.

Australian Government (2017a) *A Picture of Overweight and Obesity in Australia*. Canberra: Australian Institute of Health and Welfare. Online: <www.aihw. gov.au/getmedia/172fba28-785e-4a08-ab37-2da3bbae40b8/aihw-phe-216.pdf. aspx?inline=true> Accessed 21 February 2018.

Australian Government (2017b) *Overweight and Obesity in Australia: A Birth Cohort Analysis*. Canberra: Australian Institute of Health and Welfare. Online: <www.aihw. gov.au/getmedia/be8da99a-46d1-4d27-a391-c057e30d3299/aihw-phe-215.pdf. aspx?inline=true> Accessed 21 February 2018.

Avanceña, A.L.V., DeLuca, E.K., Lott, B. et al. (2021) Income and income inequality are a matter of life and death. What can policymakers do about it? *American Journal of Public Health*, https://ajph.aphapublications.org/doi/full/10.2105/AJPH.2021.306301.

Azzarito, L. (2009) The Panopticon of physical education: pretty, active and ideally white, *Physical Education and Sport Pedagogy*, 14(1): 19–40.

Azzarito, L. (2010) Future girls, transcendent femininities and new pedagogies: toward girls' hybrid bodies? *Sport, Education and Society*, 15(3): 261–275.

Becker, H. and Pessin, A., (2006) A dialogue on the ideas of 'world' and 'field', *Sociological Forum*, 21(2): 275–286.

Backstrom, L. (2020) Shifting the blame frame: agency and the parent-child relationship in an anti-obesity campaign, *Childhood*, 27(2): 203–219.

Bacon, L. (2006) End the war on obesity: make peace with your patients, *Medscape*. Online: <www.ncbi.nlm.nih.gov/pmc/articles/PMC1868359/> Accessed 5 April 2019.

Bacon, L. (2010) *Health at Every Size: The Surprising Truth about Your Weight*. Dallas, TX: BenBella Books, Inc.

Bacon, L. (2014a) Body trust and respect as a prescription for successful diabetes care: why it's time to ditch the diet mentality, *Canadian Diabetes Association Professional Conference*, Winnipeg, Manitoba, Canada, 23 October.

Bacon, L. (2014b) Opening remarks – Health at Every Size, *Dietitians of Canada Conference*, Toronto, Canada, 19 September.

Bacon, L. and Aphramor, L. (2011) Weight science: evaluating the evidence for a paradigm shift, *Nutrition Journal*, 10(9), https://doi.org/10.1186/1475-2891-10-9.

Bacon, L. and Aphramor, L. (2014) *Body Respect*. Dallas, TX: BenBella Books.

Bacon, L., O'Reilly, C. and Aphramor, L. (2016) Reflections on thin privilege and responsibility. In E. Cameron and C. Russell (eds), *The Fat Pedagogy Reader*. New York: Peter Lang Publishing.

Bacon, L., Stern, J.S., Van Loan, M.D. and Keim, N.L. (2005) Size acceptance and intuitive eating improve health for obese, female chronic dieters, *Journal of the American Dietetic Association*, 105(6): 929–936.

Bakare, L. (2020) A million people livestream Joe Wicks online 'PE lesson', *The Guardian*, 23 March. Online: <www.theguardian.com/world/2020/mar/23/a-million-people-livestream-joe-wicks-online-pe-lesson> Accessed 23 March 2020.

Baker, N. (2016) 25% back prosecuting parents of obese children, *Irish Examiner*, 23 September. Online: <www.irishexaminer.com/ireland/25-back-prosecuting-parents-of-obese-children-422474.html> Accessed 9 July 2018.

Banks, D. and Purdy, M. (eds) (2001) *The Sociology and Politics of Health: A Reader.* London: Routledge.

Barlow, C. and Awan, I. (2016) 'You need to be sorted out with a knife': the attempted online silencing of women and people of Muslim faith within academia, *Social Media + Society*, 2(4): 1–11.

Barnes, D., Chowkwanyun, M. and Sivaramakrishnan, K. (2020) *Pandemic Syllabus*, 29 December. Columbia University, Department of History. Online: <www.public-books.org/pandemic-syllabus/> Accessed 29 December 2020.

Barosh, L., Friel, S., Engelhardt, K. and Chan, L. (2014) The cost of a healthy and sustainable diet: who can afford it? *Australian and New Zealand Journal of Public Health*, 38(1): 7–12.

Barron, E., Bakhai, C., Kar, P. et al. (2020) *Type 1 and Type 2 Diabetes and COVID-19 Related Mortality in England: A Whole Population Study.* NHS England. Online: <www.england.nhs.uk/wp-content/uploads/2020/05/valabhji-COVID-19-and-Diabetes-Paper-1.pdf> Accessed 20 August 2020.

Bauld, L., Carters-White, L., Cerny, C. et al. (2021) Turning the tide: The Obesity Health Alliance's healthy weight strategy, *thebmjopinion*, 8 October. Online: <https://blogs.bmj.com/bmj/2021/10/08/turning-the-tide-the-obesity-health-alliances-healthy-weight-strategy/> Accessed 12 October 2021.

Baum, F. and Fisher, M. (2014) Why behavioural health promotion endures despite its failure to reduce health inequities, *Sociology of Health & Illness*, 36(2): 213–225.

BBC News (2021) Mediator drug: French pharmaceutical firm fined over weight loss pill, 29 March. Online: <www.bbc.com/news/world-europe-56562909> Accessed 31 March 2021.

Beaumont, P. and Graham-Harrison, E. (2020) 'One big wave' – why the Covid-19 second wave may not exist. *The Guardian*, 29 July.

Beausoleil, N. (2009) An impossible task: preventing disordered eating in the context of the current obesity panic. In J. Wright and V. Harwood (eds), *Biopolitics and the Obesity Epidemic: Governing Bodies.* New York: Routledge.

Beavers, K.M., Lyles, M.F., Davis, C.C. et al. (2011) Is lost lean muscle mass from weight loss recovered in weight regain in postmenopausal women? *American Journal of Clinical Nutrition*, 94(3): 767–774.

Becher, T., Palanisamy, S., Kramer, D.J. et al. (2021) Brown adipose tissue is associated with cardiometabolic health, *Nature Medicine*, 27: 58–65.

Becker, H.S. (1963) *Outsiders: Studies in the Sociology of Deviance.* New York: Free press.

Bégin, C., Carbonneau, E., Gagnon-Girouard, M.-P.. et al. (2019) Eating-related and psychological outcomes of Health at Every Size intervention in health and social services centers across the province of Québec, *American Journal of Health Promotion*, 33(2): 248–258.

Bell, K. and Green, J. (2016) On the perils of invoking neoliberalism in public health critique, *Critical Public Health*, 26(3): 239.

Bell, K. and Green, J. (2020) Premature evaluation? Some cautionary thoughts on global pandemics and scholarly publishing, *Critical Public Health*, 30(4): 379–383.

Bell, K. and McNaughton, D. (2007) Feminism and the invisible fat man, *Body & Society*, 13(1): 107–131.

Bell, K., McNaughton, D. and Salmon, A. (2009) Medicine, morality and mothering: public health discourses on foetal alcohol exposure, smoking around children and childhood overnutrition, *Critical Public Health*, 19(2): 155–170.

Belousov, K., Horlick-Jones, T. and Bloor, M. (2007) Any port in a storm: fieldwork difficulties in dangerous and crisis-ridden settings, *Qualitative Research*, 7(2): 155–175.

Berger, P. (1963) *Invitation to Sociology: A Humanistic Perspective.* Aylesbury: Penguin.

Berlant, L. (2011) *Cruel Optimism*. Durham: Duke University Press.

Berman, M.I., Morton, S.N. and Hegel, M.T. (2016) Health at Every Size and acceptance and commitment therapy for obese, depressed women: treatment development and clinical application, *Clinical Social Work Journal*, 44(3): 265–278.

Bernstein, B. (1990) *The Structuring of Pedagogic Discourse*. London: Routledge.

Bernstein, B. (1996) *Pedagogy, Symbolic Control and Identity: Theory, Research, Critique*. London and New York: Taylor and Francis.

Bernstein, B. (2000) *Pedagogy, Symbolic Control and Identity*, revised edn. New York and Oxford: Rowman & Littlefield Publishers.

Bernstein, B. (2001) From pedagogies to knowledges. In A. Morias, I. Neves, B. Davies and H. Daniels (eds), *Towards a Sociology of Pedagogy: The Contribution of Basil Bernstein to Research*. New York: Peter Lang.

Bernstein, B. and St. John, M. (2009) The Roseanne Benedict Arnolds: how fat women are betrayed by celebrity icons. In E. Rothblum and S. Solovay (eds), *The Fat Studies Reader*. New York: New York University Press.

Berwick, D.M. (2020) The moral determinants of health, *JAMA*, 324(3): 225–226.

Bhaskar, R. (1989) *Reclaiming Reality*. London: Verso.

Bienkov, A. (2020) A police chief threatened to start checking shopping trolleys for 'unnecessary' items during the UK coronavirus lockdown, *Business Insider*, 9 April.

Biesta (2012) Becoming public: public pedagogy, citizenship and the public sphere, *Social & Cultural Geography*, 13(7): 683–697.

Birch, L.L., Johnson, S.L., Andresen, G. et al. (1991) The variability of young children's energy intake, *New England Journal of Medicine*, 324(4): 232–238.

Bjørkdahl, K. and Carlsen, B. (eds) (2019) *Pandemics, Publics, and Politics: Staging Responses to Public Health Crises*. Gateway East, Singapore: Palgrave Macmillan.

Blackshaw, J., Feeley, A., Mabbs, L. et al. (2020) *Excess Weight and COVID-19: Insights from New Evidence*. London: Public Health England.

Blanchard, S. (2020) Britain is told to lose weight for the winter as deputy chief medical officer admits she is 'very concerned' about a second wave and urges people to slim down to cut their risk of dying, *MailOnline*, 8 July. Online: <www.dailymail.co.uk/news/article-8502521/Lose-weight-protect-coronavirus-deputy-chief-medical-officer-says.html> Accessed 10 July 2020.

Boero, N. (2009) Fat kids, working moms, and the 'epidemic of obesity': race, class, and mother blame. In E. Rothblum and S. Solovay (eds), *The Fat Studies Reader*. New York: New York University Press.

Boero, N. (2010) Bypassing blame; bariatric surgery and the case of biomedical failure. In A.E. Clarke, L. Mamo, J.R. Fosket et al. (eds), *Biomedicalization: Technoscience, Health, and Illness in the U.S.* Durham and London: Duke University Press.

Boero, N. (2012) *Killer Fat: Media, Medicine, and Morals in the American 'Obesity Epidemic'*. New Brunswick, NJ: Rutgers University Press.

Boero, N. (2013) Obesity in the media: social science weighs in, *Critical Public Health*, 23(3): 371–380.

Boero, N. and Thomas, P. (2016) Fat kids, *Fat Studies*, 5(2): 91–97.

Bombak, A.E. (2014a) The contribution of applied social sciences to obesity stigma-related public health approaches, *Journal of Obesity*, 2014: 267286.

Bombak, A.E. (2014b) The 'obesity epidemic': evolving science, unchanging etiology, *Sociology Compass*, 8(5): 509–524.

Bombak, A. (2014c) Obesity, Health at Every Size, and public health policy, *American Journal of Public Health*, 104(2): e60–e67.

Bombak, A. (2014d) Letters. Bombak responds to Lekkas and Stankov, *American Journal of Public Health*, 104(7): e1–e2.

Bombak, A. (2014e) *Obese Individuals' Perceptions of Health and Obesity and the Lived Experience of Weight Loss, Gain, or Maintenance over Time*. PhD dissertation. University of Manitoba. Online: <http://hdl.handle.net/1993/30076>.

Bombak, A.E. (2015) 'Obesities': experiences and perspectives across weight trajectories, *Health Sociology Review*, 24(3): 256–269.

Bombak, A.E. and Hanson, H.M. (2017) A critical discussion of patient engagement in research, *Journal of Patient-Centered Research and Reviews*, 4(1): 39–41.

Bombak, A.E., McPhail, D. and Ward, P. (2016) Reproducing stigma: interpreting 'overweight' and 'obese' women's experiences of weight-based discrimination in reproductive healthcare, *Social Science & Medicine*, 166: 94–101.

Bombak, A.E., Riediger, N.D., Bensley, J. et al. (2020) A systematic search and critical thematic, narrative review of lifestyle interventions for the prevention and management of diabetes, *Critical Public Health*, 30(1): 103–114.

Boni, Z. (2020) Slim choices: young people's experiences of individual responsibility for childhood obesity, *Critical Public Health*. Advance online publication: https://doi.org/10.1080/09581596.2020.1851655.

Booth, R. and Butler, P. (2018) UK austerity has inflicted 'great misery' on citizens, UN says, *The Guardian*, 16 November.

Bordo, S. (2003) *Unbearable Weight: Feminism, Western Culture, and the Body*, 10th anniversary edition. California: University of California Press.

Borkoles, E., Carroll, S., Clough, P. and Polman, R.C.J. (2016) Effect of a non-dieting lifestyle randomised control trial on psychological well-being and weight management in morbidly obese pre-menopausal women, *Maturitas*, 83: 51–58.

Borland, S. (2015) Obesity in women as dangerous as 'terror threat', *MailOnline*, 11 December. Online: <www.dailymail.co.uk/news/article-3355256/Obesity-women-dangerous-terror-threat-Extraordinary-claim-health-chief-uses-speech-demand-condition-added-list-public-health-threats.html> Accessed 12 December 2015.

Borland, S. (2018) Britain's child obesity disgrace, *MailOnline*, 29 May. Online: <www.dailymail.co.uk/news/article-5780597/Britains-child-obesity-disgrace-Figures-reveal-170-000-leave-primary-school-overweight.html> Accessed 27 December 2020.

Borovoy, A. and Roberto, C.A. (2015) Japanese and American public health approaches to preventing population weight gain: a role for paternalism? *Social Science & Medicine*, 143: 62–70.

Boseley, S. (2016a) Junk food shortening lives of children worldwide, data shows, *The Guardian*, 7 October.

Boseley, S. (2016b) Health chief: obesity warning letters to parents must not be watered down, *The Guardian*, 3 November.

Boseley, S. (2017) First US sugar tax sees soft drink sales fall by almost 10%, study shows, *The Guardian*, 18 April.

Boseley, S. (2018) GPs to prescribe very low calorie diets in hope of reversing diabetes, *The Guardian*, 30 November.

Bosello, O., Donataccio, M.P. and Cuzzolaro, M. (2016) Obesity or obesities? Controversies on the association between Body Mass Index and premature mortality, *Eating and Weight Disorders*, 21(2): 165–174.

Bosomworth, N.J. (2012) The downside of weight loss: realistic intervention in body-weight trajectory, *Canadian Family Physician*, 58(5): 517–523.

Boswell, J. (2016) *The Real War on Obesity: Contesting Knowledge and Meaning in a Public Health Crisis*. London: Palgrave Macmillan.

Bosy-Westphal, A. and Müller, M.J. (2021) Diagnosis of obesity based on body composition – time for a change in paradigm, *Obesity Reviews*, (Sup. 2): e13190.

Bourdieu, P. (2001) *Masculine Domination*. Cambridge: Polity Press.

Bourdieu, P., Accardo, A., Balazs, G. et al. (1999) *The Weight of the World: Social Suffering in Contemporary Society*. Stanford: Stanford University Press.

Brady, J., Gingras, J. and Aphramor, L. (2013) Theorizing Health at Every Size as a relational-cultural endeavour, *Critical Public Health*, 23(3): 345–355.

Braun, N., Gomes, F. and Schütz, P. (2015) 'The obesity paradox' in disease – is the protective effect of obesity true? *Swiss Medical Weekly*, 145: w14265.

Brewis, A.A. (2014) Stigma and the perpetuation of obesity, *Social Science & Medicine*, 118: 152–158.

Brewis, A., SturtzSreetharan, C. and Wutich, A. (2018) Obesity stigma as a globalizing health challenge, *Globalization and Health*, 14(20). https://doi.org/10.1186/s12992-018-0337-x.

Brewis, A. and Wutich, A. (2019) *Lazy, Crazy, and Disgusting: Stigma and the Undoing of Global Health*. Baltimore, MD: Johns Hopkins University Press.

Bridge, G., Lomazzi, M. and Bedi, R. (2020) Implementation of a sugar-sweetened beverage tax in low- and middle-income countries: recommendations for policy makers, *Journal of Public Health Policy*, 41(1): 84–97.

British Nutrition Foundation (1999) *Taskforce on Obesity Report*. UK Blackwell Science.

British Sociological Association (2017) *Ethics Guidelines and Collated Resources for Digital Research: Statement of Ethical Practice Annexe*. British Sociological Association. Online: <www.britsoc.co.uk/media/24309/bsa_statement_of_ethical_practice_annexe.pdf> Accessed 14 June 2021.

Brody, J.E. (2020) Half of us face obesity, dire predictions show, *The New York Times*, 10 February. Online: <www.nytimes.com/2020/02/10/well/live/half-of-us-face-obesity-dire-projections-show.html> Accessed 3 March 2020.

Brooker, P., Barnett, J., Vines, J. et al. (2018) Doing stigma: online commenting around weight-related news media, *New Media & Society*, 20(9): 3201–3222.

Brooks, B. (2020) Why is New Orleans death rate twice New York's? Obesity is a factor, *Reuters*, 2 April.

Brown, R.D. (2020) Public health lessons learned from biases in coronavirus mortality overestimation, *Disaster Medicine and Public Health Preparedness*, 14(3): 364–371.

Brown, T. (2014) Differences by degree: fatness, contagion and pre-emption, *Health*, 18(2): 117–129.

Bruce, L.J. and Ricciardelli, L.A. (2016) A systematic review of the psychosocial correlates of intuitive eating among adult women, *Appetite*, 96: 454–472.

Burdick, J. and Sandlin, J. (2013) Learning, becoming, and the unknowable: conceptualizations, mechanisms, and process in public pedagogy literature, *Curriculum Inquiry*, 43(1): 142–177.

Burgard, D. (2009) What is 'Health at Every Size'? In E. Rothblum and S. Solovay (eds), *The Fat Studies Reader*. New York: New York University Press.

Burns, M. and Gavey, N. (2004) 'Healthy weight' at what cost? 'Bulimia' and a discourse of weight control, *Journal of Health Psychology*, 9(4): 549–565.

Burrows, L. (2016) 'Obesity' warriors in the tertiary classroom. In E. Cameron and C. Russell (eds), *The Fat Pedagogy Reader: Challenging Weight-Based Oppression through Critical Education*. New York: Peter Lang.

Burrows, L. and Wright, J. (2004) The discursive production of childhood, identity and health. In J. Evans, B. Davies and J. Wright (eds), *Body Knowledge and Control: Studies in the Sociology of Physical Education and Health*. London: Routledge.

Burrows, L., Wright, J. and Jungersen-Smith, J. (2002) 'Measure your belly': New Zealand children's constructions of health and fitness. *Journal of Teaching in Physical Education*, 2(2): 39–48.

Burrows, L., Wright, J. and McCormack, J. (2009) Dosing up on food and physical activity: New Zealand children's ideas about health, *Health Education Journal*, 68: 157–169.

Cadena-Schlam, L. and Lopez-Guimera, G. (2014) Intuitive eating: an emerging approach to eating behaviour, *Nutricion Hospitalaria*, 31: 995–1002.

Caduff, C. (2020) What went wrong: corona and the world after the full stop, *Medical Anthropology Quarterly*, 34(4): 467–487.

Cahill, D. (2011) Beyond neoliberalism? Crisis and the prospects for progressive alternatives, *New Political Science*, 33(4): 479–492.

Cain, P. and Donaghue, N. (2018) Political and health messages are differently palatable: a critical discourse analysis of women's engagement with Health at Every Size and fat acceptance messages, *Fat Studies*, 7(3): 264–277.

Cain, P., Donaghue, N. and Ditchburn, G. (2017) Concerns, culprits, counsel, and conflict: a thematic analysis of 'obesity' and fat discourse in digital news media, *Fat Studies*, 6(2): 170–188.

Cale, L. and Harris, J. (2013) 'Every child (of every size) matters' in physical education! Physical education's role in childhood obesity, *Sport, Education and Society*, 18(4): 433–452.

Calnan, M., Williams, S.J. and Gabe, J. (2020) Uncertain times: trust matters during the pandemic, *Discover Society*, 1 June. Online: <https://discoversociety.org/2020/06/01/uncertain-times-trust-mattersduring-the-pandemic/> Accessed 2 June 2020.

Calogero, R.M., Tylka, T.L., Mensinger, J.L. et al. (2019) Recognizing the fundamental right to be fat: a weight-inclusive approach to size acceptance and healing from sizeism, *Women and Therapy*, 42(1–2): 22–44.

Cameron, E. (2016) Challenging 'size matters' messages: an exploration of the experiences of critical obesity scholars in Higher Education, *Canadian Journal of Higher Education*, 46(2): 111–126.

Cameron, E., Oakley, J., Walton, G. et al. (2014) Moving beyond the injustices of the schooled healthy body. In I. Bogotch and C. Shields (eds.), *The International Handbook of Social Justice and Educational Leadership*. New York: Springer Publishing.

Cameron, E. and Russell, C. (eds) (2016) *The Fat Pedagogy Reader*. New York: Peter Lang Publishing.

Campaign for Social Science (2017) Child obesity is 'national scandal', says Chair of NHS England. Online: <https://campaignforsocialscience.org.uk/news/child-obesity-national-scandal-says-chair-nhs-england/> Accessed 12 April 2017.

Campos, P. (2004) *The Obesity Myth: Why America's Obsession with Weight is Hazardous to your Health*. New York: Gotham Books.

Campos, P. (2011) Does fat kill?: A review of the epidemiological evidence. In E. Rich, L.F. Monaghan and L. Aphramor (eds), *Debating Obesity: Critical Perspectives*. Basingstoke: Palgrave MacMillan.

Campos, P., Saguy, A., Ernsberger, P. et al. (2006) The epidemiology of overweight and obesity: public health crisis or moral panic? *International Journal of Epidemiology*, 35(1): 55–60.

Carabine, J. (2001) Unmarried motherhood 1830–1990: a geneological analysis. In M. Wetherell, S. Taylor and S.J. Yates (eds), *Discourse as Data: A Guide for Analysis*. London: SAGE.

Casazza, K., Fontaine, K.R., Astrup, A. et al. (2013) Myths, presumptions, and facts about obesity, *New England Journal of Medicine*, 368(5): 446–454.

Castro-Vázquez, G. (2019) A metabolic self in contemporary Japan: a cultural reading, *Social Theory & Health*, 17(3): 367–388.

CDC (2020) Coronavirus disease 2019 (COVID-19). People of any age with underlying medical conditions, *Centers for Disease Control and Prevention*. Online: <www.cdc.gov/coronavirus/2019-ncov/need-extra-precautions/people-with-medical-conditions.html#obesity> Accessed 14 July 2020.

Chancel, L., Piketty, T., Saez, E. et al. (2022) *World Inequality Report 2022*. World Inequality Lab. Online: <https://wir2022.wid.world/> Accessed 14 February 2022.

Chou, W. S., Prestin, A. and Kunath, S. (2014) Obesity in social media: a mixed methods analysis, *Translational Behavioral Medicine*, 4(3): 314–323.

Chrisafis, A. (2013) France shaken by fresh scandal over weight-loss drug linked to deaths, *The Guardian*, 6 January.

Christensen, P. and James, A. (eds) (2008) *Research with Children: Perspectives and Practices*, 2nd edn. Abingdon: Routledge.

Clarke, A.E., Shim, J.K., Mamo, L. et al. (2003) Biomedicalization: technoscientific transformations of health, illness, and U.S. biomedicine, *American Sociological Review*, 68(2): 161–194.

Clarke, A.E., Shim, J.K., Mamo, L. et al. (2010) Biomedicalization: a theoretical and substantive introduction. In A.E. Clarke, L. Mamo, J.R. Fosket et al. (eds), *Biomedicalization: Technoscience, Health, and Illness in the U.S.* Durham and London: Duke University Press.

Cliff, K. and Wright, J. (2010) Confusing and contradictory: considering obesity discourse and eating disorders as they shape body pedagogies in HPE, *Sport, Education and Society*, 15(2): 221–233.

Clifford, D., Ozier, A., Bundros, J. et al. (2015) Impact of non-diet approaches on attitudes, behaviors, and health outcomes: a systematic review, *Journal of Nutrition Education and Behavior*, 47: 143–155.

Cohen, D. (2005) The rise of reality science, *BMJ*, 330: 1216.

Cohen, L., Perales, D. and Steadman, C. (2005) The O word: why the focus on obesity is harmful to community health, *Californian Journal of Health Promotion*, 3(3): 154–161.

Cohen, S. (2002 [1972]) *Folk Devils and Moral Panics*, 3rd edn. London: Routledge.

College of Medicine and Integrated Health (2020) Make yourself 'as fit as possible' to beat COVID-19 second wave, says deputy Chief medical Officer, 10 July. Online: <https://collegeofmedicine.org.uk/make-yourself-as-fit-as-possible-to-beat-covid-second-wave-says-deputy-chief-medical-officer/> Accessed 1 August 2020.

Collin, J., Ralston, R., Hill, S.E. and Westerman, L. (2020) *Signalling Virtue, Promoting Harm: Unhealthy Commodity Industries and COVID-19*. NCD Alliance, Spectrum. Online: <https://ncdalliance.org/sites/default/files/resource_files/SignallingVirtue%2CPromotingHarm_Sept2020_FINALv.pdf> Accessed 1 October 2020.

Collins, C., Ocampo, O. and Paslaski, S. (2020) *Billionaire Bonanza: Wealth Windfalls, Tumbling Taxes, and Pandemic Profiteers*. Institute for Policy Studies. Online: <https://inequality.org/wp-content/uploads/2020/04/Billionaire-Bonanza-2020-April-21.pdf> Accessed 1 May 2020.

Collins, H. and Evans, R., (2002) The third wave of science studies: studies of expertise and experience, *Social Studies of Science*, 32(2): 235–296.

Collins, R. (1974) Three faces of cruelty: towards a comparative sociology of violence, *Theory & Society*, 1(4): 415–440.

Colls, R. and Evans, B. (2014) Making space for fat bodies?: A critical account of 'the obesogenic environment', *Progress in Human Geography*, 38(6): 733–753.

Colucci, E. (2007) 'Focus groups can be fun': the use of activity-oriented questions in focus group discussions, *Qualitative Health Research*, 17(10): 1422–1433.

Compare, D., Rocco, A., Sanduzzi Zamparelli, M. and Nardone, G. (2016) The gut bacteria-driven obesity development, *Digestive Diseases*, 34(3): 221–229.

Connell, R. (2007) *Southern Theory: The Global Dynamics of Knowledge in Social Science*. London and New York: Routledge.

Connell, R. (2020) COVID-19/Sociology, *Journal of Sociology*, 56(4): 745–751.

Connelly, S. (2020) Universities, finance capital and the impact of COVID-19, *Discover Society*, 28 May. Online: <https://discoversociety.org/2020/05/28/universities-finance-capital-and-the-impact-of-covid-19/> Accessed 30 May 2020.

Connor, M. (2020) Coronavirus: stay fit to fight the virus, say medics, *BBC News*, 28 March. Online: <www.bbc.co.uk/news/uk-52076856> Accessed 28 March 2020.

Cooper, C. (1997) Can a fat woman call herself disabled? *Disability & Society*, 12(1): 31–42.

Cooper, C. (1998) *Fat and Proud: The Politics of Size*. London: The Women's Press.

Cooper, C. (2010) Fat studies: mapping the field, *Sociology Compass*, 4(12): 1020–1034.

Cooper, C. (2011) Fat lib: how fat activism expands the obesity debate. In E. Rich, L.F. Monaghan and L. Aphramor (eds), *Debating Obesity: Critical Perspectives*. Basingstoke: Palgrave MacMillan.

Cooper, C. (2016a) *Fat Activism: A Radical Social Movement*. Bristol: HammerOn Press.

Cooper, C. (2016b) The rhetoric around obesity is toxic. So I created a new language for fat people, *The Guardian*, 26 October. Online: <www.theguardian.com/commentisfree/2016/oct/26/rhetoric-obesity-toxic-new-language-fat-people> Accessed 28 December 2020.

Cooper Stoll, L. (2019) Fat is a social justice issue, too, *Humanity & Society*, 43(4): 421–441.

Cooper Stoll, L. and Egner, J. (2021) We must do better: fatphobia and ableism in sociology, *Sociology Compass*, 15(4): e12869.

Corbin, J. and Strauss, A.L. (1987) Accompaniments of chronic illness: changes in body, self, biography and biographical time, *Research in the Sociology of Health Care*, 6: 249–281.

Cornish, F. (2021) 'Grenfell changes everything?' Activism beyond hope and despair, *Critical Public Health*, 31(3): 293–305.

Courtney-Guy, S. (2020) Warning obesity should be tackled to help reduce coronavirus deaths, *Metro*, 25 July. Online: <https://metro.co.uk/2020/07/25/warning-obesity-should-tackled-help-reduce-coronavirus-deaths-13037996/> Accessed 26 July 2020.

Crawford, R. (1980) Healthism and the medicalization of everyday life, *International Journal of Health Services*, 10(3): 365–388.

Crossley, N. (2022) Social movements. In L.F. Monaghan and J. Gabe (eds), *Key Concepts in Medical Sociology*, 3rd edn. London: SAGE.

Croston, A. and Hills, L.A. (2017) The challenges of widening 'legitimate' understandings of ability within physical education, *Sport, Education and Society*, 22(5): 618–634.

C.S. Mott Children's Hospital (2012) School obesity programs may promote worrisome eating behaviors and physical activity in kids. *C.S. Mott Children's Hospital National Poll on Children's Health*, 14(2). Online: <https://mottpoll.org/sites/default/files/documents/012412eatingbehaviors.pdf> Accessed 28 December 2020.

Cullen, P. (2016) New strategy aims to tackle Irish obesity levels, *The Irish Times*, 16 May. Online: <www.irishtimes.com/news/health/new-strategy-aims-to-tackle-irish-obesity-levels-1.2648845> Accessed 20 May 2016.

Curty, G. (2017) Capitalism, structural crisis and contemporary social movements: an interview with Immanuel Wallerstein, *Critical Sociology*, 43(3): 331–335.

Cyr, M. and Riediger, N. (2021) (Re)claiming our bodies using a Two-Eyed Seeing approach: Health-At-Every-Size (HAES®) and Indigenous knowledge, *Canadian Journal of Public Health*, 112: 493–497.

Dallmeyer, M. (2020) Two fat professors' are afraid of COVID-19 causing 'fatphobia', *CAMPUSREFORM*, 5 April. Online: <www.campusreform.org/?ID=14656> Accessed 15 April 2020.

David, P.M. and Le Dévédec, N. (2019) Preparedness for the next epidemic: health and political issues of an emerging paradigm, *Critical Public Health*, 29(3): 363–369.

Davidson, H. (2020) Global report: virus has unleashed a 'tsunami of hate' across the world, says UN chief, *The Guardian*, 8 May. Online: <www.theguardian.com/world/2020/may/08/global-report-china-open-to-cooperate-with-who-on-virus-origin-as-trump-repeats-lab-claim> Accessed 8 May 2020.

Davis, M.D.M. (2019) Uncertainty and immunity in public communications on pandemics. In K. Bjørkdahl and B. Carlsen (eds), *Pandemics, Publics, and Politics: Staging Responses to Public Health Crises*. East Gate, Singapore: Palgrave Macmillan.

De Brún, A., McCarthy, M., McKenzie, K. and McGloin, A. (2013) 'Fat is your fault'. Gatekeepers to health, attributions of responsibility and the portrayal of gender in the Irish media representation of obesity, *Appetite*, 62: 17–26.

Dehghan, P., Farhangi, M.A., Nikniaz, Z. and Asghari-Jafarabadi, M. (2020) Gut microbiota-derived metabolite trimethylamine N-oxide (TMAO) potentially increases the risk of obesity in adults: an exploratory systematic review and dose-response meta-analysis, *Obesity Reviews*, 21(5): e12993.

Delahanty, L.M., Pan, Q., Jablonski, K.A. et al. (2014) Effects of weight loss, weight cycling, and weight loss maintenance on diabetes incidence and change in cardio-metabolic traits in the Diabetes Prevention Program, *Diabetes Care*, 37(10): 2738–2745.

Dennis, M.K. and Robin, T. (2020) Healthy on our own terms: indigenous wellbeing and the colonized food system, *Journal of Critical Dietetics*, 5(1): 1–8.

Dew, K. (2014) *The Cult and Science of Public Health: A Sociological Investigation*. New York: Berghahn.

DHSC (1980) *Inequalities in Health: Report of a Working Group* (The Black Report). London: HMSO.

DHSC (1998) *Independent Inquiry into Inequalities in Health Report* (Acheson Report). Online: <https://assets.publishing.service.gov.uk/government/uploads/system/uploads/attachment_data/file/265503/ih.pdf> Accessed 20 October 2020.

DHSC (2018) *Childhood Obesity: A Plan for Action, Chapter 2*. Online: <www.gov.uk/government/publications/childhood-obesity-a-plan-for-action-chapter-2> Accessed 20 October 2020.

DHSC (2019) *Government Response to the House of Commons Health and Social Care Select Committee Report on Childhood Obesity: Time for Action, Eighth Report of Session 2017-2019*. Online: <www.parliament.uk/documents/commons-committees/Health/Correspondence/2017-19/Childhood-obesity-Government-Response-to-eighth-report-17-19.pdf> Accessed 2 February 2020.

DHSC (2020) *Tackling Obesity: Empowering Adults and Children to Live Healthier Lives*, 27 July. Online: <www.gov.uk/government/publications/tackling-obesity-government-strategy/tackling-obesity-empowering-adults-and-children-to-live-healthier-lives> Accessed 2 August 2020.

Dickins, M., Thomas, S.L., King, B. et al. (2011) The role of the Fatosphere in fat adults' responses to obesity stigma: a model of empowerment without a focus on weight loss, *Qualitative Health Research*, 21(12): 1679–1691.

Dinerstein, A.C., Schwartz, G. and Taylor, G. (2014) Sociological imagination as social critique: interrogating the 'Global Economic Crisis', *Sociology*, 48(5): 859–868.

Dingwall, R. (2020a) Coronavirus UK – could we live with a 'second influenza'? *Social Science Space*, 22 June. Online: <www.socialsciencespace.com/2020/06/coronavirus-uk-could-we-live-with-asecond-influenza/> Accessed 28 June 2020.

Dingwall, R. (2020b) Coronavirus UK – patrician policymaking, *Social Science Space*. Online: <www.socialsciencespace.com/2020/08/coronavirus-uk-patrician-policy-making/> Accessed 20 October 2020.

Dingwall, R. (2020c) I am especially touched by this affirmation from my scholarly community at this time. Trying to be a voice for […]. *Twitter*, 31 July. <https://twitter.com/rwjdingwall/status/1289114964473544705> Accessed 31 July 2020.

Dingwall, R. (2021) No one can make all lives completely safe … we must fight the pandemic of fear, *Sunday Express*, 17 January.

Dingwall, R. (2022) Pandemics and epidemics, in L.F. Monaghan and J. Gabe (eds), *Key Concepts in Medical Sociology*. London: SAGE.

Dingwall, R., Hoffman, L.M. and Staniland, K. (eds) (2013) *Pandemics and Emerging Infectious Diseases: The Sociological Agenda*. Chichester: Wiley-Blackwell.

Dixon, H. (2013) Obesity crisis risks making Britain 'fat man of Europe', warns report, *The Telegraph*, 18 February.

Dixon, J.B., Egger, G.J., Finkelstein, E.A. et al. (2015) 'Obesity paradox' misunderstands the biology of optimal weight throughout the life cycle, *International Journal of Obesity*, 39(1): 82–84.

Dodsworth, L. (2021) *A State of Fear: How the UK Government Weaponised Fear During the COVID-19 Pandemic*. London: Pinter & Martin Ltd.

Doehner, W., Von Haehling, S. and Anker, S.D. (2015) Protective overweight in cardiovascular disease: moving from 'paradox' to 'paradigm', *European Heart Journal*, 36(40): 2729–2732.

DOH (2008) *Healthy Weight, Healthy Lives: A Toolkit for Developing Local Strategies*. London: Department of Health.

DOH (2016) *A Healthy Weight for Ireland: Obesity Policy and Action Plan*. Dublin: Stationary Office. Online: <http://health.gov.ie/wp-content/uploads/2016/09/A-Healthy-Weight-for-Ireland-Obesity-Policy-and-Action-Plan-2016-2025.pdf> Accessed 21 February 2018.

Donaghue, N. and Allen, M. (2016) 'People don't care as much about their health as they do about their looks': personal trainers as intermediaries between aesthetic and health-based discourses of exercise participation and weight management, *International Journal of Sport and Exercise Psychology*, 14(1): 42–56.

Donnelly, L. (2019) 13 million adults in the UK are obese, amid doubling in weight problems, *The Telegraph*, 14 November.

Donnelly, L. and Newey, S. (2020) Obese or overweight patients in most need of critical care, *The Telegraph*, 24 March. Online: <www.telegraph.co.uk/news/2020/03/23/obese-overweight-coronavirus-patients-need-critical-care/> Accessed 28 March 2020.

DPP Research Group (2002) The Diabetes Prevention Program (DPP): description of lifestyle intervention, *Diabetes Care*, 25(12): 2165–2171.

DPP Research Group (2009) 10-Year follow-up of diabetes incidence and weight loss in the Diabetes Prevention Program Outcomes Study, *The Lancet*, 374(9702): 1677–1686.

Drury, J., Reicher, S. and Stott, C. (2020) COVID-19 in context: why do people die in emergencies? It's probably not because of collective psychology, *British Journal of Social Psychology*, 59(3): 686–693.

Dukelow, F. (2017) 32 and 37 inches – the healthy body and the politics of waist circumference: a governmental analysis of the *Stop the Spread* campaign. In C.E. Edwards and E. Fernández (eds), *Reframing Health and Health Policy in Ireland: A Governmental Analysis*. Manchester: Manchester University Press.

Edgley, C. and Brissett, D. (1990) Health Nazis and the cult of the perfect body: some polemical observations, *Symbolic Interaction*, 13(2): 257–279.

Edgley, C. and Brissett, D. (1999) *A Nation of Meddlers*. Boulder, CO: Westview Press.

Eichelberger, L. (2007) SARS and New York's Chinatown: the politics of risk and blame during an epidemic of fear, *Social Science & Medicine*, 65: 1284–1295.

Elias, N. (2000[1939]) *The Civilizing Process: Sociogenetic and Psychogenetic Investigations*, revised edn. Oxford: Blackwell.

Ellison, J., McPhail, D. and Mitchinson, W. (eds) (2016) *Obesity in Canada: Critical Perspectives*. Toronto: University of Toronto Press.

Ernsberger, P. (2009) Does social class explain the connection between weight and health? In E. Rothblum and S. Solovay (eds), *The Fat Studies Reader*. New York: New York University Press.

Evans, B. (2006) 'Gluttony or sloth': critical geographies of bodies and morality in (anti) obesity policy, *Area*, 38(3): 259–267.

Evans, B. (2010) Anticipating fatness: childhood, affect and the pre-emptive 'war on obesity', *Transactions of the Institute of British Geographers*, 35(1): 21–38.

Evans, B. and Colls, R. (2009) Measuring fatness, governing bodies: the spatialities of the Body Mass Index (BMI) in anti-obesity politics, *Antipode*, 41(5): 1051–1083.

Evans, B. and Colls, R. (2011) Doing more good than harm? The absent presence of children's bodies in (anti-)obesity policy. In E. Rich, L.F. Monaghan and L. Aphramor (eds), *Debating Obesity: Critical Perspectives*. Basingstoke: Palgrave Macmillan.

Evans, B., Colls, R. and Hörshelmann, R. (2011a) 'Change4Life for your kids': embodied collectives and public health pedagogy, *Sport, Education and Society*, 16(3): 323–341.

Evans, B. and Cooper, C. (2016) Reframing fatness: critiquing 'obesity'. In A. Whitehead, A. Woods, S. Atkinson et al. (eds), *The Edinburgh Companion to the Critical Medical Humanities*. Edinburgh: Edinburgh University Press.

Evans, J. and Davies, B. (2017) In pursuit of equity and inclusion: populism, politics and the future of educational research in physical education, health and sport, *Sport, Education and Society*, 22(5): 684–694.

Evans, J. and Davies, B. (2020) Embodying policy concepts, *Sport, Education and Society*, 25(7): 735–751.

Evans, J., Davies, B., Rich, E. and DePian, L. (2013) Understanding policy: why health education policy is important and why it does not appear to work, *British Educational Research Journal*, 39(2): 320–337.

Evans, J., De Pian, L. and Rich, E. (2011b) Health imperatives, policy and the corporeal device: schools, subjectivity and children's health, *Policy Futures in Education*, 9(3): 328–340.

Evans, J., Rich, E., Allwood, R. and Davies, B. (2008) *Education, Disordered Eating and Obesity Discourse: Fat Fabrications*. New York: Routledge.

Evans, J., Rich, E. and Holroyd, R. (2004) Disordered eating and disordered schooling: what schools do to middle class girls, *British Journal of Sociology of Education*, 25(2): 123–142.

Farrell, A.E. (2011) *Fat Shame: Stigma and the Fat Body in American Culture*. New York: New York University Press.

Farrell, L.C., Warin, M.J., Moore, V.M. and Street, J.M. (2016) Emotion in obesity discourse: understanding public attitudes towards regulations for obesity prevention, *Sociology of Health & Illness*, 38(4): 543–558.

Featherstone, M. (1991) The body in consumer culture. In M. Featherstone, M. Hepworth and B. Turner (eds), *The Body: Social Process and Cultural Theory*. London: SAGE.

Ferguson, N.M., Laydon, D., Nedjati-Gilani, G. et al. (2020) Impact of non-pharmaceutical interventions (NPIs) to reduce COVID-19 mortality and healthcare demand,

Imperial College COVID-19 Response Team, 16 March. Online: <www.imperial.ac.uk/media/imperial-college/medicine/sph/ide/gida-fellowships/Imperial-College-COVID19-NPI-modelling-16-03-2020.pdf> Accessed 3 April.

Fikkan, J.L. and Rothblum, E.D. (2012) Is fat a feminist issue? Exploring the gendered nature of weight bias, *Sex Roles*, 66: 575–592.

Fine, G. (1980) The Kentucky fried rat: legends and modern society, *Journal of the Folklore Institute*, 17(2): 222–243.

Finkelstein, E.A., Khavjou, O.A., Thompson, H. et al. (2012) Obesity and severe obesity forecasts through 2030, *American Journal of Preventive Medicine*, 42(6): 563–570.

Fitzpatrick, K. (2014) Critical approaches to health education. In K. Fitzpatrick and R. Tinning (eds), *Health Education: Critical Perspectives*. New York: Routledge.

Fitzpatrick, K. and Tinning, R. (2014) Considering the politics and practice of health education. In K. Fitzpatrick and R. Tinning (eds), *Health Education: Critical Perspectives*. New York: Routledge.

Flegal, K.M., Kit, B.K., Orpana, H. and Graubard, B.I. (2013) Association of all-cause mortality with overweight and obesity using standard Body Mass Index categories: a systematic review and meta-analysis, *JAMA*, 309(1): 71–82.

Flew, T. (2020) Globalization, neo-globalization and post-globalization: the challenge of populism and the return of nationalism, *Global Media and Communication*, 16(1): 19–39.

Flinders, M. (2020) Coronavirus and the politics of crisis fatigue, *The Conversation*, 25 March. Online: <https://theconversation.com/coronavirus-and-the-politics-of-crisis-fatigue-134702> Accessed 5 April 2020.

Flint, S.W., Nobles, J. and Gately, P. (2018) Weight stigma and discrimination: a call to the media, *The Lancet Diabetes & Endocrinology*, 6(3): 169–170.

Food and Agriculture Organization of the United States (2021) *World Food Situation: FAO Food Price Index*. Online: <www.fao.org/worldfoodsituation/foodpricesindex/en/> Accessed 28 June 2021.

Foresight (2007) *Tackling Obesities: Future Choices Project Report*. London: HMSO

Fothergill, E., Guo, J., Howard, L. et al. (2016) Persistent metabolic adaptation 6 years after 'The Biggest Loser' competition, *Obesity*, 24(8): 1599–1821.

Foucault, M. (2008) *The Birth of Biopolitics: Lectures at the Collège de France 1978-1979*. Basingstoke: Palgrave MacMillan.

Foucault, M. (1995 [1975]) *Discipline and Punish: The Birth of the Prison*. New York: Vintage Books.

Fox, N.J. and Powell, K. (2021) Non-human matter, health disparities and a thousand tidy dis/advantages, *Sociology of Health & Illness*, 43(3): 779–795.

Francombe-Webb, J. (2016) Critically encountering exer-games and young femininity, *Television & New Media*, 17(5): 449–464.

Fraser, S., Maher, J. and Wright, J. (2010) Between bodies and collectivities: articulating the action of emotion in obesity epidemic discourse, *Social Theory & Health*, 8(2): 192–209.

Frederick, D.A., Saguy, A.C., Sandhu, G. and Mann, T. (2016) Effects of competing news media frames of weight on anti-fat stigma, beliefs about weight and support for obesity-related public policies, *International Journal of Obesity*, 40(3): 534–539.

French, J. (2011) Why nudging is not enough, *Journal of Social Marketing*, 1(2): 154–162.

French, M. and Monahan, T. (2020) Dis-ease surveillance: how might surveillance studies address COVID-19? *Surveillance & Society*, 18(1): 1–11.

Friedman, K.E., Reichmann, S.K., Constanzo, P.R. et al. (2005) Weight stigmatization and ideological beliefs: relation to psychological functioning in obese adults, *Obesity Research*, 13(5): 907–916.

Friedman, M. (2015) Mother blame, fat shame, and moral panic: 'obesity' and child welfare, *Fat Studies*, 4(1): 14–27.

Friedman, S.R., Williams, L.D., Guarino, H. et al. (2022) The stigma system: how sociopolitical domination, scapegoating, and stigma shape public health, *Journal of Community Psychology*, 50(1): 385–408.

Friere, P. (2014 [1992]) *Pedagogy of Hope: Reliving Pedagogy of the Oppressed*. London: Bloomsbury.

Fullagar, S. and Pavlidis, A. (2021) Thinking through the disruptive effects and affects of the coronavirus with feminist new materialism, *Leisure Sciences*, 43(1–2): 152–159.

Fullagar, S., Pavlidis, A. and Francombe-Webb, J. (2018) Feminist theories after the poststructuralist turn. In D. Parry (ed), *Feminisms in Leisure Studies: Advancing a Fourth Wave*. New York: Routledge.

Fullagar, S., Rich, E. and Ni Shuilleabhain, N. (2022) New materialist enactment. In M. Gard, D. Powell and J. Tenorio (eds), *Routledge Handbook of Critical Obesity Studies*. New York and London: Routledge

Gabe, J. (2022) Risk and malpractice. In L.F. Monaghan and J. Gabe (eds), *Key Concepts in Medical Sociology*, 3rd edn. London: SAGE.

Gaesser, G.A. (2002) *Big Fat Lies: The Truth About your Weight and Health*. Carlsbad, CA: Gurze Books.

Gaesser, G. (2009) Is 'permanent weight-loss' an oxymoron? The statistics on weight-loss and the national weight control registry. In E. Rothblum and S. Solovay (eds), *The Fat Studies Reader*. New York: New York University Press.

Gailey, J.A. and Harjunen, H. (2019) A cross-cultural examination of fat women's experiences: stigma and gender in North American and Finnish culture, *Feminism & Psychology*, 29(3): 374–390.

Gard, M. (2009a) Friends, enemies and the cultural politics of critical obesity research. In J. Wright and V. Harwood (eds), *Biopolitics and the Obesity Epidemic: Governing Bodies*. New York: Routledge.

Gard, M. (2009b) Book review. Men and the war on obesity, *Managing Leisure*, 14(3): 235–236.

Gard, M. (2011) *The End of the Obesity Epidemic*. New York: Routledge.

Gard, M. (2013) Disagreement, not misrecognition: a reply to Monaghan, *Social Theory & Health*, 11(1): 106–115.

Gard, M. (2016) Navigating morality, politics, and reason: towards scientifically literate and intellectually ethical fat pedagogies. In E. Cameron and C. Russell (eds), *The Fat Pedagogy Reader*. New York: Peter Lang Publishing.

Gard, M. and Pluim, C. (2014) *Schools and Public Health: Past, Present, Future*. Lanham, MD: Rowman and Littlefield.

Gard, M. and Vander Schee, C. (2011) The obvious solution. In M. Gard (ed), *The End of the Obesity Epidemic*. New York: Routledge.

Gard, M. and Wright, J. (2005) *The Obesity Epidemic: Science, Morality and Ideology*. London: Routledge.

Garfinkel, H. (1956) Conditions of successful degradation ceremonies, *American Journal of Sociology*, 61(5): 420–424.

Gaztambide-Fernández, R. and Arráiz Matute, A. (2014) 'Pushing against': relationality, intentionality, and the ethical imperative of pedagogy. In J. Burdick, J.A. Sandlin and M.P. O'Malley (eds), *Problematizing Public Pedagogy*. New York: Routledge.

Gibbs, W.W. (2005) Obesity: an overblown epidemic? *Scientific American*, 292(6): 70–77.

Gibson, K. and Malcolm, D. (2020) Theorizing physical activity health promotion: towards an Eliasian framework for the analysis of health and medicine, *Social Theory & Health*, 18(1): 66–85.

Giddens, A. (1979) *Central Problems in Social Theory*. Macmillan: London.

Gilbert, N. (2021) UK academics seethe over universities cost-cutting moves, *Nature*, 9 August.

Gill, R. (2007) Postfeminist media culture: elements of a sensibility, *European Journal of Cultural Studies*, 10(2): 147–166.

Gill, R. (2009) Breaking the silence: the hidden injuries of neo-liberal academia. In R. Flood and R. Gill (eds), *Secrecy and Silence in the Research Process: Feminist Reflections*. London: Routledge.

Gill, R. (2016) Postfeminism?: New feminist visibilities in postfeminist times, *Feminist Media Studies*, 16(4): 610–630.

Gingras, J., Asada, Y., Fox, A. et al. (2014) Critical dietetics: a discussion paper, *Journal of Critical Dietetics*, 2(1): 2–12.

Gingras, J. and Cooper, C. (2013) Down the rabbit hole: a critique of the ® in HAES®, *Journal of Critical Dietetics*, 1(3): 2–5.

Ginsberg, B. (2011) *The Fall of the Faculty: The Rise of the All-Administration University and Why It Matters*. Oxford: Oxford University Press.

Giroux, H.A. (1992) *Border Crossings*. London: Routledge.

Giroux, H.A. (2004) Public pedagogy and the politics of neo-liberalism: making the political more pedagogical, *Policy Futures in Education*, 2(3/4): 494–503.

Giroux, H.A. (2020) The Covid19 pandemic is exposing the plague of neoliberalism. *TRUTHOUT*, 7 April. Online: <https://truthout.org/articles/the-covid-19-pandemic-is-exposing-the-plague-of-neoliberalism/> Accessed 16 December 2020.

Glenn, N.M., McGannon, K.R. and Spence, J.C. (2013) Exploring media representations of weight-loss surgery, *Qualitative Health Research*, 25(5): 631–644.

Glock, S., Beverborg, A.O.G. and Müller, B.C.N. (2016) Pre-service teachers' implicit and explicit attitudes toward obesity influence their judgments of students, *Social Psychology of Education*, 19(1): 97–115.

Glonti, K., Mackenbach, J.D., Ng, J. et al. (2016) Psychosocial environment: definitions, measures and associations with weight status: a systematic review, *Obesity Reviews*, 17: 81–95.

Goffman, E. (1961) *Asylums: Essays on the Social Situation of Mental Patients and Other Inmates*. Middlesex: Penguin.

Goffman, E. (1968 [1963]) *Stigma: Notes on the Management of Spoiled Identity*. Harmondsworth: Pelican Books.

Goffman, E. (1974) *Frame Analysis: An Essay on the Organization of Experience*. Cambridge, MA: Harvard University Press.

Goodyear, V.A., Kerner, C. and Quennerstedt, M. (2019) Young people's uses of wearable healthy lifestyle technologies; surveillance, self-surveillance and resistance, *Sport, Education and Society*, 24(3): 212–225.

Gotovac, S., LaMarre, A. and Lafreniere, K. (2020) Words with weight: the construction of obesity in eating disorders research, *Health*, 24(2): 113–131.

Graeber, D. (2019) *Bullshit Jobs: A Theory*. New York: Simon & Schuster.

Graham, H. (1994) Surviving by smoking. In S. Wilkinson and C. Kitzinger (eds), *Women and Health: Feminist Perspectives*. New York: Taylor & Francis.

Graso, M., Xuan Chen, F. and Reynolds, T. (2021) Moralization of Covid-19 health response: asymmetry in tolerance for human costs, *Journal of Experimental Social Psychology*, 93: 104084.

Gray, E., Pluim, C., Pike, J. and Leahy, D. (2018) 'Someone has to keep shouting': celebrities as food pedagogues, *Celebrity Studies*, 9(1): 69–83

Greaney, M.L., Lees, F.D. and Lynch, B. (2012) Using focus groups to identify factors affecting healthful weight maintenance in Latino immigrants, *Journal of Nutrition Education & Behavior*, 44(5): 448–453.

Green, G.C. and Buckroyd, J. (2008) Disordered eating cognitions and behaviours among slimming organization competition winners, *Journal of Human Nutrition & Dietetics*, 21(1): 31–38.

Green, J. (2020) Critique, culture and crisis, *Cost of Living*, 29 July. Online: <www.cost-ofliving.net/critique-culture-and-crisis/> Accessed 16 August 2020.

Greenhalgh, S. (2015) *Fat-talk Nation: The Human Costs of America's War on Fat*. New York: Cornell University Press.

Greenhalgh, S. (2019) Soda industry influence on obesity science and policy in China, *Journal of Public Health Policy*, 40: 5–16.

Greenleaf, C., Petrie, T.A. and Martin, S.B. (2014) Relationship of weight-based teasing and adolescents' psychological well-being and physical health, *Journal of School Health*, 84(1): 49–55.

Greenway, F.L. (2015) Physiological adaptations to weight loss and factors favouring weight regain, *International Journal of Obesity*, 39(8): 1188–1196.

Gregg, E.W., Chen, H., Wagenknecht, L.E. et al. (2012) Association of an intensive life-style intervention with remission of type 2 diabetes, *Journal of the American Medical Association*, 308(23): 2489–2496.

Grønning, I., Scambler, G. and Tjora, A. (2012) From fatness to badness: the modern morality of obesity, *Health*, 17(3): 266–283.

Groven, K.S., Ahlsen, B. and Robertson, S. (2018) Stories of suffering and success: men's embodied narratives following bariatric surgery, *Indo-Pacific Journal of Phenomenology*, 18(1): 1–14.

Gujral, U.P., Vittinghoff, E., Mongraw-Chaffin, M. et al. (2017) Cardiometabolic abnormalities among normal-weight persons from five racial/ethnic groups in the United States: a cross-sectional analysis of two Cohort studies, *Annals of Internal Medicine*, 166(9): 628–636.

Gupta, P., Gonzalez, D. and Waxman, E. (2020) Forty percent of Black and Hispanic parents of school-age children are food insecure, *Urban Institute*, 8 December. Online: <https://www.urban.org/sites/default/files/publication/103335/forty_percent_of_black_and_hispanic_parents_of_school_age_children_are_food_insecure.pdf> Accessed 21 January 2021.

Guthman, J. (2009) Teaching the politics of obesity: insights into neoliberal embodiment and contemporary biopolitics, *Antipode*, 41(5): 1110–1133.

Hackman, J., Maupin, J. and Brewis, A.A. (2016) Weight-related stigma is a significant psychosocial stressor in developing countries: evidence from Guatemala, *Social Science & Medicine*, 161: 55–60.

Hajj, N.E., Schneider, E., Lehnen, H. and Haaf, T. (2014) Epigenetics and life-long consequences of an adverse nutritional and diabetic intrauterine environment, *Reproduction*, 148(6): R111–R120.

Halford, S. (2020) Sociology and the social sciences in the COVID-19 crisis, *BSA Everyday Society*, 25 March. Online: <https://es.britsoc.co.uk/sociology-and-the-social-sciences-in-the-covid-19-crisis/> Accessed 28 March 2020.

Hallissey, M. (2016) Government launches 10-year war on obesity, *Sunday Business Post*, 22 September. Online <www.businesspost.ie/government-launches-10-year-war-on-obesity/> Accessed 23 September 2016.

Hamera, J. (2019) Weighty anti-feminism, weighty contradictions: anti-fat coverage and invective in US right-wing populist outlets, *Women's Studies*, 48(2): 146–166.

Hamman, R.F., Wing, R.R., Edelstein, S.L. et al. (2006) Effect of weight loss with lifestyle intervention on risk of diabetes, *Diabetes Care*, 29(9): 2102–2107.

Hansen, P.G., Skov, L.R. and Skov, K.K. (2016) Making healthier choices easier: regulation versus nudging, *Annual Review of Public Health*, 37: 237–251

Harris, A. (2004) *Future Girl: Young Women in the Twenty-First Century*. New York: Routledge

Harris, J. (2018) The case for physical education becoming a core subject in the national curriculum, *Physical Education Matters*, 13(2): 9–12.

Harris, S. (2016) Health Canada reviewing food guide, critics demand drastic changes now, *CBC News*, 22 March. Online: <www.cbc.ca/news/business/health-canada-food-guide-1.3501318> Accessed 1 October 2016.

Harrison, L. and Leahy, D. (2006) Pursuing HPE outcomes through health education. In R. Tinning, L. McCuaig and L. Hunter (eds), *Teaching Health and Physical Education in Australian Schools*. Frenchs Forest, NSW: Pearson.

Harvey, D. (1998) The body as an accumulation strategy, *Environment and Planning D: Society and Space*, 16(4): 401–421.

Harvey, D. (2005) *A Brief History of Neoliberalism*. Oxford: Oxford University Press.

Harvie, M. and Howell, A. (2017) Potential benefits and harms of intermittent energy restriction and intermittent fasting amongst obese, overweight and normal weight subjects – a narrative review of human and animal evidence, *Behavioral Sciences*, 7(1): 4, https://doi.org/10.3390/bs7010004.

Harwood, V. and Wright, J. (2012) Editorial: policy, schools and the new health imperatives, *Discourse: Studies in the Cultural Politics of Education*, 33(5): 611–615.

Hass, M. (2017) After the after: The Biggest Loser and post-makeover narrative trajectories in digital media, *Fat Studies*, 6(2): 135–151.

Haugue, M.-I. (2009) Bodily practices and discourses of hetero-femininity: girls' constitution of subjectivities in their social transition between childhood and adolescence, *Gender and Education*, 21: 293–307.

Hebert, J.R., Allison, D.B., Archer, E. et al. (2013) Scientific decision making, policy decisions, and the obesity pandemic, *Mayo Clinic Proceedings*, 88(6): 593–604.

Heindel, J.J., Newbold, R. and Schug, T.T. (2015) Endocrine disruptors and obesity, *Nature Reviews Endocrinology*, 11(11): 653–661.

Helm, T. and Campbell, D. (2020) Doctors to prescribe bike rides to tackle UK obesity crisis, *The Guardian*, 26 July. Online: <www.theguardian.com/politics/2020/jul/26/doctors-to-prescribe-bike-rides-to-tackle-uk-obesity-crisis-amid-coronavirus-risk> Accessed 26 July.

Herndon, A.M. (2005) Collateral damage from friendly fire?: Race, nation, class and the 'war against obesity', *Social Semiotics*, 15(2): 127–141.

Herndon, A.M. (2014) *Fat Blame: How the War on Obesity Victimizes Women and Children*. Kansas: University Press of Kansas.

Heuer, C.A. (2010) 'Fattertainment' – obesity in the media, *The Obesity Action Coalition*. Online: <www.obesityaction.org/community/article-library/fattertainment-obesity-in-the-media/> Accessed 19 April 2021.

Heyes, C.J. (2006) Foucault goes to weight watchers, *Hypatia*, 21(2): 126–149.

Heyes, C.J. (2007) *Self-transformations: Foucault, Ethics, and Normalized Diets*. New York: Oxford University Press.

Hickey-Moody, A., Palmer, H. and Sayers, E. (2016) Diffractive pedagogies: dancing across new materialist imaginaries, *Gender and Education*, 28(2): 213–229.

Hickey-Moody, A., Savage, G.C. and Windle, J. (2010) Pedagogy writ large: public, popular and cultural pedagogies in motion, *Critical Studies in Education*, 51(3): 227–236.

Hillier-Brown, F.C., Bambra, C.L., Cairns, J.M. et al. (2014) A systematic review of the effectiveness of individual, community and societal level interventions at reducing socioeconomic inequalities in obesity amongst children, *BMC Public Health*, 14, 834.

Himmelstein, M.S., Puhl, R.M. and Quinn, D.M. (2019) Overlooked and understudied: health consequences of weight stigma in men, *Obesity*, 27(10): 1598–1605.

Hine, C. (2000) *Virtual Ethnography.* London: SAGE.

Ho, J.Y. and Hendi, A.S. (2018) Recent trends in life expectancy across high income countries: retrospective observational study, *BMJ*, 362: k2562.

Holland, K.E., Blood, R.W., Thomas, S.L. et al. (2011) 'Our girth is plain to see': an analysis of newspaper coverage of *Australia's Future 'Fat Bomb'*, *Health, Risk & Society*, 13(1): 31–46.

Holland, K.E., Blood, R.W., Thomas, S.L. and Lewis, S. (2015) Challenging stereotypes and legitimating fat: an analysis of obese people's views on news media reporting guidelines and promoting body diversity, *Journal of Sociology*, 51(2): 431–455.

Holman, D., Lynch, R. and Reeves, A. (2018) How do health behaviour interventions take account of social context? A literature trend and co-citation analysis, *Health*, 22(4): 389–410.

Hughes, V. (2013) The big fat truth, *Nature*, 497(7450): 428–430.

Humphrey, L., Clifford, D. and Morris, M.N. (2015) Health at Every Size college course reduces dieting behaviors and improves intuitive eating, body esteem, and anti-fat attitudes, *Journal of Nutrition Education and Behavior*, 47(4): 354–360.

Hunger, J.M., Major, B., Blodorn, A. and Miller, C.T. (2015) Weighed down by stigma: how weight-based social identity threat contributes to weight gain and poor health, *Social and Personality Psychology Compass*, 9(6): 255–268.

Hynnä, K. and Kyrölä, K. (2019) 'Feel in your body': fat activist affects in blogs, *Social Media + Society*, 5(4): 1–11.

Independent Auditor's Report (2019) *Leadership Institute Audited Financial Statements Years Ended December 31, 2018 and 2017.* Online: <www.leadershipinstitute.org/aboutus/Files/2018Audit.pdf> Accessed 17 April 2020.

Inthorn, S. and Boyce, T. (2010) 'It's disgusting how much salt you eat!' Television discourses of obesity, health and morality, *International Journal of Cultural Studies*, 13(1): 83–100.

Ioannidis, J.P.A. (2020a) Global perspective of COVID-19 epidemiology for a full-cycle pandemic, *European Journal of Clinical Investigation*, 50(12): e13423.

Ioannidis, J.P.A. (2020b) Coronavirus disease 2019: the harms of exaggerated information and non-evidence-based measures, *European Journal of Clinical Investigation*, 50(4): e13222.

Isono, M., Watkins, P.L. and Lian, L.E. (2009) Bon bon fatty girl: a qualitative exploration of weight bias in Singapore. In E. Rothblum and S. Solovay (eds), *The Fat Studies Reader.* New York: New York University Press.

James, A. and Hockey, J. (2007) *Embodying Health Identities.* Palgrave MacMillan, Basingstoke.

Janesick, A.S. and Blumberg, B. (2016) Obesogens: an emerging threat to public health, *American Journal of Obstetrics and Gynecology*, 214(5): 559–565.

Jayawardena, R., Sooriyaarachchi, P., Chourdakis, M. et al. (2020) Enhancing immunity in viral infections, with special emphasis on COVID-19: a review, *Diabetes & Metabolic Syndrome: Clinical Research and Reviews*, 14(4): 367–382.

Jendrzyca, A. and Warschburger, P. (2016) Weight stigma and eating behaviours in elementary school children: a prospective population-based study, *Appetite*, 102: 51–59.

Jensen, T. (2018) *Parenting the Crisis: The Cultural Politics of Parent-Blame*. Bristol: Polity.

John, G.K. and Mullin, G.E. (2016) The gut microbiome and obesity, *Current Oncology Reports*, 18(45).

Johnson, I. (2014) Children taken into care for being too fat, *Independent*, 28 February.

Joy, P.J. and Numer, M. (2018) Constituting the ideal body: a poststructural analysis of 'obesity' discourses among gay men, *Journal of Critical Dietetics*, 4(1): 47–58.

Kamola, I. (2019) Dear administrators: to protect your faculty from right-wing attacks, follow the money, *Journal of Academic Freedom*, 10: 1–24.

Kanagasingam, D., Norman, M. and Hurd, L. (2021) Illuminating the ethical tensions in the obesity Canada website: a transdisciplinary social justice perspective, *Journal of Critical Realism*, 20(5): 474–490.

Kannen, V. (2016) 'How can you be teaching this?' Tears, fears, and fat. In E. Cameron and C. Russell (eds), *The Fat Pedagogy Reader*. New York: Peter Lang Publishing.

Kapilashrami, A., Otis, M., Omodara, D. et al. (2021) Ethnic disparities in health & social care workers' exposure, protection, and clinical managements of the COVID-19 pandemic in the UK, *Critical Public Health*. Advance online publication: https://doi.org/1 0.1080/09581596.2021.1959020.

Kassirer, J.P. and Angell, M. (1998) Losing weight – an ill-fated New Year's resolution? *New England Journal of Medicine*, 338: 52–54.

Keane, H. (2005) Diagnosing the male steroid user: drug use, body image and disordered masculinity, *Health*, 9(2): 189–208.

Kearnes, M., Cook, B.R., Kuch, D. et al. (2020) We should listen to coronavirus experts, but local wisdom counts too, *The Conversation*, 1 April. Online: <https://theconversation.com/we-should-listen-to-coronavirus-experts-but-local-wisdom-counts-too-134034> Accessed 2 April 2020.

Kehler, M. and Atkinson, M. (eds) (2010) *Boys' Bodies: Speaking the Unspoken*. New York: Peter Lang.

Keith, S.W., Redden, D.T., Katzmarzyk, P.T. et al. (2006) Putative contributors to the secular increase in obesity: exploring the roads less travelled, *International Journal of Obesity*, 30(11): 1585–1594.

Keleman Saxena, A. and Johnson, J.L. (2020) Cues for ethnography in pandamning times: thinking with digital sociality in the Covid-19 pandemic, *Somatosphere*, 31 May.

Kelly, M.P. and Barker, M. (2016) Why is changing health-related behaviour so difficult? *Public Health*, 136: 109–116.

Kelly, M.P. and Russo, F. (2018) Causal narratives in public health: the difference between mechanisms of aetiology and mechanisms of prevention in non-communicable diseases, *Sociology of Health & Illness*, 40(1): 82–99.

Kirk, D. (2006) The 'obesity crisis' and school physical education, *Sport, Education and Society*, 11(2): 121–133.

Kirkland, A. (2011) The environmental account of obesity: a case for feminist scepticism, *Signs*, 36(2): 463–485.

Kirkup, K. (2016) Senate report warns of obesity crisis in Canada, *CTV News*, 1 March. Online: <www.ctvnews.ca/health/senate-report-warns-of-obesity-crisis-in-canada-1.2799035> Accessed 1 October 2016.

Kivisto, P. (2019) The politics of cruelty, *The Sociological Quarterly*, 60(2): 191–200.

Klein, N. (2007) *The Shock Doctrine: The Rise of Disaster Capitalism*. London: Penguin.

Klein, N. (2020) Coronavirus capitalism – and how to beat it, *The Intercept*, 16 March. Online: <https://theintercept.com/2020/03/16/coronavirus-capitalism/> Accessed 18 March 2020.

Knibbs, J. (2019) Boris Johnson health: how Tory leader hopeful was pushed to lose weight by doctors, *Express*, 18 June.

Krueger, R.A. and Casey, M.A. (2000) *Focus Groups: A practical Guide for Applied Research*, 3rd edn. Thousand Oaks, CA: SAGE.

Kuczmarski, R.K., Flegal, K.M., Campbell, S.M. and Johnson, C.L. (1994) Increasing prevalence of overweight among US adults: the National Health and Nutrition Examination Surveys, 1960-1991, *JAMA*, 272: 205–211.

Kuk, J.L., Rotundi, M., Sui, X. et al. (2018) Individuals with obesity but no other metabolic risk factors are not at significantly elevated all-cause mortality risk in men and women, *Clinical Obesity*, 8(5): 305–312.

Kwan, S. and Graves, J. (2013) *Framing Fat: Competing Constructions in Contemporary Culture*. New Brunswick, NJ: Rutgers University Press.

Lakoff, A. (2007) Preparing for the next emergency, *Public Culture*, 19(2): 247–271.

Land, N. (2018) Fat knowledges and matters of fat: towards re-encountering fat(s). *Social Theory & Health*, 16(1): 77–93.

Larkin, J. and Rice, C. (2005) Beyond 'healthy eating' and 'healthy weights': harassment and the health curriculum in middle schools, *Body Image*, 2(3): 219–232.

Latour, B. (2004) Why has critique run out of steam? From matters of fact to matters of concern, *Critical Inquiry*, 30(2): 225–248.

Lavie, C.J., De Schutter, A. and Milani, R.V. (2015) Healthy obese versus unhealthy lean: the obesity paradox, *Nature Reviews Endocrinology*, 11(1): 55–62.

Lavie, C.J. and Loberg, K. (2014) *The Obesity Paradox: When Thinner Means Sicker and Heavier Means Healthier*. New York: Hudson Street Press.

Lawson, V. and Wardle, J. (2013) A qualitative exploration of the health promotion effects of varying body size in photographs analyzed using interpretative phenomenological analysis, *Body Image*, 10(1): 85–94.

Leadership Institute (2020) About the Leadership Institute. Online: <www.leadershipinstitute.org/aboutus/> Accessed 20 April 2020.

Leahy, D. (2009) Disgusting pedagogies. In J. Wright and V. Harwood (eds), *Biopolitics and the Obesity Epidemic*. New York: Routledge.

Leahy, D., O'Flynn, G. and Wright, J. (2013) A critical 'critical inquiry' proposition in health and physical education, *AsiaPacific Journal of Health, Sport and Physical Education*, 4(2): 175–187.

LeBesco, K. (2004) *Revolting Bodies? The Struggle to Redefine Fat Identity*. Boston, MA: University of Massachusetts Press.

LeBesco, K. (2010) Fat panic and the new morality. In J.M. Metzl and A. Kirkland (eds), *Against Health: How Health Became the New Morality*. New York: New York University Press.

LeBesco, K. (2011) Neoliberalism, public health, and the moral perils of fatness, *Critical Public Health*, 21(2): 153–164.

Leder, D. (1990) *The Absent Body*. Chicago, IL: University of Chicago Press.

Lee, J.A. and Pausé, C. (2016) Stigma in practice: barriers to health for fat women, *Frontiers in Psychology*, 7: 2063, https://www.frontiersin.org/articles/10.3389/fpsyg.2016.02063/full.

Lee, M., Ata, R.N. and Brannick, M.T. (2014) Malleability of weight-biased attitudes and beliefs: a meta-analysis of weight bias reduction interventions, *Body Image*, 11(3): 251–259.

Levay, C. (2014) Obesity in organizational context, *Human Relations*, 67(5): 565–585.

Lewis, S, Thomas, S.L., Blood, R.W. et al. (2011) How do obese individuals perceive and respond to the different types of obesity stigma that they encounter in their daily lives? A qualitative study, *Social Science & Medicine*, 73(9): 1349–1356.

Limatius, H. (2019) 'I'm a fat bird and I just don't care': a corpus-based analysis of body descriptors in plus-size fashion blogs, *Discourse, Context & Media*, 31: 100316.

Lipman, P. (2011) *The New Political Economy of Urban Education: Neoliberalism, Race, and the Right to the City*. New York: Routledge.

Liu, X., Guo, L., Xiao, K. et al. (2020) The obesity paradox for outcomes in atrial fibrillation: evidence from an exposure-effect analysis of prospective studies, *Obesity Reviews*, 21(3): e12970.

Lobstein, T. and Brinsden, H. (2020) *Obesity: Missing the 2025 Targets. Trends, Costs and Country Reports*. London: WOF.

Loke, Y.K. and Heneghan, C. (2020) Why nobody can ever recover from COVID-19 in England – a statistical anomaly, *CEBM*, 18 July. Online: <www.cebm.net/covid-19/why-no-one-can-ever-recover-from-covid-19-in-england-a-statistical-anomaly/> Accessed 20 July 2020.

Longhurst, R. (2012) Becoming smaller: autobiographical spaces of weight loss, *Antipode*, 44(3): 871–888.

Loughland, T. and Sriprakash, A. (2016) Bernstein revisited: the recontextualisation of equity in contemporary Australian school education, *British Journal of Sociology of Education*, 37(2): 230–247.

Lown, B., Cash, R.A. and Rohde, J.E. (2021) Renewed threat of nuclear holocaust requires physician activism, *New England Journal of Medicine*, 384: 292.

Lozano-Sufrategui, L., Carless, D., Pringle, A. et al. (2016) 'Sorry mate, you're probably a bit too fat to be able to do any of these': men's experiences of weight stigma, *International Journal of Men's Health*, 15(1): 4–23.

Lupton, D. (1995) *The Imperative of Health: Public Health and the Regulated Body*. London: SAGE.

Lupton, D. (1996) *Food, the Body and the Self*. London: SAGE.

Lupton, D. (2012) A sociological critique of the Health at Every Size movement, *This Sociological Life: A Blog by Sociologist Deborah Lupton*. Online: <https://simplysociology.wordpress.com/2012/09/24/a-sociological-critique-of-the-health-at-every-size-movement/#comments> Accessed 28 December 2016.

Lupton, D. (2013) *Fat*. New York: Routledge.

Lupton, D. (2014) 'How do you measure up?' Assumptions about 'obesity and health-related behaviors and beliefs in two Australian 'obesity' prevention campaigns, *Fat Studies*, 3(1): 32–44.

Lupton, D. (2015) The pedagogy of disgust: the ethical, moral and political implications of using disgust in public health campaigns, *Critical Public Health*, 25(1): 4–14.

Lupton, D. (2017) Digital media and body weight, shape, and size: an introduction and review, *Fat Studies*, 6(2): 119–134.

Lupton, D. (2018) *Fat*, 2nd edn. New York: Routledge.

Lupton, D. (2020) Social research for a COVID and post-COVID world: an initial research agenda, *Medium*, 29 March. Online: <https://medium.com/@deborahalupton/social-research-for-a-covid-and-post-covid-world-an-initial-agenda-796868f1fb0e> Accessed 30 March 2020.

Lupton, D., Southerton, C., Clark, M. and Watson, A. (2021) *The Face Mask in COVID Times: A Sociomaterial Analysis*. Berlin/Boston, MA: Walter de Gruyter.

Lupton, D. and Willis, K. (eds) (2021) *The COVID Crisis: Social Perspectives*. London and New York: Routledge.

Lusted, D. (1986) Why pedagogy? *Screen*, 27(5): 2–14.

MacBride-Stewart, S. (2022) Environment. In L.F. Monaghan and J. Gabe (eds), *Key Concepts in Medical Sociology*, 3rd edn. London: SAGE.

MacGregor, H., Leach, M., Wilkinson, A. and Parker, M. (2020) COVID-19 – a social phenomenon requiring diverse expertise. Institute of Development Studies, 20 March. Online: <www.ids.ac.uk/opinions/covid-19-a-social-phenomenon-requiring-diverse-expertise/> Accessed 1 August 2020.

Mackenbach, J.D., Rutter, H., Compernolle, S. et al. (2014) Obesogenic environments: a systematic review of the association between the physical environment and adult weight status, the SPOTLIGHT project, *BMC Public Health*, 14(233), https://doi.org/10.1186/1471-2458-14-233.

MacLean, P.S., Bergouignan, A., Cornier, M.A. and Jackman, M.R. (2011) Biology's response to dieting: the impetus for weight regain, *American Journal of Physiology – Regulatory Integrative and Comparative Physiology*, 301(3): R581–R600.

MacNeill, M. and Rail, G. (2010) The visions, voices and moves of young 'Canadians': exploring diversity, subjectivity and cultural constructions of fitness and health. In J. Wright and D. Macdonald (eds), *Young People, Physical Activity and the Everyday*. London: Routledge.

MacPhail, A. and Kinchin, G. (2004) The use of drawings as an evaluative tool: students' experiences of sport education, *Physical Education and Sport Pedagogy*, 9(1): 87–108.

Madigan, C.D., Pavey, T., Daley, A.J. et al. (2018) Is weight cycling associated with adverse health outcomes? A cohort study, *Preventive Medicine*, 108: 47–52.

Maguire, M., Braun, A. and Ball, S. (2015) 'Where you stand depends on where you sit': the social construction of policy enactments in the (English) secondary school, *Discourse: Studies in the Cultural Politics of Education*, 36(4): 485–499.

Maher, J., Fraser, S. and Wright, J. (2010) Framing the mother: childhood obesity, maternal responsibility and care, *Gender Studies*, 19(3): 233–247.

Maidment, J. (2020a) Lose weight, save the NHS: Boris Johnson reveals his fight to diet as government launches anti-obesity drive, *Daily Mail*, 27 July.

Maidment, J. (2020b) Michael Gove reveals that police have imposed more than 3,200 fines on 'Covidiots' for flouting coronavirus lockdown rules, *MailOnline*, 28 April.

Malhotra, A. (2020) Absolutely disgraceful. Feeding junk food to already overweight and obese NHS staff? [...] *Twitter*, 22 April. Online: <https://twitter.com/draseemmalhotra/status/1252861958652452864?lang=en> Accessed April 23 2020.

Mann, T., Tomiyama, A.J., Westling, E. et al. (2007) Medicare's search for effective obesity treatments: diets are not the answer, *American Psychologist*, 62(3): 220–233.

Mannion, R. and Small, N. (2019) On folk devils, moral panics and new wave public health, *International Journal of Health Policy Management*, 18(2): 678–683.

Mansfield, L. and Rich, E. (2003) Public health pedagogy, border crossings and physical activity at every size, *Critical Public Health*, 23(3): 356–370.

Mansnerus, E. (2013) Using model-based evidence in the governance of pandemics, *Sociology of Health & Illness*, 35(2): 280–291.

Marmot, M. (2004a) *The Status Syndrome: How Your Social Standing Directly Affects Your Health*. London: Bloomsbury.

Marmot, M. (2004b) Evidence based policy or policy based evidence?: Willingness to take action influences the view of the evidence – look at alcohol, *BMJ*, 328(7445): 906–907.

Marmot, M., Allen, J., Boyce, T. et al. (2020a) *Heath Equity in England: The Marmot Review 10 Years On*. London: Institute of Health Equity.

Marmot, M., Allen, J., Goldblatt, P. et al. (2020b) *Build Back Fairer: The COVID-19 Marmot Review. The Pandemic, Socioeconomic and Health Inequalities in England*. London: Institute of Health Equity.

Martin, G.P., Hanna, E., McCartney, M. and Dingwall, R. (2020a) Science, society, and policy in the face of uncertainty: reflections on the debate around face coverings for the public during COVID-19, *Critical Public Health*, 30(5): 501–508.

Martin, G.P., Hanna, E. and Dingwall, R. (2020b) Response to Greenhalgh et al.: face masks, the precautionary principle, and evidence-informed policy, *BMJ*, 369: m1435.

Martínez-Rodríguez, F.M. and Fernández-Herrería, A. (2017) Is there life beyond neo-liberalism? Critical socio-educational alternatives for civic construction, *Globalisation, Societies and Education*, 15(2): 135–146.

Mata, J. and Hertwig, R. (2018) Public beliefs about obesity relative to other major health risks: representative cross-sectional surveys in the USA, the UK, and Germany, *Annals of Behavioral Medicine*, 52(4): 273–286.

Mauro, M., Taylor, V., Wharton, S. and Sharma, A.M. (2008) Barriers to obesity treatment, *European Journal of Internal Medicine*, 19(3): 173–180.

Mayer, K. (2004) An unjust war: the case against the government's war on obesity, *Georgetown Law Journal*, 92(5): 999–1031.

McAuley, P.A. and Blair, S.N. (2011) Obesity paradoxes, *Journal of Sports Sciences*, 29(8): 773–782.

McCartney, G., Dickie, E., Escobar, O. and Collins, C. (2021) Health inequalities, fundamental causes and power: towards the practice of good theory, *Sociology of Health & Illness*, 43(1): 20–39.

McCurry, J. (2008) Japanese firms face penalties for overweight staff, *The Guardian*, 19 March.

McEvilly, N. (2015) Investigating the place and meaning of 'physical education' to pre-school children: methodological lessons from a research study, *Sport, Education and Society*, 20(3): 340–360.

McGoey, L. (2019) *The Unknowers: How Strategic Ignorance Rules the World*. London: Zed Books.

McKelvie, G. (2020) NHS staff fighting coronavirus war are 'suicidal and afraid to hug their kids', *Mirror*, 18 April.

McLeod, J. and Yates, L. (2006) *Making Modern Lives: Subjectivity, Schooling and Social Change*. New York: SUNY Press.

McNaughton, D. (2013) 'Diabesity' down under: overweight and obesity as cultural signifiers for type 2 diabetes mellitus, *Critical Public Health*, 23(3): 274–288.

McPhail, D. (2010) 'This is the face of obesity': gender and the production of emotional obesity in 1950s and 1960s Canada, *Radical Psychology*, 8(1).

McPhail, D. (2013) Resisting biopedagogies of obesity in a problem population: understandings of healthy eating and healthy weight in a Newfoundland and Labrador community, *Critical Public Health*, 23(3): 289–303.

McPhail, D. (2017) *Contours of the Nation: Making Obesity and Imagining Canada 1945-1970*. Toronto: University of Toronto Press.

McPhail, D. and Bombak, A.E. (2015) Fat, queer and sick? A critical analysis of 'lesbian obesity' in public health discourse, *Critical Public Health*, 25(5): 539–553.

McPhail, D., Bombak, A., Ward, P. and Allison, J. (2016) Wombs at risk, wombs as risk: fat women's experiences of reproductive care, *Fat Studies*, 5(2): 98–115.

McVey, G., Gusella, J., Tweed, S. and Ferrari, M. (2009) A controlled evaluation of web-based training for teachers and public health practitioners on the prevention of eating disorders, *Eating Disorders*, 17(1): 1–26.

Meadows, A. and Bombak, A.E. (2019) Yes, we can (no you can't): weight stigma, exercise self-efficacy, and active fat identity development, *Fat Studies*, 8(2): 135–153.

Meadows, A. and Daníelsdóttir, S. (2016) What's in a word? Weight stigma and terminology, *Frontiers in Psychology*, 7: 1527, https://www.frontiersin.org/articles/10.3389/fpsyg.2016.01527/full.

Mediouni, M., Madiouni, R. and Kaczor-Urbanowicz, K.E. (2020) COVID-19: how the quarantine could lead to the depreobesity, *Obesity Medicine*, 19(100255): 1–2.

Medvedyuk, S., Ahmednur, A. and Raphael, D. (2018) Ideology, obesity and the social determinants of health: a critical analysis of the obesity and health relationship, *Critical Public Health*, 28(5): 573–585.

Mehta, T., Smith, D.L. Jr., Muhammad, J. and Casazza, K. (2014) Impact of weight cycling on risk of morbidity and mortality, *Obesity Reviews*, 15(11): 870–881.

Meleo-Erwin, Z. (2012) Disrupting normal: towards the 'ordinary and familiar' in fat politics, *Feminism and Psychology*, 22(3): 388–402.

Meleo-Erwin, Z.C. (2019) 'No-one is as invested in your continued good health as you should be': an exploration of the post-surgical relationships between weight-loss surgery patients and their home bariatric clinics, *Sociology of Health & Illness*, 41(2): 285–302.

Mendoza, K.R. (2009) Seeing through the layers: fat suits and thin bodies in *The Nutty Professor* and *Shallow Hal*. In E. Rothblum and S. Solovay (eds), *The Fat Studies Reader*. New York: New York University Press.

Mennell, S. (1991) On the civilizing of appetite. In M. Featherstone, M. Hepworth and B. Turner (eds), *The Body: Social Process and Cultural Theory*. London: SAGE.

Mensinger, J.L., Calogero, R.M. and Tylka, T.L. (2016) Internalized weight stigma moderates eating behavior outcomes in women with high BMI participating in a healthy living program, *Appetite*, 102: 32–43.

Mensinger, J.L. and Meadows, A. (2017) Internalized weight stigma mediates and moderates physical activity outcomes during a healthy living program for women with high Body Mass Index, *Psychology of Sport and Exercise*, 30: 64–72.

Mensinger, J.L., Tylka, T.L. and Calamari, M.E. (2018) Mechanisms underlying weight status and healthcare avoidance in women: a study of weight stigma, body-related shame and guilt, and healthcare stress, *Body Image*, 25: 139–147.

Metzl, J.M. and Hansen, H. (2014) Structural competency: theorizing a new medical engagement with stigma and inequality, *Social Science & Medicine*, 103: 126–133.

Metzl, J.M. and Kirkland, A.K. (eds) (2010) *Against Health: How Health Became the New Morality*. New York: New York University Press.

Miah, A. and Rich, E. (2008) *The Medicalization of Cyberspace*. Abingdon: Routledge.

Miller, L.J. and Lu, W. (2019) These are the healthiest nations, *Bloomberg*, 24 February. Online: <www.bloomberg.com/news/articles/2019-02-24/spain-tops-italy-as-world-s-healthiest-nation-while-u-s-slips> Accessed 16 March 2019.

Miller, S.A., Wu, R.K.S. and Oremus, M. (2018) The association between antibiotic use in infancy and childhood overweight or obesity: a systematic review and meta-analysis, *Obesity Reviews*, 19(11): 1463–1475.

Mills, C.W. (1959) *The Sociological Imagination*. New York: Oxford University Press.

Mitchell, A. (2005) Pissed off. In D. Kulick and A. Meneley (eds), *Fat: The Anthropology of an Obsession*. New York: Penguin.

Mitha, K., Quereshi, K., Adatia, S. and Dodhia, H. (2020) Racism as a social determinant: COVID-19 and its impacts on racial/ethnic minorities, *Discover Society*, 22 December. Online: <https://discoversociety.org/2020/12/22/racism-as-a-social-determinant-covid-19-and-its-impacts-on-racial-ethnic-minorities/> Accessed 16 January 2021.

Monaghan, L.F. (2001) *Bodybuilding, Drugs and Risk*. London: Routledge.

Monaghan, L.F. (2002) Hard men, shop boys and others: embodying competence in a masculinist occupation, *The Sociological Review*, 50(3): 334–355.

Monaghan, L.F. (2005a) Discussion piece: a critical take on the obesity debate, *Social Theory & Health*, 3(4): 302–314.

Monaghan, L.F. (2005b) Big handsome men, bears and others: virtual constructions of 'fat male embodiment', *Body & Society*, 11(2): 81–111.

Monaghan, L.F. (2006) Corporeal indeterminacy: the value of embodied, interpretive sociology. In D. Waskul and P. Vannini (eds), *Body/Embodiment: Symbolic Interactionism and the Sociology of the Body*. Aldershot: Ashgate.

Monaghan, L.F. (2007a) McDonaldizing men's bodies? Slimming, associated (ir)rationalities and resistances, *Body & Society*, 13(2): 67–93.

Monaghan, L.F. (2007b) Body Mass Index, masculinities and moral worth: men's critical talk about 'appropriate' weight-for-height, *Sociology of Health & Illness*, 29(4): 584–609.

Monaghan, L.F. (2008) *Men and the War on Obesity: A Sociological Study*. New York: Routledge.

Monaghan, L.F. (2009) Commentary on Kanayama et al.: the normalization of steroid use, *Addiction*, 104: 1979–1980.

Monaghan, L.F. (2010a) 'Physician heal thyself' part 1: a qualitative analysis of a Medscape debate on clinicians' bodyweight, *Social Theory & Health*, 8(1): 1–27.

Monaghan, L.F. (2010b) 'Physician heal thyself' part 2: debating clinicians' bodyweight, *Social Theory & Health*, 8(1): 28–50.

Monaghan, L.F. (2013) Extending the obesity debate, repudiating misrecognition: politicising fatness and health (practice), *Social Theory & Health*, 11(1): 81–105.

Monaghan, L.F. (2014a) Civilising recalcitrant boys' bodies: pursuing social fitness through the anti-obesity offensive, *Sport, Education and Society*, 19(6): 691–711.

Monaghan, L.F. (2014b) Debating, theorising and researching 'obesity' in challenging times, *Social Theory & Health: Inaugural Virtual Special Issue on Obesity*. Online: <https://link.springer.com/article/10.1057/sth.2014.10>.

Monaghan, L.F. (2015) Critiquing masculinity myths: rethinking male bodies, obesity and health in context, *International Journal of Men's Health*, 14(3): 250–266.

Monaghan, L.F. (2017) Re-framing weight-related stigma: from spoiled identity to macro-social structures, *Social Theory & Health*, 15(2): 182–205.

Monaghan, L.F. (2020) Coronavirus (COVID-19), pandemic psychology and the fractured society: a sociological case for critique, foresight and action, *Sociology of Health & Illness*, 42(8): 1982–1995.

Monaghan, L.F., Bombak, A.E. and Rich, E. (2018) Obesity, neoliberalism and epidemic psychology: critical commentary and alternative approaches to public health, *Critical Public Health*, 28(5): 498–508.

Monaghan, L.F., Colls, R. and Evans, R. (eds) (2014) *Obesity Discourse and Fat Politics: Research, Critique and Interventions*. New York: Routledge.

Monaghan, L.F. and Gabe, J. (2016) Embodying health identities: a study of young people with asthma, *Social Science & Medicine*, 160: 1–8.

Monaghan, L.F. and Hardey, M. (2011) Bodily sensibility: vocabularies of the discredited male body. In E. Rich, L.F. Monaghan and L. Aphramor (eds), *Debating Obesity: Critical Perspectives*. London: Palgrave MacMillan.

Monaghan, L.F., Hollands, R. and Pritchard, G. (2010) Obesity epidemic entrepreneurs: types, practices and interests, *Body & Society*, 16(2): 37–71.

Monaghan, L.F. and Malson, H. (2013) 'It's worse for women and girls': negotiating embodied masculinities through weight-related talk, *Critical Public Health*, 23(3): 304–319.

Monaghan, L.F. and O'Flynn, M. (2017) The Madoffization of Irish society: from Ponzi finance to sociological critique, *The British Journal of Sociology*, 68(4): 670–692.

Monaghan, L.F., Rich, E. and Bombak, A.E. (2019) Media, 'fat panic' and public pedagogy: mapping contested terrain, *Sociology Compass*, 13(1): 1–17. e12651.

Montani, J.P., Viecelli, A., Prevot, A. and Dulloo, A. (2006) Weight cycling during growth and beyond as a risk factor for later cardiovascular diseases: the 'repeated overshoot' theory, *International Journal of Obesity*, 30: S58–S66.

Moore, R. (2013) *Basil Bernstein: The Thinker and the Field*. New York: Routledge.

Moss, N. and Petherick, L. (2016) The enemy within: teaching 'hard knowledges' about 'soft bodies in a Kinesiology faculty. In E. Cameron and C. Russell (eds), *The Fat Pedagogy Reader*. New York: Peter Lang Publications.

Moynihan, R. (2006a) Expanding definitions of obesity may harm children, *BMJ*, 332: 1412.

Moynihan, R. (2006b) Obesity taskforce linked to WHO takes 'millions' from drugs firms, *BMJ*, 332: 1412.

Mulderrig, J. (2017) Reframing obesity: a critical discourse analysis of the UK's first social marketing campaign, *Critical Policy Studies*, 11(4): 455–476.

Mulderrig, J. (2019) The language of 'nudge' in health policy: pre-empting working class obesity through 'biopedagogy', *Critical Policy Studies*, 13(1): 101–121.

Murray, S. (2005a) Doing politics or selling out? Living the fat body, *Women's Studies*, 34(3–4): 265–277.

Murray, S. (2005b) Introduction to 'Thinking Fat'. Special issue of Social Semiotics, *Social Semiotics*, 15(2): 111–112.

Murray, S. (2008) *Fat Female Body*. London: Palgrave Macmillan.

Mykhalovskiy, E., Frohlich, K.L., Poland, B. et al. (2019) Critical social science *with* public health: agonism, critique and engagement, *Critical Public Health*, 29(5): 522–533.

Nash, M. and Warin, M. (2017) Squeezed between identity politics and intersectionality: a critique of 'thin privilege' in Fat Studies, *Feminist Theory*, 18(1): 69–87.

National Preventative Health Taskforce (2009) *Australia: The Healthiest Country by 2020. National Preventative Health Strategy – Overview*. Canberra: Australian Government.

Nazroo, J. (2013) Ethnicity. In J. Gabe and L.F. Monaghan (eds), *Key Concepts in Medical Sociology*, 2nd edn. London: SAGE.

Nettleton, S. and Watson, J. (eds) (1998) *The Body in Everyday Life*. London: Routledge.

Newhook, J., Gregory, D. and Twells, L. (2015) 'Fat girls' and 'big guys': gendered meanings of weight loss surgery, *Sociology of Health & Illness*, 37(5): 653–667.

Ng Tang Fui, M., Hoermann, R., Dupuis, P. et al. (2016) Effect of testosterone therapy combined with a very low caloric diet on fat mass in obese men with a low- to low-normal testosterone level: a randomized controlled trial. Poster presented at *Endocrine Society's 98th Annual Meeting and Expo*, 2 April, Boston.

Ni Shuilleabhain, N., Rich, E. and Fullagar, S. (2021) Rethinking digital media literacy to address body dissatisfaction in schools: lessons from feminist new materialism, *New Media & Society*. Advance online publication: https://doi.org/10.1177/14614448211041715.

Obesity Action Coalition (2018) About the OAC. Online: <www.obesityaction.org/our-purpose/about-us/> Accessed 8 February 2019.

Obesity Canada (2020) <https://obesitycanada.ca/>.

Obesity Health Alliance (2021) *Turning the Tide: A 10-Year Healthy Weight Strategy*. Online: <https://aso.org.uk/sites/default/files/news/2021-09/Turning-the-Tide-Strategy-Report.pdf> Accessed 12 October 2021.

O'Connell, L., Quigley, F., Williams, O. et al. (2021) 'It's all right for you thinnies': 'obesity', eating disorders, and COVID-19. In P. Beresford, M. Farr, G. Hickey et al. (eds), *COVID-19 and Co-Production in Health and Social Care Research, Policy and Practice, Volume 1: The Challenges and Necessity of Co-Production*. Bristol: Policy Press.

O'Dea, J. (2004) Child obesity prevention: first, do no harm, *Health Education Research: Theory and Practice*, 20(2): 259–265.

OECD (2017) *Obesity Update 2017*. Online: <www.oecd.org/els/health-systems/Obesity-Update-2017.pdf> Accessed 5 February 2019.

Office for National Statistics (2020) *Coronavirus (COVID-19) Related Deaths by Ethnic Group, England and Wales: 2 March 2020 to 10 April 2020*. ONS. Online: <www.ons.gov.uk/

peoplepopulationandcommunity/birthsdeathsandmarriages/deaths/articles/corona
virusrelateddeathsbyethnicgroupenglandandwales/2march2020to10april2020> Accessed
7 May 2020.

O'Flynn, M., Monaghan, L.F. and Power, M.J. (2014) Scapegoating during a time of
crisis: a critique of post 'Celtic Tiger' Ireland, *Sociology, Special Issue: Sociology and the
Global Economic Crisis*, 48(5): 921–937.

Ogden, C.L., Carroll, M.D., Fryar, C.D. and Flegal, K.M. (2015) Prevalence of obesity among adults and youth: United States, 2011-2014. *NCHS Data Brief*, No. 219.
Online: <www.cdc.gov/nchs/data/databriefs/db219.pdf> Accessed 21 February 2018.

Ogden, L.G., Stroebele, N., Wyatt, H.R. et al. (2012) Cluster analysis of the National
Weight Control Registry to identify distinct subgroups maintaining successful weight
loss, *Obesity*, 20(10): 2039–2047.

O'Hara, L. and Gregg, J. (2012) Human rights casualties from the 'war on obesity': why
focusing on body weight is inconsistent with a human rights approach to health, *Fat
Studies*, 1(1): 32–46.

O'Hara, L. and Taylor, J. (2014) Health at Every Size: a weight neutral approach for
empowerment, resilience and peace, *International Journal of Social Work and Human
Services Practice*, 2(6): 272–282.

O'Hara, L. and Taylor, J. (2018) What's wrong with the 'war on obesity?' A narrative
review of the weight-centered health paradigm and the development of the 3C framework to build critical competency for a paradigm shift, *SAGE Open*, 8(2), https://doi.
org/10.1177/2158244018772888.

Oliver, E. (2006) *Fat Politics: The Real Story Behind America's Obesity Epidemic*. New York:
Oxford University Press.

Olshansky, S.J., Passaro, D.J., Hershow, R.C. et al. (2005) A potential decline in life
expectancy in the United States in the 21st century, *New England Journal of Medicine*,
352: 1138–1145.

Orbach, S. (2020) Britain's obesity strategy ignores the science: dieting doesn't work, *The
Guardian*, 28 July.

Orchard, T.J., Temprosa, M., Barrett-Connor, E. et al. (2013) Long-term effects of the
Diabetes Prevention Program Interventions on cardiovascular risk factors: a report
from the DPP Outcomes Study, *Diabetic Medicine*, 30(1): 46–55.

O'Regan, E. (2016) Revealed: new plan to stop Ireland becoming the fattest country in
Europe. *Independent.ie*, 23 September. <www.independent.ie/life/health-wellbeing/
healthy-eating/revealed-new-plan-to-stop-ireland-becoming-the-fattest-country-
in-europe-35069347.html> Accessed 23 September 2016.

O'Reilly, C. and Sixsmith, J. (2012) From theory to policy: reducing harms associated
with the weight-centered health paradigm, *Fat Studies*, 1(1): 97–113.

O'Toole, J. (2019) Crafting weight stigma in slimming classes: a case study in Ireland, *Fat
Studies*, 8(1): 10–24.

Overend, A., Bessey, M., Hite, A. et al. (2020) Introduction to against healthisms: challenging the paradigm of 'eating right', *Journal of Critical Dietetics*, 5(1): 1–3.

Paine, E.A. (2021) 'Fat broken arm syndrome': negotiating risk, stigma, and weight bias
in LGBTQ healthcare, *Social Science & Medicine*, 270: 113609.

Parliament of Canada (2016) *Obesity in Canada: A Whole-of-Society Approach for a
Healthier Canada*. Online: <https://sencanada.ca/content/sen/committee/421/SOCI/
Reports/2016-02-25_Revised_report_Obesity_in_Canada_e.pdf> Accessed 10
December 2018.

Parsons, A.A., Walsemann, K.M., Jones, S.J., et al. (2016) The influence of dominant obesity discourse on child health narratives: a qualitative study, *Critical Public Health*, 26(5): 602–614.

Patel, S.L. and Holub, S.C. (2012) Body size matters in provision of help: factors related to children's willingness to help overweight peers, *Obesity*, 20(2): 382–388.

Pausé, C. (2015) Rebel heart: performing fatness wrong online, *M/C Journal*, 18(3), https://doi.org/10.5204/mcj.977.

Pausé, C., Parker, G. and Gray, L. (2021) Resisting the problematisation of fatness in COVID-19: in pursuit of health justice, *International Journal of Disaster Risk Reduction*, 54: 102021.

Pearl, R.L. and Puhl, R.M. (2018) Weight bias internalization and health: a systematic review, *Obesity Reviews*, 19(8): 1141–1163.

Pedersen, M. (2012) A day in the Cadillac: the work of hope in urban Mongolia, *Social Analysis*, 56(2): 136–151.

Peeters, A. (2018) Journals should no longer accept 'obesity paradox' articles, *International Journal of Obesity*, 42: 584–585.

Pegington, M., French, D.P. and Harvie, M.N. (2020) Why young women gain weight: a narrative review of influencing factors and possible solutions, *Obesity Reviews*, 21(5): e13002.

Perreault, L., Pan, Q. Mather, K.J. et al. (2012) Effect of regression from prediabetes to normal glucose regulation on long-term reduction in diabetes risk: results from the Diabetes Prevention Program Outcomes Study, *The Lancet*, 379(9833): 2243–2251.

Pescosolido, B.A. and Martin, J.K. (2015) 'The stigma complex', *Annual Review of Sociology*, 41: 87–116.

Peters, M.A., Rizvi, F., McCulloch, G. et al. (2020) Reimagining the new pedagogical possibilities for universities post-Covid-19, *Educational Philosophy and Theory*. Advance online publication: https://doi.org/10.1080/00131857.2020.1777655.

Petersen, A. and Lupton, D. (1996) *The New Public Health and Self in the Age of Risk*. London: SAGE.

Petersen, A. and Wilkinson, I. (2015) Editorial introduction: the sociology of hope in contexts of health, medicine, and healthcare, *Health*, 19(2): 113–118.

Peterson, J.L., Puhl, R.M. and Luedicke, J. (2012) An experimental assessment of physical educators' expectations and attitudes: the importance of student weight and gender, *Journal of School Health*, 82(9): 432–440.

Petherick, L. (2013) Producing the young biocitizen: secondary school students' negotiation of learning in physical education, *Sport, Education and Society*, 18(6): 711–730.

Petherick, L. (2015) Shaping the child as a healthy child: health surveillance, schools, and biopedagogies, *Cultural Studies ↔ Critical Methodologies*, 15(5): 361–370.

Phelan, S.M., Burgess, D.J., Yeazel, M.W. et al. (2015) Impact of weight bias and stigma on quality of care and outcomes for patients with obesity, *Obesity Reviews*, 16(4): 319–326.

PHSA (2013) Technical Report: From Weight to Well-Being: Time for a Shift in Paradigms? Provisional Health Service Authority. Online: <www.phsa.ca/Documents/w2wbtechnicalreport_20130208final.pdf> Accessed 14 February 2019.

Pickersgill, M. (2020) Pandemic sociology, *Engaging Science, Technology, and Society*, 6: 347–350.

Pidd, H. (2018) Couples being denied IVF on NHS over man's age or weight, *The Guardian*, 29 October.

Platt, L. and Warwick, R. (2020) Are some ethnic groups more vulnerable to COVID-19 than others? *Institute for Fiscal Studies*. Online: <www.ifs.org.uk/inequality/chapter/are-some-ethnic-groups-more-vulnerable-to-covid-19-than-others/> Accessed 20 October 2020.

Poole, M.K., Fleischhacker, S.E. and Bleich, S.N. (2021) Addressing child hunger when school is closed — considerations during the pandemic and beyond, *New England Journal of Medicine*, 384: e35.

Popay, J., Whitehead, M. and Hunter, D.J. (2010) Injustice is killing people on a large scale – but what is to be done about it? *Journal of Public Health*, 32(2): 148–149.

Popkin, B.M., Du, S., Green, W.D. et al. (2020) Individuals with obesity and COVID-19: a global perspective on the epidemiology and biological relationships, *Obesity Reviews*, 21(11): e13128.

Popkin, B.M., Du, S., Green, W.D. et al. (2021) Reply to the John Speakman critique of 'impact of obesity on COVID-19 related mortality: a comment on estimates in Popkin et al (2020)', *Obesity Reviews*, 22(8): e13259.

Powell, D. and Fitzpatrick, K. (2015) 'Getting fit basically just means, like, nonfat': children's lessons in fitness and fatness, *Sport, Education and Society*, 20(4): 463–484.

Porter, S. (1993) Critical realist ethnography: the case of racism and professionalism in a medical setting, *Sociology*, 27(4): 591–609.

Prado, C.M., Purcell, S.A., Alish, C. et al. (2018) Implications of low muscle mass across the continuum of care: a narrative review, *Annals of Medicine*, 50(8): 675–693.

Preston, J. and Firth, R. (2020) *Coronavirus, Class and Mutual Aid in the United Kingdom*. Cham: Palgrave Macmillan.

Pringle, R. and Pringle, D. (2012) Competing obesity discourses and critical challenges for health and physical educators, *Sport, Education and Society*, 17(2): 143–161.

Puhl, R.M. (2011) Weight stigmatization toward youth: a significant problem in need of societal solutions, *Childhood Obesity*, 7(5): 359–363.

Puhl, R.M. (2020) What words should we use to talk about weight? A systematic review of quantitative and qualitative studies examining preferences for weight-related terminology, *Obesity Reviews*, 21(6): e13008.

Puhl, R.M. and Heuer, C.A. (2009) The stigma of obesity: a review and update, *Obesity*, 17(5): 941–964.

Puhl, R.M. and Heuer, C.A. (2010) Obesity stigma: important considerations for public health, *American Journal of Public Health*, 100(6): 1019–1028.

Puhl, R.M., Latner, J.D., O'Brien, K. et al. (2015) A multinational examination of weight bias: predictors of anti-fat attitudes across four countries, *International Journal of Obesity*, 39(7): 1166–1173.

Puhl, R.M., Luedicke, J. and Heuer, C. (2011) Weight-based victimization toward overweight adolescents: observations and reactions of peers, *Journal of School Health*, 81(11): 696–703.

Puhl, R.M., Peterson, J.L. and Luedicke, J. (2013) Weight-based victimization: bullying experiences of weight loss treatment-seeking youth, *Pediatrics*, 131(1): e1–e9.

Quigley, M. (2013) Nudging for health: on public policy and designing choice architecture, *Medical Law Review*, 21: 588–621.

Quinlan, A. (2018) A weighty problem: how Ireland is on course to be the fattest nation in Europe, *Independent.ie*, 19 May.

Quintáns, J.M. (2019) 80% of men and 55% of women in Spain will be overweight by 2030: study, *El País*, 10 January. Online: <https://elpais.com/elpais/2019/01/10/inenglish/1547131751_501777.html> Accessed 16 March 2019.

Quirke, L. (2016) 'Fat-proof your child': parenting advice and child obesity', *Fat Studies*, 5(2): 137–155.

Raffoul, A. and Williams, L. (2021) Integrating Health at Every Size principles into adolescent care, *Current Opinion in Pediatrics*, 33(4): 361–367.

Rahman, S.Y. (2020) 'Social distancing' during COVID-19: the metaphors and politics of pandemic response in India, *Health Sociology Review*, 29(2): 131–139.

Rail, G. (2009) Canadian youth's discursive constructions of health in the context of obesity discourse. In J. Wright and V. Harwood (eds), *Biopolitics and the 'Obesity Epidemic': Governing Bodies*. London: Routledge.

Rail, G. (2012) The birth of the obesity clinic: confessions of the flesh, biopedagogies and physical culture, *Sociology of Sport Journal*, 29(2): 227–253.

Rail, G., Holmes, D. and Murray, S.J. (2010) The politics of evidence on 'domestic terrorists': obesity discourses and their effects, *Social Theory & Health*, 8(3): 259–279.

Raisborough, J. (2016) *Fat Bodies, Health and the Media*. London: Palgrave Macmillan.

Raisborough, J., Ogden, C. and Stone de Guzman, V. (2019) When fat meets disability in poverty porn: exploring the cultural mechanisms of suspicion in *Too Fat to Work*, *Disability & Society*, 34(2): 276–295.

Rasmussen, S.H., Shrestha, S. and Bjerregaard, L.G. et al. (2018) Antibiotic exposure in early life and childhood overweight and obesity: a systematic review and meta-analysis, *Diabetes, Obesity and Metabolism*, 20(6): 1508–1514.

Ravussin, E. and Ryan, D.H. (2016) Energy expenditure and weight control: is the biggest loser the best loser? *Obesity*, 24(8): 1607–1608.

Rebughini, P. (2021) A sociology of anxiety: Western modern legacy and the Covid-19 outbreak, *International Sociology*, 36(4): 554–568.

Reid, M., Worsley, A. and Mavondo, F. (2015) The obesogenic household: factors influencing dietary gatekeeper satisfaction with family diet, *Psychology and Marketing*, 32(5): 544–557.

Reidinger, B. (2020) The elephant in the room: a fat woman in academe, *Inside Higher Ed*, 17 January.

Rhodes, T., Lancaster, K. and Rosengarten, M. (2020) A model society: maths, models and expertise in viral outbreaks, *Critical Public Health*, 30(3): 253–256.

Rice, C. (2007) Becoming 'the fat girl': acquisition of an unfit identity, *Women's Studies International Forum*, 30(2): 158–174.

Rice, C. (2015) Rethinking fat: from bio-to body-becoming pedagogies. *Cultural Studies ↔ Critical Methodologies*, 15(5): 387–397.

Rich, E. (2010) Editorial: body pedagogies, education and health, *Sport, Education and Society*, 15(2): 147–150.

Rich, E. (2011) 'I see her being obesed': public pedagogy, reality media and the obesity crisis, *Health*, 15(1): 3–21.

Rich, E. (2012) Beyond school boundaries: new health imperatives, families and schools, *Discourse: Studies in the Cultural Politics of Education*, 33(5): 635–654.

Rich, E. (2016) Troubling obesity discourse through public pedagogy. In E. Cameron and C. Russell (eds), *The Fat Pedagogy Reader: Challenging Weight-Based Oppression in Education*. New York: Peter Lang Publishers.

Rich, E. (2018) Gender, health and physical activity in the digital age: between post-feminism and pedagogical possibilities, special issue 'Gender, PE and Active Lifestyles', *Sport, Education and Society*, 23(8): 736–747.

Rich, E., De Pian, L. and Francombe-Webb, J. (2015) Physical cultures of stigmatisation: health policy and social class, *Sociological Research Online*, 20(2): 10, http://www.socresonline.org.uk/20/2/10.html.

Rich, E. and Evans, J. (2005) 'Fat Ethics' – the obesity discourse and body politics, *Social Theory & Health*, 3(4): 341–358.

Rich, E. and Evans, J. (2009) Performative health in schools: welfare policy, neoliberalism and social regulation? In J. Wright and V. Harwood (eds), *Biopolitics and the 'Obesity Epidemic': Governing Bodies*. New York: Routledge.

Rich, E. and Evans, J. (2013) Changing times, future bodies? The significance of health in young women's imagined futures, *Pedagogy, Culture & Society*, 21(1): 5–22.

Rich, E., Holroyd, R. and Evans, J. (2004) 'Hungry to be noticed': young women, anorexia and schooling. In J. Evans and B. Davies (eds), *Body Knowledge and Control: Studies in the Sociology of Physical Education and Health*. London: Routledge.

Rich, E. and Mansfield, L. (2019) Fat and physical activity: understanding and challenging weight stigma, *Fat Studies*, 8(2): 99–109.

Rich, E. and Miah, A. (2014) Understanding digital health as public pedagogy: a critical framework, *Societies*, 4(2): 296–315.

Rich, E. and Miah, A. (2017) Mobile, wearable and ingestible health technologies: towards a critical research agenda, *Health Sociology Review*, 26(1): 84–97.

Rich, E., Monaghan, L.F. and Aphramor, L. (eds) (2011) *Debating Obesity: Critical Perspectives*. Basingstoke: Palgrave Macmillan.

Rickett, O. (2020) Coronawashing: for big, bad businesses, it's the new greenwashing, *The Guardian*, 11 May. Online: <www.theguardian.com/commentisfree/2020/may/11/coronawashing-big-business-greenwashing-polluters-tax> Accessed 1 July 2020.

Riediger, N. (2016) Why a 'pop tax' is the wrong weapon to fight obesity, *Globe & Mail*, 22 May.

Riediger, N.D. and Bombak, A.E. (2018) Sugar-sweetened beverages as the new tobacco: examining a proposed tax policy through a Canadian social justice lens, *Canadian Medical Association Journal*, 190(11): E327–E330.

Riediger, N.D., Bombak, A.E., Mudryj, A. et al. (2018) A systematic search and qualitative review of reporting bias of lifestyle interventions in randomized controlled trials of diabetes prevention and management, *Nutrition Journal*, 17(1): 83.

Ries, N., Rachul, C. and Caulfield, T. (2011) Newspaper reporting on legislative policy interventions to address obesity: United States, Canada and the United Kingdom, *Journal of Public Health Policy*, 32(1): 73–90.

Riley, S., Evans, A. and Robson, M. (2019) *Postfeminism and Health: Critical Psychology and Media Perspectives*. New York: Routledge.

Ringrose, J. (2013) *Postfeminist Education? Girls and the Sexual Politics of Schooling*. New York: Routledge.

Ritzer, G. (ed) (2010) *McDonaldization: The Reader*, 3rd edn. California: Pine Forge Press & SAGE.

Rizvi, F. and Lingard, B. (2010) *Globalizing Education Policy*. London and New York: Routledge.

Rizvi, F. and Lingard, B. (2011) Social equity and the assemblage of values in Australian higher education, *Cambridge Journal of Education*, 41(1): 5–22.

Roberts, A. and Muta, S. (2017) Representations of female body weight in the media: an update of *Playboy* magazine from 2000 to 2014, *Body Image*, 20: 16–19.

Robertson, L. and Thomson, D. (2014) Giving permission to be fat? Examining the impact of body-based belief systems, *Canadian Journal of Education*, 37(4): 1–25.

Robison, J. (2005) Health at Every Size: toward a new paradigm of weight and health, *Medscape General Medicine*, 7(3): 13.

Roehling, P.V. (2012) Fat is a feminist issue, but it is complicated: commentary on Fikkan and Rothblum, *Sex Roles*, 66(9–10): 593–599.

Rogge, M.M., Greenwald, M. and Golden, A. (2004) Obesity, stigma and civilized oppression, *Advanced Nursing Studies*, 27(4): 301–315.

Rosenbaum, M., Hirsch, J., Gallagher, D.A. and Leibel, R.L. (2008) Long-term persistence of adaptive thermogenesis in subjects who have maintained a reduced body weight, *American Journal of Clinical Nutrition*, 88(4): 906–912.

Rosenbaum, M. and Leibel, R.L. (2016) Models of energy homeostasis in response to maintenance of reduced body weight, *Obesity*, 24(8): 1620–1629.

Rothblum, E. (2018) Slim chance for permanent weight loss, *Archives of Scientific Psychology*, 6: 63–69.

Rothblum, E. and Solovay, S. (eds) (2009) *The Fat Studies Reader*. New York: New York University Press.

RTÉ (2016) Obesity problem focus of new government plan, *RTÉ News*. Online: <www.rte.ie/news/2016/0922/818313-obesity-health-weight/> Accessed 23 September 2016.

Ruiz, M.C., Devonport, T.J., Chen-Wilson, C.-H. et al. (2021) A cross-cultural exploratory study of health behaviours and wellbeing during COVID-19, *Frontiers in Psychology*, 11: 608216, https://doi.org/10.3389/fpsyg.2020.608216.

Rundle, A.G., Park, Y., Herbstman, J.B. et al. (2020) COVID-10-related school closings and risk of weight gain among children, *Obesity*, 28(6): 1008–1009.

Russell-Mayhew, S., Nutter, S., Ireland, A. et al. (2015) Pilot testing a professional development model for preservice teachers in the area of health and weight: feasibility, utility, and efficacy, *Advances in School Mental Health Promotion*, 8(3): 176–186.

Ryan, D.H., Ravussin, E. and Heymsfield, S. (2020) COVID 19 and the patient with obesity – the editors speak out, *Obesity*, 28(5): 847.

Rychter, A.M., Zawada, A., Ratajczak, A.E. et al. (2020) Should patients with obesity be more afraid of COVID-19? *Obesity Reviews*, 21(9): e13083.

Saad, M.J.A., Santos, A. and Prada, P.O. (2016) Linking gut microbiota and inflammation to obesity and insulin resistance, *Physiology*, 31(4): 283–293.

Saguy, A.C. (2012) Why fat is a feminist issue, *Sex Roles*, 66(9–10): 600–607.

Saguy, A.C. (2013) *What's Wrong With Fat?* New York: Oxford University Press.

Saguy, A.C. and Almeling, R. (2005) Fat panic! The obesity epidemic as moral panic. *Paper presented at the Annual Meeting of the American Sociological Association*, 12 August, Philadelphia, PA.

Saguy, A.C. and Almeling, R. (2008) Fat in the fire? Science, the news media and the obesity epidemic, *Sociological Forum*, 23(1): 53–83.

Saguy, A.C., Frederick, D. and Gruys, K. (2014) Reporting risk, producing prejudice: how news reporting on obesity shapes attitudes about health risk, policy, and prejudice, *Social Science & Medicine*, 111: 125–133.

Saguy, A.C. and Gruys, K. (2010) Morality and health: news media constructions of overweight and eating disorders, *Social Problems*, 57(2): 231–250.

Saguy, A., Gruys, K. and Gong, S. (2010) Social problem construction and national context: news reporting on 'overweight' and 'obesity' in the United States and France, *Social Problems*, 57(4): 586–610.

Sainsbury, A. and Hay, P. (2014) Call for an urgent rethink of the 'Health at Every Size' concept, *Journal of Eating Disorders*, 2(8), https://doi.org/10.1186/2050-2974-2-8.

Saguy, A.C. and Riley, K. (2005) Weighing both sides: morality, mortality and framing contests over of obesity, *Journal of Health Politics, Policy and Law*, 30(5): 869–921.

Salas, X.R., Kirk, S., Alberga, S. et al. (2020) *Weight Bias, Obesity Stigma and COVID-19: Call to Action*. Obesity Canada, 25 May. Online: <http://obesitycanada.ca/wp-content/uploads/2020/05/WeightBias-Stigma-Covid-9.pdf> Accessed 28 May.

Saldaña, J. (2003) *Longitudinal Qualitative Research: Analyzing Change through Time.* California: AltaMira Press.

Sandberg, S. and Fondevila, G. (2020) Corona crimes: how pandemic narratives change criminal landscapes, *Theoretical Criminology*. Advance online publication: https://doi.org/10.1177/1362480620981637.

Sandlin, J., O'Malley, M.P. and Burdick, J. (2011) Mapping the complexity of public pedagogy scholarship: 1894-2010, *Review of Educational Research*, 81(3): 338–375.

Sanyaolu, A., Okorie, C., Marinkovic, A. et al. (2019) Measles outbreak in unvaccinated and partially vaccinated children and adults in the United States and Canada (2018-2019): a narrative review of cases, *INQUIRY: The Journal of Health Care, Organization, Provision, and Financing*, 56, https://doi.org/10.1177/0046958019894098.

Sarlio-Lähteenkorva, S. and Winkler, J.T. (2015) Could a sugar tax help combat obesity? *BMJ*, 351: h4047.

Scally, G. (2021) England's new office for health improvement and disparities, *BMJ*, 375: n2323.

Scambler, G. (2001) Critical realism, sociology and health inequalities: social class as a generative mechanism and its media of enactment, *Journal of Critical Realism*, 4(1): 35–42.

Scambler, G. (2006) Jigsaws, models and the sociology of stigma, *Journal of Critical Realism*, 5(2): 273–289.

Scambler, G. (2012) Health inequalities, *Sociology of Health & Illness*, 34(1): 130–146.

Scambler, G. (2013a) Material and cultural factors. In J. Gabe and L.F. Monaghan (eds), *Key Concepts in Medical Sociology*, 2nd edn. London: SAGE.

Scambler, G. (2013b) Resistance in unjust times: Archer, structured agency and the sociology of health inequalities, *Sociology*, 47(1): 142–156.

Scambler, G. (2018) *Sociology, Health and the Fractured Society: A Critical Realist Account.* New York: Routledge.

Scambler, G. (2020a) The fractured society: structures, mechanisms, tendencies, *Journal of Critical Realism*, 19(1): 1–13.

Scambler, G. (2020b) Covid-19 as a 'breaching experiment': exposing the fractured society, *Health Sociology Review*, 29(2): 140–148.

Schaefer, J.T. and Magnuson, A.B. (2014) A review of interventions that promote eating by internal cues, *Journal of the Academy for Nutrition and Dietetics*, 114: 734–760.

Scheindlin, B. (2005) 'Take one more bite for me': Clara Davis and the feeding of young children, *Gastronomica*, 5(1): 65–69.

Schorb, F. (2013) Fat politics in Europe: theorizing on the premises and outcomes of European anti-'obesity-epidemic' policies, *Fat Studies*, 2(1): 3–16.

Schorb, F. (2021) Fat as a neoliberal epidemic; analyzing fat bodies through the lens of political epidemiology, *Fat Studies*. Advance online publication: https://doi.org/10.1080/21604851.2021.1906524.

Schrecker, T. and Bambra, C. (2015) *How Politics Makes us Sick: Neoliberal Epidemics.* Basingstoke: Palgrave MacMillan.

Schrempft, S., van Jaarsveld, C.H.M., Fisher, A. and Wardle, J. (2015) The obesogenic quality of the home environment: associations with diet, physical activity, TV viewing, and BMI in preschool children, *PLoS ONE*, 10(8): e0134490, https://doi.org/10.1371/journal.pone.0134490.

Schulz, M., Liese, A.D., Boeing, H. et al. (2005) Associations of short-term weight changes and weight cycling with incidence of essential hypertension in the EPIC-Potsdam Study, *Journal of Human Hypertension*, 19(1): 61–67.

Schwartz, H. (1986) *Never Satisfied: A Cultural History of Diets, Fantasies and Fat.* New York: Free Press.

Schwartz, M.B., Chambliss, H.O., Brownell, K.D. et al. (2003) Weight bias among health professionals specializing in obesity, *Obesity Research*, 11(9): 1033–1039.

Schwartz, M.W., Seeley, R.J., Zeltser, L.M. et al. (2017) Obesity pathogenesis: an endocrine society scientific statement, *Endocrine Reviews*, 38(4): 267–296.

Scott-Samuel, A., Bambra, C., Collins, C. et al. (2014) The impact of Thatcherism on health and well-being in Britain, *International Journal of Health Services*, 44(1): 53–71.

Selinger, E. and Whyte, K. (2011) Is there a right way to nudge? The practice and ethics of choice architecture, *Sociology Compass*, 5(10): 923–935.

Setälä, V. and Väliverronen, E. (2014) 'Fighting fat: the role of "field experts" in mediating science and biological citizenship', *Science as Culture*, 23(4): 517–536.

Share, M. and Share, P. (2017) Doing the 'right thing'? Children, families and fatness in Ireland. In C.E. Edwards and E. Fernández (eds), *Reframing Health and Health Policy in Ireland: A Governmental Analysis*. Manchester: Manchester University Press.

Sheach Leith, V.M. (2015) An autoethnography of fat and weight loss: becoming the BwO with Deleuze and Guattari, *Sociological Research Online*, 21(3): 7, <http://www.socresonline.org.uk/21/3/7.html>.

Sheldrick, G. (2020) We must win obesity war for the NHS: third of COVID-19 deaths linked to diabetes, *Express*, 21 May. Online: <www.express.co.uk/news/uk/1285168/covid-1obesity-nhs-fat-diabetes> Accessed 1 August 2020.

Sherlaw, W. and Raude, J. (2013) Why the French did not choose to panic: a dynamic analysis of the public response to the influenza pandemic, *Sociology of Health & Illness*, 35(2): 332–344.

Shilling, C. (2005) *The Body in Culture, Technology & Society*. London: SAGE.

Shilling, C. (2008) *Changing Bodies: Habit, Crisis and Creativity*. London: SAGE.

Shilling, C. (2010) Exploring the society-body-school nexus: theoretical and methodology issues in the study of body pedagogics, *Sport, Education and Society*, 15(2): 151–167.

Shilling, C. (2012) *The Body and Social Theory*, 3rd edn. London: SAGE.

Siddique, H. (2016) Childhood obesity 'an exploding nightmare', says health expert. *The Guardian*, 25 January. Online: <www.theguardian.com/society/2016/jan/25/childhood-obesity-commission-world-health-organisation> Accessed 27 January 2016.

Simandan, D., Rinner, C. and Capurri, V. (in press) Confronting the rise of authoritarianism during the COVID-19 pandemic should be a priority for critical geographers and social scientists, *ACME: An International Journal for Critical Geographies*.

Singh, P. (2015) Performativity and pedagogising knowledge: globalising educational policy formation, dissemination and enactment, *Journal of Education Policy*, 30(3): 363–384.

Singh, P., Thomas, S. and Harris, J. (2013) Recontextualising policy discourses: a Bernsteinian perspective on policy interpretation, translation, enactment, *Journal of Education Policy*, 28(4): 465–480.

Sinha, R. (2018) Role of addiction and stress neurobiology on food intake and obesity, *Biological Psychology*, 131: 5–13.

Skeggs, B. (1997) *Formations of Class and Gender*. London: Sage.

Smith, G.J.D. (2016) Surveillance, data and embodiment: on the work of being watched, *Body & Society*, 22(2): 108–139.

Smith, R. (2020) The faults and dangers of iatrocracy, *thebmjopinion*, 11 August. Online: <https://blogs.bmj.com/bmj/2020/08/11/richard-smith-the-faults-and-dangers-of-an-iatrocracy/>.

So, J., Prestin, A., Lee, L., et al. (2016) What do people like to 'share' about obesity? A content analysis of frequent retweets about obesity on Twitter, *Health Communication*, 31(2), 193–206.

Sojka, C.J. and Sanchez, S. (2019) All people deserve a voice in reproductive care: trans-inclusion in fat studies, *Women's Reproductive Health*, 6(4): 259–264.

Solovay, S. (2000) *Tipping the Scales of Justice: Fighting Weight-Based Discrimination*. New York: Prometheus Books.

Sookoian, S., Gianotti, T.F., Burgueño, A.L. and Pirola, C.J. (2013) Fetal metabolic programming and epigenetic modifications: a systems biology approach, *Pediatric Research*, 73(4–2): 531–542.

Speakman, J.R. (2021) Impact of obesity on COVID-19 related mortality: a comment on estimates in Popkin et al 2020, *Obesity Reviews*, 22(8): e13250.

Sponholz, L. and Christofoletti, R. (2019) From preachers to comedians: ideal types of hate speakers in Brazil, *Global Media and Communication*, 15(1): 67–84.

Sport England (2020) *COVID-19 Briefing: Exploring Attitudes and Behaviours in England during the COVID-19 Pandemic*. Online: <https://data.londonsport.org/dataset/ep5kd/covid19-briefing-exploring-attitudes-and-behaviours-in-england-during-the-covid19-pandemic> Accessed 10 February 2021.

Stanford, F.C., Tauqeer, Z. and Kyle, T.K. (2018) Media and its influence on obesity, *Current Obesity Reports*, 7(2): 186–192.

Staniland, K. and Smith, G. (2013) Flu frames, *Sociology of Health & Illness*, 35(2): 309–324.

Stearns, P.N. (2002) *Fat History: Bodies and Beauty in the Modern West*. New York: New York University Press.

Stephenson, E. and Harris-Rimmer, S. (2020) Covid-19 responses: why feminist leadership matters in a crisis, *The Interpreter*. Lowry Institute, 31 March. Online: <www.lowyinstitute.org/the-interpreter/covid-19-responses-why-feminist-leadership-matters-crisis> Accessed 9 July.

Stevens, J., Bradshaw, P.T., Truesdale, K.P. and Jensen, M.D. (2015) Obesity paradox should not interfere with public health efforts, *International Journal of Obesity*, 39(1): 80–81.

Stewart, H. and Walker, P. (2020) Labour welcomes PM's 'conversion' on obesity after coronavirus scare, *The Guardian*, 15 May.

Stinson, K. (2001) *Women and Dieting Culture: Inside a Commercial Weight Loss Group*. New Brunswick, NJ: Rutgers University Press.

Stirrup, J., Hooper, O., Sandford, R. et al. (2020) 'PE' with Joe (Bloggs): the rise and risks of celebrity 'teachers', *British Educational Research Association Blog*, 20 July. Online: <www.bera.ac.uk/blog/pe-with-joe-bloggs-the-rise-and-risks-of-celebrity-teachers> Accessed 27 August 2020.

Strauss, R.S. and Pollack, H.A. (2003) Social marginalization of overweight children, *Archives of Pediatrics and Adolescent Medicine*, 157(8): 746–752.

Streeck, W. (2016) *How Will Capitalism End? Essays on a Failing System*. London and New York: Verso.

Strong, P. (1990) Epidemic psychology: a model, *Sociology of Health & Illness*, 12(3): 249–259.

Stunkard, A.J. (1958) The management of obesity, *New York State Journal of Medicine*, 58: 79–87.

Sturm, R. (2002) The effects of obesity, smoking, and drinking on medical problems and costs, *Health Affairs*, 21(2): 245–253.

Sumithran, P., Prendergast, L.A., Delbridge, E. et al. (2011) Long-term persistence of hormonal adaptations to weight loss, *New England Journal of Medicine*, 365(17): 1597–1604.

Sun, Y., Wang, Q., Yang, G. et al. (2016) Weight and prognosis for influenza A (H1N1) pdm09 infection during the pandemic period between 2009 and 2011: a systematic review of observational studies with meta-analysis, *Infectious Diseases*, 48(11–12): 813–822.

Swinburn, B.A., Kraak, V.I., Allender, S. et al. (2019) The global syndemic of obesity, undernutrition, and climate change: *The Lancet* Commission report, *The Lancet*, 393(10173): 791–846.

Sykes, H. and McPhail, D. (2008) Unbearable lessons: contesting fat phobia in physical education, *Sociology of Sport Journal*, 25(1): 66–96.

Szymczak, J.E. (2016) Infections and interaction rituals in the organisation: clinician accounts of speaking up or remaining silent in the face of threats to patient safety, *Sociology of Health & Illness*, 38(2): 325–339.

Tamarkin, S. (2016) 26 people share the important reasons they stopped dieting and how they found self-acceptance, *Buzzfeed*, 19 May. Online: <www.buzzfeed.com/sallyta-markin/why-people-stopped-dieting> Accessed 31 December 2016.

Tan, C.K.K. (2016) Gaydar: using skilled vision to spot gay 'Bears' in Taipei, *Anthropological Quarterly*, 89(3): 841–864.

Tan, M., Feng, J.H. and MacGregor, G.A. (2020) Obesity and covid-19: the role of the food industry, *BMJ*, 369: m2237.

Tartof, S.Y., Qian, L., Hong, V. et al. (2020) Obesity and mortality among patients diagnosed with COVID-19: results from an integrated health care organization, *Annals of Internal Medicine*, https://doi.org/10.7326/M20-3742.

Taylor, E.H., Marson, J., Elhadi, M. et al. (2021) Factors associated with mortality in patients with COVID-19 admitted to intensive care: a systematic review and meta-analysis, *Anaesthesia*, 76(9): 1224–1232.

The Lancet (2020) Editorial: medicine and medical science, Black Lives must matter more, *The Lancet*, 395(10240): 1813.

The Nutrire CoLab (2020) Letter to the editor: anthropologists respond to the Lancet EAT Commission, *Bionatura*, 5(1), https://doi.org/10.21931/RB/2020.05.01.2.

The Report of the National Taskforce on Obesity (2005) *Obesity – The Policy Challenges*. Online: <www.hse.ie/eng/health/child/healthyeating/taskforceonobesity.pdf> Accessed 10 October 2016.

Theodosius, C. (2022) Formal divisions in healthcare. In L.F. Monaghan and J. Gabe (eds), *Key Concepts in Medical Sociology*, 3rd edn. London: SAGE.

Thille, P. (2019) Managing anti-fat stigma in primary care: an observational study, *Health Communication*, 34(8): 892–903.

Thomas, P. (2016) Doing it for the children, *Fat Studies*, 5(2): 203–209.

Thomas, S.L., Hyde, J., Karunaratne, A. et al. (2008) Being 'fat' in today's world: a qualitative study of the lived experiences of people with obesity in Australia, *Health Expectations*, 11(4): 321–330.

Thoune, D. (2020) Diet culture at the end of the world, *Two Fat Professors*, 1 April. Online: <www.twofatprofessors.com/post/diet-culture-at-the-end-of-the-world> Accessed 15 April 2020.

Throsby, K. (2008a) Happy re-birthday: weight loss surgery and the 'new me', *Body & Society*, 14(1): 117–133.

Throsby, K. (2008b) 'That's a bit drastic': risk and blame in accounts of obesity surgery. In F. Alexander and K. Throsby (eds), *Gender and Interpersonal Violence: Language, Action and Representation*. Basingstoke: Palgrave MacMillan.

Throsby, K. (2009) The war on obesity as a moral project: weight loss drugs, obesity surgery and negotiating failure, *Science as Culture*, 18(2): 201–216.

Throsby, K. (2012) Obesity surgery and the management of excess: exploring the body multiple, *Sociology of Health & Illness*, 34(1): 1–15

Throsby, K. (2020) Pure, white and deadly: sugar addiction and the cultivation of urgency, *Food, Culture & Society*, 23(1): 11–29.

Throsby, K. and Gimlin, D. (2010) Critiquing thinness and wanting to be thin. In R. Ryan-Flood and R. Gill (eds), *Secrecy and Silence in the Research Process: Feminist Reflections*. Abingdon: Routledge.

Tiggemann, M. (2004) Body image across the adult life span: stability and change, *Body Image*, 1(1): 29–41.

Timmermans, S. and Tavory, I. (2012) Theory construction in qualitative research: from grounded theory to abductive analysis, *Sociological Theory*, 30(3): 167–186.

Tinning, R (2014) Getting which message across? The (H)PE teacher as health educator. In K. Fitzpatrick and R. Tinning (eds), *Health Education: Critical Perspectives*. Abingdon: Taylor and Francis.

Tischner, I. (2013) *Fat Lives: A Feminist Psychological Exploration*. New York: Routledge.

Tischner, I. and Malson, H. (2011) 'You can't be supersized?' Exploring femininities, body size and control within the obesity terrain. In E. Rich, L.F. Monaghan and L. Aphramor (eds), *Debating Obesity: Critical Perspectives*. Basingstoke: Palgrave Macmillan.

Toffoletti, K., Thorpe, H. and Francombe-Webb, J. (2018) *New Sporting Femininities: Embodied Politics in Postfeminist Times*. Basingstoke: Palgrave Macmillan.

Tomiyama, A.J. (2014) Weight stigma is stressful. A review of evidence for the cyclic obesity/weight-based stigma model, *Appetite*, 82: 8–15.

Tomiyama, A.J., Ahlstrom, B., Mann, T. (2013) Long-term effects of dieting: is weight-loss related to health? *Social and Personality Psychology Compass*, 7(12): 861–877.

Tomiyama, A.J., Hunger, J.M., Nguyen-Cuu, J. and Wells, C. (2016) Misclassification of cardiometabolic health when using Body Mass Index categories in NHANES 2005-2012, *International Journal of Obesity*, 40(5): 883–886.

Tooze, A. (2020) How coronavirus almost brought down the global financial system, *The Guardian*, 14 April.

Tremblay, A. (2016) Metabolic adaptation: here to stay? *Obesity*, 24(8): 1609–1610.

Turner, B.S. (1992) *Regulating Bodies: Essays in Medical Sociology*. London: Routledge.

Turner, B.S. (1996) *The Body and Society*, 2nd edn. London: SAGE.

Tyler, I. (2013) *Revolting Subjects: Social Abjection and Resistance in Neoliberal Britain*. London: Zed Books.

Tyler, I. (2020) *Stigma: The Machinery of Inequality*. London: Zed Books.

Tylka, T.L., Annunziato, R.A., Burgard, D. et al. (2014) The weight-inclusive versus weight-normative approach to health: evaluating the evidence for prioritizing well-being over weightloss, *Journal of Obesity*, 2014, 983495.

Ulijaszek, S. (2014) Obesity, government and the media. In K. Eli and S. Ulijaszek (eds), *Obesity, Eating Disorders and the Media*. Farnham: Ashgate.

Ulijaszek, S.L. and McLennan, A.J. (2016) Framing obesity in UK policy from the Blair years, 1997–2015: the persistence of individualistic approaches despite overwhelming evidence of societal and economic factors, and the need for collective responsibility, *Obesity Reviews*, 17: 397–411.

United Nations (2020) *Policy Brief: The Impact of COVID-19 on Women*, 9 April. Online: <www.un.org/sexualviolenceinconflict/wp-content/uploads/2020/06/report/policy-brief-the-impact-of-covid-19-on-women/policy-brief-the-impact-of-covid-19-on-women-en-1.pdf> Accessed 23 April 2020.

Urquhart, M. (2020) 'Emotional hangover' predicted when busy complain line's days are over, *CBC News*, 23 April.

US DHHS (2014) *Healthy People 2020*. US Department of Health and Human Services. Online: <www.healthypeople.gov/2020/topics-objectives/topic/nutrition-and-weight-status/objectives> Accessed 1 October 2014.

US DHHS (2020) *Healthy People 2030*. US Department of Health and Human Services. Online: <https://health.gov/healthypeople/objectives-and-data/browse-objectives/overweight-and-obesity> Accessed 10 October 2020.

Van Amsterdam, N. and Knoppers, A. (2018) Healthy habits are no fun: how Dutch youth negotiate discourses about food, fit, fat and fun, *Health*, 22(2): 128–146.

Vander Schee, C. and Kline, K. (2013) Neoliberal exploitation in reality television: youth, health and the spectacle of celebrity 'concern', *Journal of Youth Studies*, 16(5): 565–578.

Vighi, F. (2021) A self-fulfilling prophecy: systemic collapse and pandemic simulation, *The Philosophical Salon*, 16 August. Online: <https://thephilosophicalsalon.com/a-self-fulfilling-prophecy-systemic-collapse-and-pandemic-simulation> Accessed 8 January 2022.

Villalon, K.L., Gozansky, W.S., Van Pelt, R.E. et al. (2011) A losing battle: weight regain does not restore weight loss-induced bone loss in postmenopausal women, *Obesity*, 19(12): 2345–2350.

Vogel, E. (2018) Operating (on) the self: transforming agency through obesity surgery and treatment, *Sociology of Health & Illness*, 40(3): 508–522.

Walby, S. (2015) *Crisis*. Cambridge: Polity Press.

Walker, C., Eustice, P. and Baxter, C. (2020) It's time to trust hungry people, *Cost of Living*, 26 May. Online: <www.cost-ofliving.net/its-time-to-trust-hungry-people/> Accessed 30 May 2020.

Walker, P. (2020a) No 10 plans weight loss drive to ready UK for expected Covid-19 second wave, *The Guardian*, 11 July.

Walker, P. (2020b) Boris Johnson: obesity drive will not be 'bossy or nannying', *The Guardian*, 27 July.

Walkerdine, V. (2009) Biopedagogies and beyond. In J. Wright and V. Walkerdine (eds.), *Biopolitics and the 'Obesity Epidemic': Governing Bodies*. New York: Routledge.

Wallerstein, I. (2011) Dynamics of (unresolved) global crisis. In C. Calhoun and G. Derluguian (eds), *Business as Usual: The Roots of the Global Financial Meltdown*. New York: New York University Press.

Wann, M. (1998) *Fat!So? Because you Don't Have to Apologize for your Size*. Berkeley, CA: Ten Speed Press.

Wann, M. (2009) Foreword: fat studies: an invitation to revolution. In E. Rothblum and S. Solovay (eds), *The Fat Studies Reader*. New York: New York University Press.

Ward, P., Beausoleil, N. and Heath, O. (2016) Creating space for a critical examination of weight-centered approaches in health pedagogy and health professions. In E. Cameron and C. Russell (eds), *The Fat Pedagogy Reader*. New York: Peter Lang Publishing.

Ward, P. and McPhail, D. (2019) Fat blame and shame in reproductive care: implications for ethical healthcare interactions, *Women's Reproductive Health*, 6(4): 225–241.

Ward, P.R. (2020) A sociology of the Covid-19 pandemic: a commentary and research agenda for sociologists, *Journal of Sociology*, 56(4): 726–735.

Ward, Z.J., Bleich, S.N., Cradocl, A.L. et al. (2019) Projected U.S. state-level prevalence of adult obesity and severe obesity, *New England Journal of Medicine*, 381: 2440–2450.

Warin, M. (2010) Foucault's progeny: Jamie Oliver and the art of governing obesity, *Social Theory & Health*, 9(1): 24–40.

Warin, M. (2015) Material feminism, obesity science and the limits of discursive critique, *Body & Society*, 21(4): 48–76.

Warin, M. (2020) The 'gentle and invisible' violence of obesity prevention, *American Anthropologist*, 122(3): 672–673.

Warin, M., Kowal, E. and Meloni, M. (2020) Indigenous knowledge in a postgenomic landscape: the politics of epigenetic hope and reparation in Australia, *Science, Technology, & Human Values*, 45(1): 87–111.

Warin, M. and Moore, V. (2021) Epistemic conflicts and Achilles' heels: constraints of a university and public sector partnership to research obesity in Australia, *Critical Public Health*, 31(5): 617–628.

Warin, M., Turner, K., Moore, V. and Davies, M. (2008) Bodies, mothers and identities: rethinking obesity and the BMI, *Sociology of Health & Illness*, 30(1): 97–111.

Warin, M. and Zivkovic, T. (2019) *Fatness, Obesity, and Disadvantage in the Australian Suburbs: Unpalatable Politics*. Cham: Palgrave Macmillan.

Warin, M., Zivkovic, T., Moore, V. and Davies, M. (2012) Mothers as smoking guns: fetal overnutrition and the reproduction of obesity, *Feminism & Psychology*, 22(3): 360–375.

Warkentin, L.M., Das, D., Majumdar, S.R. et al. (2014) The effect of weight loss on health-related quality of life: systematic review and meta-analysis of randomized trials, *Obesity Reviews*, 15: 169–182.

Waskul, D. and Vannini, P. (eds) (2006) *Body/Embodiment: Symbolic Interaction and the Sociology of the Body*. Aldershot: Ashgate.

Watson, J. (2000) *Male Bodies: Health, Culture and Identity*. Buckingham: Open University Press.

Webb, J.B., Vinoski Thomas, E., Rogers, C.B. et al. (2019) Fitspo at Every Size? A comparative content analysis of #curvyfit versus #curvyyoga Instagram images, *Fat Studies*, 19(2): 154–172.

Webb, J.B., Vinoski Thomas, E., Warren-Findlow, J. et al. (2017) Is the 'Yoga Bod' the new skinny?: A comparative content analysis of mainstream Yoga Lifestyle Magazine covers, *Body Image*, 20: 87–98.

Webb, J.B., Warren-Findlow, J., Chou, Y. and Adams, L. (2013) Do you see what I see?: An exploration of inter-ethnic ideal body size comparisons among college women, *Body Image*, 10(3): 369–379.

Weedon, C. (1997) *Feminist Practice and Poststructuralist Theory*. Oxford: Blackwell.

Weinstock, J. and Krehbiel, M. (2009) Fat youth as common targets for bullying. In E. Rothblum and S. Solovay (eds), *The Fat Studies Reader*. New York: New York University Press.

Welsh, T. (2011) Healthism and the bodies of women: pleasure and discipline in the war against obesity, *Journal of Feminist Scholarship*, 1: 33–48.

Whitesel, J. (2014) *Fat Gay Men: Girth, Mirth and the Politics of Stigma*. New York: New York University Press.

WHO (1998) *Obesity: Preventing and Managing the Global Epidemic*. Geneva: WHO Press.

WHO (2016) *Report of the Commission on Ending Childhood Obesity*. Geneva: WHO Press.

WHO (2017) *Weight Bias and Obesity Stigma: Considerations for the European Region*. Online: <www.euro.who.int/__data/assets/pdf_file/0017/351026/WeightBias.pdf?ua=1> Accessed 18 March 2019.

WHO (2018) *Obesity and Overweight*. Online: <www.who.int/news-room/fact-sheets/detail/obesity-and-overweight> Accessed 25 February 2020.

WHO (2021) *Controlling the Global Obesity Epidemic*. Online: <www.who.int/activities/controlling-the-global-obesity-epidemic> Accessed 4 January 2021.

Wildman, R.P., Muntner, P., Reynolds, K. et al. (2008) The obese without cardiometabolic risk factor clustering and the normal weight with cardiometabolic risk factor clustering: prevalence and correlates of 2 phenotypes among the US population (NHANES 1999-2004), *Archives of Internal Medicine*, 168(15): 1617–1624.

Will, C.M. (2020) 'And breathe…'? The sociology of health and illness in COVID-19 time. *Sociology of Health & Illness*, 42(5): 967–971.

Will, C.M. and Bendelow, G. (2020) Processing the pandemic, *Sociology of Health & Illness*, 42(8): e1–e3.

Williams, G.H., Elliott, E. and Popay, J. (2022) Lay knowledge, in L.F. Monaghan and J. Gabe (eds), *Key Concepts in Medical Sociology*. London: SAGE.

Williams, O. and Annandale, E. (2019) Weight bias internalization as an embodied process: understanding how obesity stigma gets under the skin, *Frontiers in Psychology*, 10: 953, https://doi.org/10.3389/fpsyg.2019.00953.

Williams, O. and Annandale, E. (2020) Obesity, stigma and reflexive embodiment: *feeling the 'weight' of expectation*, *Health*, 24(4): 421–441.

Williams, O. and Fullagar, S. (2019) Lifestyle drift and the phenomenon of 'citizen shift' in contemporary UK health policy, *Sociology of Health & Illness*, 41(1): 20–35.

Williams, S.J. (1999) Is anybody there? Critical realism, chronic illness and the disability debate, *Sociology of Health & Illness*, 21(6): 797–819.

Williams, S.J. (2003) Beyond meaning, discourse and the empirical world: critical realist reflections on health, *Social Theory & Health*, 1(1): 42–71.

Williams, S.J. (2004) Bioattack or panic attack? Critical reflections on the ill-logic of bioterrorism and biowarfare in late/postmodernity, *Social Theory & Health*, 2(1): 67–94.

Williams, S.J. and Bendelow, G. (1998) *The Lived Body: Sociological Themes, Embodied Issues*. London: Routledge.

Williams, S.J., Birke, L. and Bendelow, G. (eds) (2003) *Debating Biology: Sociological Reflections on Health, Medicine and Society*. London: Routledge.

Williams, S.J. and Monaghan, L.F. (2022) Embodiment, in L.F. Monaghan and J. Gabe (eds), *Key Concepts in Medical Sociology*. London: SAGE.

Williams, S.N. (2008) 'Plausible uncertainty': the negotiated indeterminacy of pandemic influenza in the UK, *Critical Public Health*, 18(1): 77–85.

Williamson, B., Eynon, R. and Potter, J. (2020a) Pandemic politics, pedagogies and practices: digital technologies and distance education during the coronavirus emergency, *Learning, Media and Technology*, 45(2): 107–114.

Williamson, K., Nimegeer, A. and Lean, M. (2020b) Rising prevalence of BMI ≥40 kg/m²: a high-demand epidemic needing better documentation, *Obesity Reviews*, 21(4): e12986.

Wing, R.R. and Hill, J.O. (2001) Successful weight loss maintenance, *Annual Review of Nutrition*, 21: 323–341.

Wing, R.R., Tate, D.F., Espeland, M.A. et al. (2016) Innovative self-regulation strategies to reduce weight gain in young adults: the Study of Novel Approaches to Weight Gain Prevention (SNAP) randomized clinical tria, *JAMA Internal Medicine*, 176(6): 755–762.

Wise, J. (2016) Sugar tax could stop 3.7 million UK people becoming obese, claims report, *BMJ*, 352: i1064.

Wisniewski, A.E. (2013) The weight of communication: The Canadian Medical Association Journal's discourse on obesity, *Public Understanding of Science*, 22(3): 351–364.

WOF (2016) *World Obesity Day 2016*. World Obesity. Online: <www.obesityday.worldobesity.org/world-obesity-day-2016> Accessed 17 August 2018.

WOF (2018) *World Obesity Day 2018. End Weight Stigma*. World Obesity. Online: <www.obesityday.worldobesity.org/world-obesity-day-2018> Accessed 17 August 2018.

WOF (2019) *About us*. World Obesity. Online: <www.worldobesity.org/about/about-us> Accessed 31 December 2021.

WOF (2020) *Obesity and COVID-19 Policy Statement*. World Obesity, 27 March. Online <http://s3-eu-west-1.amazonaws.com/wof-files/Obesity_and_COVID-19_policy_statement.pdf> Accessed 14 July 2020.

Wood, H. and Skeggs, B. (2008) Spectacular morality: reality television, individualisation and the remaking of the working class. In D. Hesmondhalgh and J. Toynbee (eds), *The Media and Social Theory*. London: Routledge.

World Obesity Day (2020) *The Roots of Obesity Run Deep*. Online: <www.worldobesity-day.org/> Accessed 21 February 2020.

World Population Review (2021) Most obese countries 2021. Online: <https://world-populationreview.com/country-rankings/most-obese-countries> Accessed 7 January 2022.

Wright, J. (2004) Post-structural methodologies: the body, schooling and health. In J. Evans, B. Davies and J. Wright (eds), *Body Knowledge and Control: Studies in the Sociology of Physical Education and Health*. London: Routledge.

Wright, J. (2009) Biopower, biopedagogies and the obesity epidemic. In J. Wright and V. Harwood (eds), *Biopolitics and the Obesity Epidemic: Governing Bodies*. New York: Routledge.

Wright, J. and Harwood, V. (eds) (2009) *Biopolitics and the Obesity Epidemic: Governing Bodies*. New York: Routledge.

Wright, J. and Leahy, D. (2016) Moving beyond body image: a socio-critical approach to teaching about health and body size. In E. Cameron and C. Russell (eds), *The Fat Pedagogy Reader*. New York: Peter Lang Publishing.

Wynne, B.E. (1998) May the sheep safely graze? A reflexive view of the expert-lay knowledge divide. In S. Lash, B. Szerszynski and B. Wynne (eds), *Risk, Environment and Modernity: Towards a New Ecology*. London: SAGE.

Yager, Z., Diedrichs, P.C., Ricciardelli, L.A. and Halliwell, E. (2013) What works in secondary schools? A systematic review of classroom-based body image programs, *Body Image*, 10(3): 271–281.

Yoshizawa, R.S. (2012) The Barker hypothesis and obesity: connections for transdisciplinarity and social justice, *Social Theory & Health*, 10(4): 348–367.

Youdell, D. (2005) Sex-gender-sexuality: how sex, gender and sexuality constellations are constituted in secondary schools, *Gender and Education*, 17: 249–270.

Zannettino, L. (2008) Imagining womanhood: psychodynamic processes in the 'textual' and discursive formation of girls' subjectivities and desires for the future, *Gender and Education*, 20: 465–479.

Zhang, N., Wang, L., Zhang, M. and Nazroo, J. (2019a) Chronic exposure to ambient air pollution and obesity among older adults in China. Paper presented at *Healthy Cities: Urbanisation, Infrastructures and Everyday Life*. University of Manchester, 1–3 May.

Zhang, X., Rhoades, J., Caan, B.J. et al. (2019b) Intentional weight loss, weight cycling, and endometrial cancer risk: a systematic review and meta-analysis, *International Journal of Gynecological Cancer*, 29(9): 1361–1371.

Zhu, Y., Liu, J., Jiang, H. et al. (2020) Are long working hours associated with weight-related outcomes? A meta-analysis of observational studies, *Obesity Reviews*, 21(3): e12977.

Žižek, S. (2020) *Pandemic! COVID-19 Shakes the World*. New York: OR Books.

Zou, H., Yin, P., Liu, L. et al. (2019) Body-weight fluctuation was associated with increased risk for cardiovascular disease, all-cause and cardiovascular mortality: a systematic review and meta-analysis, *Frontiers in Endocrinology*, 10, https://doi.org/10.3389/fendo.2019.00728.

Zou, H., Yin, P., Liu, L. et al. (2021) Association between weight cycling and risk of developing diabetes in adults: a systematic review and meta-analysis, *Journal of Diabetes Investigation*, 12(4): 625–632.

INDEX

Note: Page numbers in **bold** refer to tables